Fair Resource Allocation and Rationing at the Bedside

T0201884

Fair Resource Allocation and Rationing at the Bedside

EDITED BY

Marion Danis, Samia A. Hurst,
Leonard M. Fleck, Reidun Førde,
and Anne Slowther

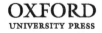
OXFORD
UNIVERSITY PRESS

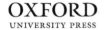

OXFORD
UNIVERSITY PRESS

Oxford University Press is a department of the University of Oxford. It furthers
the University's objective of excellence in research, scholarship, and education
by publishing worldwide. Oxford is a registered trade mark of Oxford University
Press in the UK and certain other countries.

Published in the United States of America by Oxford University Press
198 Madison Avenue, New York, NY 10016, United States of America.

Library of Congress Cataloging-in-Publication Data
Fair resource allocation and rationing at the bedside / edited by Marion Danis,
Samia Hurst, Len Fleck, Reidun Førde, and Anne Slowther.
    p. ; cm.
Includes bibliographical references.
ISBN 978–0–19–998944–7 (hardcover); 978–0–19–088213–6 (paperback);
I. Danis, Marion, editor.   II. Hurst, Samia, editor.   III. Fleck, Leonard M., editor.
IV. Førde, Reidun, editor.   V. Slowther, Anne, editor.
[DNLM: 1. Health Care Rationing—methods.   2. Resource Allocation—methods.
3. Ethics, Clinical.   4. Health Care Rationing—ethics.   5. Resource Allocation—
ethics. WA 525]
RA971.3
362.1068′1—dc23
2014011619

■ DISCLAIMER

The views expressed here are those of the authors and do not necessarily reflect the policies of the US Department of Health and Human Services or the National Institutes of Health.

Dedicated to the physicians in Italy, Norway, Switzerland, and the United Kingdom who participated in the Values at the Bedside Study and taught us so much about what physicians think and do about resource allocation and rationing at the bedside.

■ ACKNOWLEDGMENTS

Along the way many individuals and organizations helped to make this book and the research, commentaries, and analyses contained in it a reality. While we were developing the Values at the Bedside study, Stella Reiter-Theil, Renzo Pegoraro, and Arnaud Perrier were valuable collaborators without whom we could not have performed such a multi-country study as we did. Ole Norheim and Rein Vos provided expert review of the Values at the Bedside survey instrument. Bruce Brinkley, Timothy Carey, Marie Neeser, Marc-Andre Raetzo, and Dan Sulmasy piloted the survey and gave useful feedback about how to improve it. MEDTAP International provided excellent data collection. Following the survey, Elizabeth Garrett-Mayer provided invaluable statistical support, and the NIH Clinical Center Library translation service contributed by translating responses of Norwegian, Italian, Swiss, and British physicians.

We conceived of this book during the course of a symposium sponsored by the Brocher Foundation, so we are particularly appreciative of the Foundation and its staff, Marie Grosclaude, Anyck Gérard, and Raji Sultan. Several scholars who participated in our Brocher symposium influenced our thinking about how to frame the analysis as a whole in this book. They include several commentators from Switzerland: Prof. Olivier Guillod, University of Neuchatel; Dr. Markus Zimmermann-Acklin, University of Lucerne; Anna Sax, Swiss Society for Health Policy; Prof. Claudine Jeangros, University of Geneva; and Prof. Peter Suter, University of Geneva; as well as several commentators from other countries: Prof. Paul Wolpe, University of Pennsylvania, USA; Prof. Peter Ubel, Duke University, USA; Prof. Soren Holm, University of Cardiff, UK; Prof. Ole Norheim, University of Bergen, Norway; Prof. Georg Marckmann, University of Tuebingen, Germany; Dr. Daniel Strech, Hannover Medical School, Germany; and Dr. Susan Goold, University of Michigan, USA.

And, of course, most of all we want to acknowledge that we could not have prepared this book without the thoughtful contribution of our authors, whose chapters create a mosaic of ideas that we hope readers will find quite interesting and useful. Several anonymous reviewers of our book proposal offered critiques that helped to round out the topics we covered. Ben Bennett spent many hours reading and editing drafts of book chapters with the careful perspective of a serious undergraduate philosophy major during his summer internship at the NIH Department of Bioethics. Lastly, we appreciate our editors at Oxford University Press, Peter Ohlin and Lucy Randall, for their belief that our ideas for this book were worthwhile and for helping us bring them to publication.

Samia Hurst was supported by several grants over the years from the Geneva University Hospitals, the Oltramare Foundation, and from the Swiss National Science Foundation (3233B0-107266. /.1-2, and PP00P3_123340.). This project received support from the Intramural Program at the National Institutes of Health and particularly from the Department of Bioethics in the National Institutes of Health Clinical Center.

■ CONTENTS

Contributors   xv

Introduction   1
MARION DANIS, REIDUN FØRDE, LEONARD M. FLECK,
SAMIA A. HURST, AND ANNE SLOWTHER

PART ONE ■ A European Survey of Bedside Rationing

1. The Values at the Bedside Study: Bedside Rationing
   by Physicians   19
   SAMIA A. HURST, ANNE SLOWTHER, REIDUN FØRDE,
   AND MARION DANIS

2. The Interaction of Bedside Rationing and the Fairness
   of Health Care Systems: Physicians' Views   29
   SAMIA A. HURST, REIDUN FØRDE, ANNE SLOWTHER,
   AND MARION DANIS

PART TWO ■ The Societal Context

3. The Swiss Context   43
   SAMIA A. HURST

4. The United Kingdom Context   56
   ANNE SLOWTHER

5. The Norwegian Context   71
   REIDUN FØRDE

6. The Italian Context   88
   RENZO PEGORARO AND ALESSANDRA BERNARDI

PART THREE ■ Analysis of Bedside Rationing

7. How Do Economic Incentive Schemes Influence Rationing
Decisions by Primary Care Physicians?   105
THOMAS ALLEN, MATT SUTTON, AND RICHARD COOKSON

8. The Legal Context of Bedside Rationing   125
KEITH SYRETT

9. Bedside Rationing or Rational Planning: In Search
of Perspective on Medical Benefit and Safety   145
YECHIEL MICHAEL BARILAN

10. Just Caring: The Ethics Challenges of Bedside Rationing   171
LEONARD M. FLECK

11. Overdiagnosis and Overtreatment: Implications for Bedside
Rationing   204
HOWARD BRODY

12. How Can Bedside Rationing Be Justified despite Coexisting
Inefficiency? The Need for "Benchmarks of Efficiency"   211
DANIEL STRECH AND MARION DANIS

13. The Collective Action Problem   224
ROBERT E. GOODIN

14. Statistical versus Identified Lives: Why Not
to Use the "R" Word   238
PAUL T. MENZEL

15. Give to the Doctor What Is Due to the Doctor! Why "Fair
Rationing at the Bedside" Is Impossible   253
VEGARD BRUUN WYLLER

PART FOUR ■ Strategies for Promoting Fair Bedside Rationing

16. Priority Setting in Hospital Care: Implementing National
Legislation and Guidelines in a Hospital Trust   265
ODD SØREIDE, STENER KVINNSLAND,
AND TORHILD HEGGESTAD

17. Rationing by Clinical Judgment   284
    SAMIA A. HURST AND MARION DANIS

18. Fairness and Transparency in Bedside Micro-allocation:
    Improving the Ethical Competence of Clinical Staff   301
    JAN SCHÜRMANN, BARBARA MEYER-ZEHNDER,
    MARCEL MERTZ, HEIDI ALBISSER SCHLEGER,
    MATHIAS SCHLÖGL, RETO W. KRESSIG, HANS PARGGER,
    AND STELLA REITER-THEIL

19. Fair Resource Allocation in Clinical Care for Socially
    Disadvantaged Groups and Health Disparity Populations:
    Issues and Strategies   323
    IRENE DANKWA-MULLAN, PAULA Y. GOODWIN,
    AND MATTHEW WYNIA

20. Bedside Rationing After Health Care Reform in the United
    States: The Emergence of Accountable Care Organizations   356
    STEVEN D. PEARSON

21. Priority Setting Through Clinical Practice Guidelines:
    Lessons Learned   373
    OLE FRITHJOF NORHEIM

22. Physicians as Bellwethers   387
    SUSAN DORR GOOLD

23. Moving Away from Silent Trepidation: Changing the
    Discussion of Rationing and Resource Allocation   395
    MARION DANIS, GREER DONLEY, AND REIDUN FØRDE

24. Priority Setting As a Clinical Skill: How Do We Educate
    Physicians?   423
    ANNE SLOWTHER AND BENJAMIN P. BENNETT

    Afterword   439
    Index   443

■ CONTRIBUTORS

Thomas Allen, PhD
Manchester Centre for Health Economics
Institute for Population Health
University of Manchester

Yechiel Michael Barilan, MD
Associate Professor of Medical Education and Bioethics
Sackler School of Medicine
Tel Aviv University

Benjamin P. Bennett, BA
Corps Member
Avodah: The Jewish Service Corps

Alessandra Bernardi, PharmD
European Master of Bioethics (Leuven et al)
Scientific Secretary of the Local Ethics Committee
Istituto Oncologico Veneto IOV-IRCCS

Howard Brody, MD, PhD
Director, Institute for the Medical Humanities
Professor, Family Medicine
John P. McGovern Centennial Chair
University of Texas Medical Branch at Galveston

Richard Cookson, MPhil, DPhil
Reader
Centre for Health Economics
University of York

Marion Danis, MD
Head, Section on Ethics and Health Policy
and Chief, Bioethics Consultation Service
Department of Bioethics
National Institutes of Health Clinical Center

Irene Dankwa-Mullan, MD, MPH
Director
Office of Innovation and Program
Coordination
Division of Scientific Programs
National Institute on Minority Health and Health Disparities
National Institutes of Health

Greer Donley, JD
Michigan Law School
University of Michigan

Leonard M. Fleck, PhD
Professor of Philosophy and Medical Ethics
Center for Ethics and Humanities in the Life Sciences
College of Human Medicine
Michigan State University

Reidun Førde, MD
Professor of Medicine
Center for Medical Ethics
University of Oslo

Robert E. Goodin, PhD
Professor
Department of Government
University of Essex
and School of Philosophy
Australian National University

Paula Y. Goodwin, PhD
Public Health Analyst
Division of State and Community Systems Development
Center for Mental Health Services
Substance Abuse and Mental Health Services Administration (SAMHSA)

Susan Dorr Goold, MD, MHSA, MA
Professor of Internal Medicine and Health
Management and Policy
Center for Bioethics and Social Sciences in Medicine
University of Michigan

Torhild Heggestad, MD, PhD
Advisor
Research and Development
Haukeland University Hospital

Samia A. Hurst, MD, PhD
Professor
Institute for Ethics, History, and Humanities—.UNIGE
Consultant—.Conseil d'éthique clinique HUG
University of Geneva

Reto W. Kressig, MD
Professor
Chair of Geriatrics
University of Basel
and Department Head, University Center for Medicine of Aging
University Hospital Basel

Stener Kvinnsland, MD
CEO
Bergen Hospital Trust
Former Professor of Medical Oncology
University of Oslo and University of Bergen

Paul T. Menzel, PhD
Professor of Philosophy Emeritus
Department of Philosophy
Pacific Lutheran University

Marcel Mertz, MA
Chair of Philosophy III
Department of Philosophy
University of Mannheim
and Institute for History, Ethics and Philosophy of Medicine
Hannover Medical School

Barbara Meyer-Zehnder, MD
Clinical Ethics
Department of Anesthesia and Intensive Care Medicine
University Hospital Basel

Ole Frithjof Norheim, MD, PhD
Professor
Department of Public Health and Primary Health Care
University of Bergen

Hans Pargger, MD
Professor and Head Physician
Department of Anesthesia and Intensive Care Medicine
University Hospital Basel

Steven D. Pearson, MD, MSc
Visiting Scientist
Department of Bioethics
National Institutes of Health Clinical Center
Bethesda, Maryland
and President
Institute for Clinical and Economic Review

Renzo Pegoraro, MD, PhD
Scientific Director
Fondazione Lanza

Stella Reiter-Theil, PhD
Professor and Director of Clinical Ethics
University Hospital Basel, Psychiatric Hospitals of the University
    Basel/IBMB
University of Basel

Heidi Albisser Schleger, PhD
Clinical Ethics, University Hospital Basel/IBMB
University of Basel

Mathias Schlögl, MD
University Center for Medicine of Aging
University Hospital Basel

Jan Schürmann, BA
Clinical Ethics, University Hospital Basel, Psychiatric Hospitals of the
    University Basel/ IBMB

Anne Slowther, MD
Masters in Medical Ethics, DPhil in Medical Ethics
Associate Professor of Clinical Ethics
Division of Health Sciences
Warick Medical School
University of Warwick
Chair, UK Clinical Ethics Network

Odd Søreide, MD, FRCS, FACS
Medical Director (Retired), Western Norway Regional Health Authority
Former Professor of Surgery, University of Oslo and University of Bergen

Daniel Strech, MD, PhD
Professor
Centre for Ethics and Law in the Life Sciences
Institute for History and Medical Ethics
Hannover Medical School

Matt Sutton, MSc, PhD
Professor of Economics and Econometrics
Centre for Health Economics
Institute of Population Health
University of Manchester

Keith Syrett, LLB
Professor
Cardiff Law School
Cardiff University

Vegard Bruun Wyller, MD, PhD
Professor
Institute of Clinical Medicine
University of Oslo and
Pediatric Cardiologist
Deptartment of Pediatrics
Akershus University Hospital

Matthew Wynia, MD, MPH, FACP
Director
The Institute for Ethics and The Center for Patient Safety
American Medical Association
and Clinical Assistant Professor
University of Chicago

Introduction

■ MARION DANIS, REIDUN FØRDE,
LEONARD M. FLECK, SAMIA A. HURST,
AND ANNE SLOWTHER

Contemporary medicine has much to offer in efforts to promote health, prevent illness, diagnose and manage disease, and stave off death. As the populations of all countries age and the armamentarium of medicine expands, the opportunities and choices about what to provide to a given patient in pursuit of these efforts are increasingly costly and complicated. The clinician who provides care for a patient has among the most influential roles in determining the resources that are brought to bear in the effort to maintain that person's health. The clinician's judgments largely determine who receives a diagnosis and who does or does not receive surgery, a specific drug, extra days in the ICU, home health services, or any other prescribed interventions. This book will examine how physicians and other clinicians carry out this role and will explore strategies to promote their doing so as fairly and cost-consciously as possible; it will bring to your attention systems that some countries have developed to support clinicians' efforts to prioritize health care resources fairly.

The notions of containing health care costs, carefully allocating resources, and rationing medical care evokes very negative reactions in most people. The possibility that one's own doctor might limit care in order to save money seems even more dismaying. Yet the need to control medical spending, and the need to do so at least in part by rationing, seems inescapable. So as we set out to edit and author a book on resource allocation and rationing, we aimed to offer suggestions for doing so in a way that is fair and practicable with the hope of providing a countervailing perspective to the usual reaction.

Some may think that preparing a book that addresses rationing by physicians is a hardhearted pursuit. But that is not how we see it. We were motivated by the aspiration to make health promotion and the achievement of health equity sustainable endeavors and by the belief that to accomplish these goals, health care systems and all those who work in them must prioritize the interventions they provide. They must give careful thought to using cost-effective strategies, and sometimes this will require forgoing some beneficial interventions because they cost too much.

Some may imagine that we envision rationing as being foisted upon patients while they are either unaware or unwilling. But again, we do not see it this way. We believe that rationing will be more justifiable if the public recognizes the fact that health care is expensive and that costs must be constrained. We anticipate that priority setting will be more accommodating of the point of view of patients if their personal providers make them aware of and involve them in the process.

We must acknowledge that some health policy experts see little need to ration. This view is common among health policy experts in the United States who argue that, particularly in that country, overutilization and wildly excessive pricing are driving health care costs (Anderson, 2003; Oberlander & White, 2009). We do not deny that these problems contribute to health care costs. We also do not deny the general point that many powerful "actors" other than health care personnel influence costs and resource allocation. But addressing these problems and calling attention to other sources of health care costs does not obviate the need for health care systems to set priorities and for clinicians at the bedside to provide care to their patients that is efficient and fair.

We believe that a focus on factors that drive health care costs is necessary but not sufficient to address the problem regarding financial and fiscal sustainability of health care in every country. We share the view emphasized by experts at the European Observatory on Health Systems and Policies that the need for sustainability must be thought of as a problem where health system revenue is insufficient to meet health system obligations. They clarify two notions that are often confused: economic sustainability and fiscal sustainability (Thompson et al., 2007). As they argue:

> Economic sustainability refers to growth in health spending as a proportion of gross domestic product (GDP). Spending on health is economically sustainable up to the point at which the social cost of health spending exceeds the value produced by that spending. If health spending sufficiently threatens other valued areas of economic activity, health spending may come to be seen as economically unsustainable. Growth in health spending is more likely to threaten other areas of economic activity in an economy that is stagnant or shrinking than it is in an economy that is growing…
>
> Concern regarding the fiscal sustainability of a health system relates specifically to public expenditure on health care. A health system may be economically sustainable and yet fiscally unsustainable if public revenue is insufficient to meet public expenditure. There are three broad approaches to addressing the problem of fiscal sustainability: (1) increase public revenue to the point at which health system obligations can be met; (2) lessen those obligations to the point at which they can be met from existing (or projected) revenue; (3) improve the capacity of the health system to convert resources into value.

In our view, public concern should focus on both types of sustainability. Citizens have a valuable stake in having a national economy that promotes their health, and excessive spending in the health sector at the expense of other sectors does not effectively promote their health. Citizens also have a valuable stake in controlling government costs to avoid public debt that becomes increasingly paralyzing to effective public governance (Nautet & Van Meensel, 2011).

The aim of this book is thus to consider ways to foster cost-conscious care at the bedside as a feasible and ethically sound practice that can contribute to the economic and fiscal sustainability of health care. We bring together both empirical evidence about the way doctors tell us they take cost into account in their practices, along with analyses from recognized scholars from various disciplines and in different countries. Here in the introduction we begin by defining resource allocation and bedside rationing as we use the terms. We describe the origins of the book. We then outline how the book is organized and give an overview of the text.

■ DESCRIBING AND DEFINING RESOURCE ALLOCATION AND BEDSIDE RATIONING

In their very useful book, *The Global Challenge of Health Care Rationing*, Angela Coulter and Chris Ham explain how they use the word *rationing* (Coulter & Ham, 2000). They note that *rationing* has a variety of connotations and is often used interchangeably with the term *priority setting*.

> While some authors prefer to use rationing to refer only to decisions that affect individual patients (Klein et al 1996), in our view it has come to be employed to describe a variety of ways in which choices in health care are made whether they affect individuals, communities or countries. There seems little point in view of this in drawing hard and fast distinctions between rationing and priority setting. It is for this reason that throughout this book the terms are used synonymously to refer to the allocation of resources in health care both in terms of the relative priority to be attached to different demands and needs and to decisions that are made not to fund treatment for individuals or groups.

In their introduction to the book, which includes experiences with rationing in countries around the world, Coulter and Ham go on to write,

> ...it is clear that responsibility for rationing rests at a number of levels in regulated health care systems. At the macro level, politicians determine the level of funding to be allocated to the health services and how this should be distributed between areas and services. At the meso level, intermediate bodies such as sickness funds, health authorities and insurance companies make decisions on the allocation of resources to particular forms of treatment. At the micro level, clinicians use their judgement and experience to decide which patients should receive treatment and how much should be done for individual patients. Each level impacts on the

others, with clinicians retaining considerable discretion, even though politicians and managers at the macro and meso levels have increasingly questioned implicit decision making.

We agree with these descriptions of resource allocation and rationing. Indeed, the need to improve these processes at the bedside and transform them from implicit and inadequately reasoned endeavors lies at the heart of our book.

We would also agree with Peter Ubel and Susan Goold regarding the definition of bedside rationing that they used in their important article in 1997, "Recognizing bedside rationing: Clear cases and tough calls." To label a physician's decision an example of bedside rationing:

> The physician must 1) withhold, withdraw, or fail to recommend a service that, in the physician's best clinical judgment, is in the patient's best medical interests; 2) act primarily to promote the financial interests of someone other than the patient (including an organization, society at large, or the physician himself or herself)[1]; and 3) have control over the use of the beneficial service (Ubel & Goold 1997).

We recognize that the mere term *bedside rationing* is contentious. Indeed, Paul Menzel argues, in his contribution to this book, that the term *priority setting* ought to be used instead, contending that when physicians decide to withhold an intervention there is not necessarily any certainty that the patient will incur less benefit and face a worse outcome than he would have had the intervention been used.

■ ORIGINS OF THIS BOOK

The seeds of this book began in 2002 when Samia Hurst was a fellow in the Department of Bioethics at the National Institutes of Health Clinical Center. She and Marion Danis began an international collaborative project with European colleagues Anne Slowther from the United Kingdom, Reidun Forde from Norway, Stella Reiter-Theil of Switzerland, and Renzo Pegoraro of Italy to explore the experiences and attitudes of primary care providers with regard to bedside rationing. We conducted a survey entitled *Values at the Bedside*, a National Institutes of Health (NIH)–funded survey of physicians in the United Kingdom, Norway, Switzerland, and Italy that explored physicians' self-reported experience with rationing, their perception of scarcity and

---

1. We should note that while we agree with this definition of rationing, we would not consider the aim of withholding beneficial treatments from patients for the sake of profiting other parties as an ethically acceptable reason for rationing.

fairness in their health care systems, and their attitudes toward both clinical rationing and various other cost-containment strategies. (Hurst et al., 2006, 2007a, 2007b)

While it might seem odd that this project grew out of a survey initiated in the US regarding rationing practices in Europe, it becomes more understandable when one reflects on how difficult it has been to discuss resource allocation and rationing explicitly and directly in the US (Ubel, 1995; Brock, 2007). The opportunity to approach the topic in a more round-about way through initiation of a dialogue across countries, some of which are much more at ease with discussion of priority setting (Mørland, Ringard, & Røttingen, 2010), seemed like a more felicitous approach.

We should note that in the Values at the Bedside survey we did not use the term "bedside rationing," preferring to simply ask clinicians whether they took cost into account in deciding whether or not to offer a clinical intervention to a patient. We took this approach to avoid the possibility that responding clinicians might find the concept of rationing anathema, or might have biases that would lead them to answer questions about their attitudes and behaviors regarding rationing in a way that they perceived as socially acceptable. We would suggest, however, that in taking this approach in the wording of the survey we were likely to get responses from clinicians that meet the definition of bedside rationing used by Ubel and Goold.

In responding to the survey, physicians reported that they do indeed take cost into account in deciding whether or not to offer a clinical intervention to patients, and analysis of the responses revealed a number of factors associated with limit-setting in clinical care. In gathering and reporting the results of our study, we began to consider how to go beyond this empirical project. Could we take some steps toward fostering fairness in the kinds of decisions that clinicians make? Fairness and equity are key concerns in the debate surrounding the allocation of health care resources as the rise of health care costs drives attempts to contain expenditures. The issue of limiting potentially beneficial interventions on the grounds that their cost is too high is, of course, controversial (Relman, 1990; Asch & Ubel, 1997), as is the role that physicians should play in this type of cost-containment effort. (Sulmasy, 1992; Morreim, 1991; Ubel, 2001; Daniels, 1985; Bloche, 1999; Hall, 1997) We knew from an earlier survey of clinicians in the United States that clinicians do not think about the matter of fairness very explicitly when dealing with resource constraints (Hurst et al., 2005).

Thus, we proposed to hold a symposium to elicit commentary on the findings of the Values at the Bedside study at the Brocher Foundation near Geneva, Switzerland, in July 2010.

We hoped to explore what kind of bedside rationing decisions would and *should* be acceptable to reasonable people and how it might be possible to help physicians and other clinicians reach such decisions. We believed these questions were difficult, since the study results suggested that there are complex interactions between macro and meso level policy decisions and clinical rationing decisions at the micro level of patient care, just as experts such as Coulter and Ham had claimed (Coulter & Ham, 2000). By putting the study into context and understanding its implications for questions of fair clinical rationing (Carlsen & Norheim, 2005; Fleck, 2002a), along with allocation decisions at the level of health care systems, (Cappelen & Norheim, 2005; Fleck, 2002b; Holm, 1998; Emanuel & Wertheimer, 2006) we intended to bring the international discussion on health care allocation a significant step forward.

■ AN OVERVIEW OF THE BOOK

We have organized the book in four sections. We begin in the first part with a description of findings in the Values at the Bedside study. The second part elaborates on the four health care systems in which the study was conducted, to put the study findings into context. The third part provides commentaries on the study results and analyses that illuminate the ethics and practice of resource allocation and rationing at the bedside. The fourth part shifts away from a theoretical approach to offer practical strategies for promoting fair resource allocation and rationing at the bedside. Here we preview the chapters in each of these sections.

Part I. Results of the Values at the Bedside Study

In chapter 1 the authors of the Values at the Bedside study describe the extent to which doctors in the study considered limiting care because of concerns about costs and examine what forms of bedside rationing these doctors considered compatible with their role. The chapter describes the diverse criteria and strategies doctors used in rationing care. The study revealed several determinants of bedside rationing by doctors: the perception of scarcity, direct and indirect pressures exerted on doctors to ration, and country of practice. The latter likely reflects differences in the incentive structures provided by different health care systems.

Chapter 2 turns the lens in another direction and focuses on the perceptions of doctors who participated in the study regarding the health care systems in which they practice. It highlights what doctors had to say about the allocation processes at the macro and meso levels in their countries. In so doing, it provides a picture of the interactions of priority setting at various levels in each of the study countries. It also offers insights about physicians' views of the fairness of their health care systems.

Part II. The Societal Context

In this part of the book we take a detailed look at the health care system of each of the four countries in which the Values at the Bedside study was conducted. The study investigators from Switzerland, the United Kingdom, Norway, and Italy each in turn profile their health care systems and consider how their systems' characteristics may have contributed to the survey findings about doctors' attitudes and behavior toward rationing. The chapters outline the overall organization of health care in the country at the time of the study, including arrangements for funding and models for setting priorities in the allocation of health care resources. The chapters also reflect on changes to health care organization and public policy on resource allocation that have taken place in their countries in years subsequent to the study and the possible future implications for resource allocation and rationing by physicians.

Part III. Analysis of Bedside Rationing

While the challenges of fair resource allocation unfold in the context of local health care systems, decisions, and policies, ethical questions about bedside rationing are ubiquitous and transcend national boundaries. Thus the third part of the book shifts to analyses that are germane across health care systems. Contributors in this part represent a variety of disciplines including medicine, health policy, moral philosophy, and law.

We begin in chapter 7 with a review by Thomas Allen, Matt Sutton, and Richard Cookson of the results of primary care incentive schemes in the United Kingdom and consider what they can teach us about the effectiveness of such schemes for promoting rationing by practitioners. One such scheme was budget holding, which was intended to contain costs by encouraging general practitioners (GPs) to do *more* rationing, in particular by reducing prescribing and specialist referral rates, and to do so more fairly and effectively by reducing prescribing and referral for relatively unnecessary and low-benefit interventions while potentially releasing funds to increase prescribing and referral for more important interventions. A second scheme involved pay for performance, which was intended to improve quality—in particular prescribing quality—and again, to do so more fairly and effectively by targeting prescribing effort on "high-risk" patients who benefit more from a given prescribing intervention than "low-risk" patients (as the pay-for-performance targets all focused on "high-risk" patients). More recent UK National Health Service (NHS) reform proposals have a similar rationale to the first scheme, but at the "meso" level of local health care purchasing organizations called *GP consortia,* and subsequently clinical commissioning groups, rather than the "bedside" level of individual GPs or GP practices, although no doubt they have implications for the bedside level.

In chapter 8, Keith Syrett writes about the importance of the legal context of bedside rationing. Health care rationing, whether by individual clinicians or policymakers, requires balancing of competing rights, interests, and conceptions of justice. As allocation and rationing of health care resources have become more explicit, and as the public has become more informed about health care decisions, the legitimacy of these decisions has been challenged in several countries. To date the main challenges have been in relation to macro or meso level decisions; for example in the United Kingdom, challenges to central (National Institute of Health and Care Excellence) or local clinical commissioning group decisions on specific treatments. But their impact on individual clinicians' decisions at the bedside can be significant. Challenges to decision making by public bodies or public servants inevitably look to the law for guidance and adjudication. Legal judgments in such cases shape future policy and individual practice. While taking many examples from the UK context, the chapter also explores the interface between law and health care rationing from other national jurisdictions, drawing on and contrasting these examples. Syrett argues that the law has a significant contribution to make to the question of legitimacy of rationing decisions in the area of public policy, which in turn has implications for bedside rationing.

In chapter 9, Michael Barilan argues that to the extent that rationing involves forgoing of possible benefit, how benefits are defined is crucial. He links the definition of benefit to questions of flourishing and explores who should define what counts as a benefit. Should the prerogative of determining what counts as benefit be the province of medical experts, either individually or collectively? Or is defining what counts as beneficial health care in specific clinical circumstances part of a patient's right of autonomy? Some patients might demand extraordinarily aggressive and expensive care near the end of life, although most physicians and most other reasonable patients in similar circumstances would see that as a net harm. From the perspective of health care justice—fair use of limited health care resources—it seems such patients are demanding something, on the basis of a highly subjective sense of benefit, to which they have no just claim. This chapter explores when personal judgment of benefit must be respected and when it may be overridden for the sake of a more just distribution of health care resources.

In chapter 10, Leonard Fleck starts us off with the key question: Is it is ever morally permissible for physicians to make bedside rationing decisions with regard to their own patients, thereby compromising what might be regarded as those patients' "best interests"? He argues that physicians who must work within global budgets or other financial constraints are responsible for large numbers of patients, not simply the patient in the clinic at any given moment.

Fairness, compassion and loyalty to each patient require that broader perspective. He argues that bedside rationing is not avoidable, nor is it intrinsically morally objectionable. A range of clinical scenarios are considered to identify and distinguish morally permissible from morally impermissible forms of bedside rationing. He then proposes that bedside rationing is more likely to be fair if the basic rules regarding such rationing are a product of a public democratic deliberative process conducted by healthy individuals regarding their future possible seriously ill selves. In this way individuals choose for themselves whether certain beneficial health care is worth the high cost to them in the form of higher taxes or insurance premiums. This reduces considerably the moral burden of disloyalty by physicians, since patients will have collectively conveyed to physicians what care they are willing to deny themselves as "not worth it." Fleck concludes that clinical complexity can never be perfectly managed by such rules, that some flexibility must be accorded to physicians at the bedside in interpreting and applying rationing guidelines, and consequently some burden of moral judgment remains for physicians in a cost-conscious clinical environment.

Chapters 11 and 12 focus on a key issue regarding resource allocation—the inefficiency stemming from the overuse of ineffective interventions. In chapter 11, Howard Brody argues that overdiagnosis and overtreatment account for such a large part of health care expenditures that physician attention to reducing such overuse might in and of itself provide a sufficient solution to the problem of unsustainable health care costs. Part and parcel of his view is the idea that the common assumption that there is a continuum of more and less efficient medical interventions is not accurate or useful. Rather, parsing out the ineffective from effective interventions and eliminating the former would suffice. In chapter 12, Daniel Strech and Marion Danis take a contrasting approach and assume that treatments that are ineffective and treatments with a prospect of some benefit will both need to be addressed to adequately control health care costs. They consider whether rationing can be justifiable when inefficiency has not been eliminated. This chapter aims to clarify under what conditions rationing can be justified despite imperfect efficiency and concludes that if rationing is avoidable through improved efficiency at the macro or micro level of health systems (theoretically and practically), rationing cannot be justified in those cases where the rationing agent is at the same time aware that improved efficiency in her work is possible.

In chapter 13, Bob Goodin offers an analysis of the collective action problem that is posed by limited health care resources. Collective action problems occur in circumstances when individuals would all benefit from a certain action, which, however, has an associated cost making it implausible that anyone individually will undertake it. The rational choice is then to undertake this as a collective action, the cost of which is shared. This chapter explores whether it is useful to consider the need to control health care costs through rationing as a collective action problem and, if so, how one might proceed to do so. Alternatively, if not, how can we expect clinicians and patients to shoulder this responsibility as individuals?

In chapter 14, Paul Menzel focuses on the dilemma posed by the differing perspectives of statistical and identified lives. When experts write guidelines for patient care for a given health condition, they write them with a statistical perspective in mind, related to a population of patients. Yet, when clinicians care for patients with these conditions they have an identified person in front of them. Menzel argues that the statistical/identifiable distinction is easily confused and misapplied in clinical settings and that speaking of "rationing" instead of "prioritizing," as alluded to earlier, badly exacerbates these confusions. While bedside prioritizing decisions deny a potentially beneficial item to an identifiable patient for the benefit of those who are not identifiable, it is often still not known that the identifiable recipient of care will actually benefit; at this point in time in a clinical decision the *beneficiaries* of treatment are thus also significantly "statistical." The other potential beneficiaries—those who will benefit from a decision to deny treatment to a given patient now—are really no more "statistical," although they are more distant and tend to become invisible. The chapter considers how physicians may ethically prioritize lives in this complex mixture of identifiable and statistical dimensions and whether understanding and accommodating these dimensions can allow experts to write guidelines that better assist clinicians in that task.

We complete this part of the book with chapter 15, where Vegard Bruun Wyller brings to the reader a contrary view—an argument against bedside rationing. Clinical decision making might be based on moral principles focusing exclusively on the individual patient, such as the principles of beneficence, autonomy, and nonmaleficence. Alternatively, clinical decisions might include considerations in which the individual patient is seen in relation to *others*: either concomitantly diseased persons or society in general. Such considerations draw upon the moral principles of justice or solidarity as well as empirical knowledge from health economic studies. Only when one diverges from a strictly individual focus is it necessary to be concerned about sharing resources. While the need to think about sharing resources is regarded as inevitable or even suitable, Wyller considers the negative side effects of a clinical practice that pays increased attention to prioritizing and less to the classical, individually focused virtues. Three fundamental premises constitute a starting point for the discussion: (a) that prioritizing always implies *general* moral considerations, although they might be based on expert medical knowledge; (b) that prioritizing usually concerns the total usage of resources in society, not only the health budget; (c) that prioritizing, given points (a) and (b), principally belongs to the political sphere rather than the medical one. He argues that contemporary medicine neglects these premises. As a consequence, the dilemma of prioritizing is regarded as a medical dilemma rather than a political one. This exemplifies a transfer of power from the political level to the expert or bureaucratic level and hence to doctors and other health care professionals. This essay explores the disadvantages of this shift in responsibilities and concludes by urging a return to the classical medical virtues as illustrated in the parable of the Good Samaritan, who offers his entire resources for the benefit of the one individual he meets accidentally—and in that regard, he constitutes a perpetual ideal for the health care worker.

Part IV. Strategies for Promoting Fair Bedside Rationing

This last part of the book takes a more practical turn and offers some concrete suggestions and proposals for enhancing the fairness of rationing by clinicians.

In chapter 16, Odd Soreide, Stener Kvinnsland, and Torhild Heggestad from Norway describe their experience with the use of guidelines for managing bedside rationing fairly that might serve as a useful model for others. The authors suggest that while Norway has a long tradition of discussing the need for rationing both in public and among health care personnel, there has been little application of theory in practice. The authors and their colleagues, physicians who have been active in transforming the national guidelines into explicit prioritization decisions in Bergen, one of Norway's largest health care trusts, report their experience and describe the challenges they have faced and their attempts to overcome them. Of particular interest is how this work has affected hospital reimbursements and the quality of the health care delivered.

In chapter 17, a paper published by Samia Hurst and Marion Danis entitled "Rationing by clinical judgment" is reprinted from the *Kennedy Institute of Ethics Journal*. The argument is put forward that while rationing by clinical judgment is controversial, its acceptability partly depends on how it is practiced. After defining a range of circumstances in which rationing by clinical judgment are likely to take place, a framework of requirements for procedural fairness is offered to facilitate fair bedside rationing: (1) a closed system that offers reciprocity, (2) attention to general concerns of justice, (3) respect for individual variations, (4) application of a consistent process, (5) explicitness and, (6) review of decisions. The process could be monitored for its applicability and appropriateness.

In chapter 18, Jan Schurmann and colleagues describe a project intended to design various types of assistance to clinicians to help them practice fair resource micro-allocation in patient care and improve the quality of patient care. An evidence-oriented *guideline* is at the heart of the project, paying particular attention to avoid discrimination against vulnerable patient groups such as critically ill or incapacitated persons. A 4-level model is described, involving increasingly extensive solutions to match the intensity of the problem. Some difficulties may require a brief clarification by searching for and sharing relevant information; others will need a more substantial case discussion or ethics consultation. Clinical staff can choose solutions ranging from a brief clarification of issues to a full ethics consultation whenever someone feels a patient is at risk of being put at a disadvantage. Development of the guideline was based on research and consensus building, evaluation, and modification with active involvement of clinical partners. The chapter reports on the development of the guideline and its implementation in six clinical institutions.

In chapter 19, Irene Dankwa-Mullan, Paula Goodwin, and Matthew Wynia from the United States consider how bedside rationing can be carried out with sufficiently fair consideration of socially disadvantaged groups who face health disparities. They consider what constitutes fair rationing when providing clinical care for socially disadvantaged groups, particularly racial and ethnic minorities, and impoverished populations. The authors argue that the limits of evidence-based medicine due to underrepresentation of these groups in clinical trials, perceptions of nonadherence, and assumptions about stigmatized patient groups need to become a part of the dialogue to address health care disparities. The authors assess effectiveness studies for reducing intentional or unintentional bias, stigma, and discrimination against various disadvantaged groups. They then consider the value of physician–patient concordance and cultural competence as strategies for how bedside rationing in limited resource settings can be carried out fairly for all patients, including those in disadvantaged groups.

In chapter 20, Steve Pearson from the United States considers how healthcare reform under the Affordable Care Act modifies the way doctors are compensated by the public insurers, Medicare, and Medicaid. This promotes a shift from fee-for-service payments to clinicians toward global payments to existing or new accountable care organizations (ACOs)—combinations of hospitals, physician groups, and even private insurers—that function as integrated systems to provide all necessary care. The shift to ACOs is intended to bring greater coordination of care while changing the underlying financial incentive for physicians, so that they are rewarded for prevention of illness and for more efficient, less costly care overall. Pearson considers whether the financial rewards for less costly care lead to pressures on individual doctors to ration at the bedside or whether there are conceptual frameworks for larger groups of physicians to ration care in ways that will be viewed as more acceptable to patients and the public. In so doing he suggests that the term *bedside rationing* obscures the important distinction between the random variation in rationing possible across individual physicians and a more organized approach to making allocation decisions and treatment guidelines for the population being cared for by a physician organization.

In chapter 21, Ole Norheim makes the case for the importance of empirically modeling the consequences of resource allocation and rationing strategies. He argues that as with all medical practices, it is important to examine the consequences of decisions. Resource allocation and rationing practices of physicians should be no different in this regard. Yet, little research has been done to examine what the consequence of rationing guidelines would be. Following this argument, he provides an example of such modeling. A Norwegian rationing strategy for management of cardiovascular disease is put to the test to see what its impact would be. The guideline is quantitatively modeled to examine the distributional consequences for various segments of the population. Subsequently these consequences are analyzed from a normative standpoint to consider whether the guidelines are just.

In chapter 22, Susan Goold examines the possibility that doctors can serve as bellwethers of rationing. She examines the value of physicians' experience in calling attention to rationing and its effects on the practice of medicine and the quality of patient care. Physicians' role in providing direct patient care places them in a unique position to indicate when resources are too scarce, when the health care system becomes discriminatory or unjust, and when pressures brought to bear on them excessively compromise patient advocacy or excessively constrain their freedom to use resources to meet patients' needs. Acting as a bellwether for such aspects, however, requires physicians to overcome several conceptual and practical difficulties.

In chapter 23, Marion Danis, Greer Donley, and Reidun Forde explore whether it is possible to change the language about rationing to have a constructive discussion with patients. Although there is variation from country to country, there is fairly universal public antipathy to rationing. This chapter examines the basis for this antipathy and consider strategies for overcoming it. The antipathy to rationing must be overcome by means of two different strategies: by giving the issue more public attention, but also by addressing it explicitly and systematically in health care organizations and in the clinical encounter. The chapter considers two aspects of the cost of care that might be discussed in the clinical encounter: (1) the shared costs of health care that are borne collectively as insurance premiums and taxes, and (2) the costs that individuals incur personally at the time of illness. Addressing both aspects are warranted, although the justification for and approach to discussing these aspects differ. It is possible for clinicians to discuss costs with patients in a respectful manner that promotes fairness, respect for patient autonomy, and sensitivity to the needs of the patient. Such discussions can be useful with patients regarding care at any point, including care at the end of life.

In chapter 24, Anne Slowther and Ben Bennett consider how to educate future doctors and other clinicians to prepare them to participate in fair rationing or priority setting at the bedside (Weinberger, 2011). Traditionally, medical education at both an undergraduate and postgraduate level has focused on clinical competence providing doctors with the knowledge and skills to diagnose, treat, and prevent disease. The inclusion of medical ethics teaching in the curricula of medical schools in recent years has mirrored this focus, emphasizing the professional and moral obligations of physicians to respect their patients' autonomy and act in their patients' best interests. Physicians at all levels of their profession are ill-equipped to make decisions about fair allocation of resources because their training does not usually include consideration of health economics, distributive justice, or models of decision making in priority setting. Involvement in rationing creates conflict for clinicians with their core professional duty of care to do what is best for their individual patient. Slowther and Bennett consider what might be the content and format of appropriate training for clinicians in relation to health care allocation and rationing.

We wrap up in the Afterword with an overview of the book. We have made the case that clinicians do worry about cost and take it into account in their clinical decisions and that it is preferable that they do so explicitly and fairly. We suggest that this is an issue of international relevance and that while countries differ in their solutions, these solutions can be mutually instructive. We suggest that a full understanding of bedside allocation and rationing entails appreciation of the roles and interactions of health care systems and individual practitioners.

While we have highlighted this interaction, we should also say a word about how much discretion regarding resource allocation and rationing should be at the level of the physician. The prospect of increasingly expensive treatments that may yield substantial benefit, not merely marginal gains, but are too expensive for a sustainable health care system to manage, requires highly contentious priority setting. This is not the sort of decision we envision being left to the discretion of the individual physician. A fully fair arrangement of resource allocation requires system-level decisions with public engagement and leaves the more marginal decisions to providers where clinical discretion is needed. We hope that readers come away with suggestions for how health care systems and individual clinicians can effectively and ethically function in tandem to accomplish the task of delivering affordable health care. We also hope that readers come away with pointers for altering the discussion so that the public and its leadership can address the issue more openly. Having aimed to advance interdisciplinary discussion in a complex area of study, without fully resolving the issues, we hope we have contributed to the capacity of clinicians and those who partner with them to deliver affordable and fair health care.

REFERENCES

Anderson, G. F., et al. (2003). It's the prices, stupid: Why the United States is so different from other countries. *Health Affairs*, 22(3):89–105.

Asch, DA., Ubel, PA. (1997). Rationing by any other name. *New England Journal of Medicine*, 336(23):1668–1671.

Bloche, M. G. (1999). Clinical loyalties and the social purposes of medicine. *JAMA*, 281(3):268–274.

Brock, D. (2007). Health care resource prioritization and rationing: Why is it so difficult? *Social Research: An International Quarterly*, 74:125–148.

Cappelen, A. W., & Norheim, O. F. (2005). Responsibility, fairness and rationing in health care. *Health Policy*, 76(3):312–319.

Carlsen, B., & Norheim, O. F. (2005). Saying no is no easy matter: a qualitative study of competing concerns in rationing decisions in general practice. *BMC Health Services Research*, Nov 9;5:70.

Coulter, A., & Ham, C. (2000). *The Global Challenge of Health Care Rationing*. Buckingham: Open University Press.

Daniels, N. (1985). *Just Health Care*: Cambridge: Cambridge University Press.

Emanuel, E. J., & Wertheimer, A. (2006). Public health. Who should get influenza vaccine when not all can? *Science*, 312(5775):854–855.

Fleck, L. M. (2002a). Rationing: don't give up. *Hastings Center Report*, 32(2):35–36.

Fleck, L. M. (2002b). Last chance therapies: can a just and caring society do health care rationing when life itself is at stake? *Yale Journal of Health Policy, Law & Ethics*, 2(2):255–298.

Hall, M. A. (1997). *Making Medical Spending Decisions*. Oxford: Oxford University Press.

Holm, S. (1998). The second phase of priority setting. Goodbye to the simple solutions: the second phase of priority setting in health care. *British Medical Journal*, 317(7164):1000–1002.

Hurst S., Slowther A., Forde R., Pegoraro R., Reiter-Theil S., Perrier A., Garrett-Mayer E., Danis M. (2006). Prevalence and Determinants of Physician Bedside Rationing in Four European Countries. *Journal of General Internal Medicine*, 1(11):1138–1143.

Hurst, S. A., Forde, R., Reiter-Theil, S., Pegoraro, R., Perrier, A., Slowther, A., & Danis, M. (2007a). Ethical difficulties in clinical practice: experiences of European doctors. *Journal of Medical Ethics*, 33:51–57.

Hurst, S. A., Forde, R., Reiter-Theil, S., Slowther, A. M., Perrier, A., Pegoraro, R., & Danis, M. (2007b). Physicians' views on resource availability and equity in four European health care systems. *BMC Health Services Research*,7(1):137.

Hurst, S. A., & Danis, M. (2007). A framework for rationing by clinical judgment. *Kennedy Institute of Ethics Journal*,17(3):247–266.

Hurst, S. A., Hull, S. C., DuVal, G., & Danis, M. Physicians' responses to resource constraint. *Archives of Internal Medicine*, 165(6):639–644.

Mørland, B., Ringard, A., & Røttingen, J. A. (2010). Supporting tough decisions in Norway: a healthcare system approach. *International Journal of Technology Assessment in Health Care*, 26(4):398–404.

Morreim, E. (1991). *Balancing Act; The New Medical Ethics of Medicine's New Economics*. Dordrecht, Boston, London: Kluwer Academic Publishers.

Nautet, M., Van Meensel, L. (2011). Economic impact of the public debt. *Economic Review*, 2:7–19. Available at http://www.nbb.be/doc/oc/repec/ecrart/ecorevII2011_H1.pdf.

Oberlander, J. & White, J. (2009). Public attitudes toward health care spending aren't the problem; prices are. *Health Affairs, 28*(5):1285–1293.

Relman, A. (1990). Use of medical resources—overview. *Preventive Medicine,19*(6): 688–692.

Sulmasy, D. P. (1992). Physicians, cost control, and ethics. *Annals of Internal Medicine, 116*(11):920–926.

Swiss Academy of Medical Sciences. (2007). *Rationing in the Swiss health-care system: analysis and recommendations.* Available at: http://www.samw.ch/docs/Publikationen/e_Bericht.pdf.

Thompson, S., Foubister, T., & Mossialos E. (2007). *Financing Health Care in the European Union: Challenges and Policy Responses.* Observatory Series No 17. European Observatory on Health Systems and Policies. World Health Organization. Available at: http://www.euro.who.int/__data/assets/pdf_file/0009/98307/E92469.pdf.

Ubel, P. A., & Arnold, R. M. (1995). The unbearable rightness of bedside rationing: physician duties in a climate of cost containment. *Archives of Internal Medicine, 155*:1837–1842.

Ubel, P. A, & Goold, S. (1997). Recognizing bedside rationing: Clear cases and tough calls. *Annals of Internal Medicine, 126*:74–80.

Ubel, P. (2001). *Pricing Life: Why It's Time for Health Care Rationing.* Cambridge, MA: The MIT Press.

Weinberger, S. E. (2011). Providing high-value, cost-conscious care: a critical seventh general competency for physicians. *Annals of Internal Medicine, 155*(6):386–388.

PART ONE

A European Survey of Bedside Rationing

1 The Values at the Bedside Study

Bedside Rationing by Physicians

■ SAMIA A. HURST, ANNE SLOWTHER,
REIDUN FØRDE, AND MARION DANIS

In this chapter we present results from the *Values at the Bedside* study, an international, NIH-funded, European survey of physicians exploring their reported experience with rationing, their perception of scarcity and fairness in their health care systems, and their attitudes toward clinical rationing and various other cost-containment strategies. Some of the results from this study have been published elsewhere (Hurst, Slowther, et al., 2006; Hurst, Forde, et al., 2007). Based on this study we know that physicians do report bedside rationing, and we know that there are a number of factors associated with the likelihood that they do so (Hurst, Forde, et al., 2007).

When we started this international four-country study, data suggested that physicians accepted prioritization decisions, for example when faced with hypo-thetical scenarios (see for example Ryynanen, Myllykangas, et al., 1997; Cooke & Hutchinson, 2001; Rosen & Karlberg, 2002; Escher, Perneger, et al., 2004) but also as reported in their practice (Arnesen & Fredriksen, 1995; Ryynanen, Myllykangas, et al., 1999; Hurst, Hull, et al., 2005). In one study, Ayres (1996) had looked at attitudes of general practitioners in the United Kingdom regarding the relevance and impact of rationing and the strategies they would advocate for resolving rationing dilemmas, both at the individual and population level. The attitudinal data, however, and the focus on acceptable policies for resource allo-cation at the macro level, meant that their experience of day-to-day clinical strat-egies used in dealing with scarce resources was incompletely described. Three key aspects had not been explored. First, we did not know how often physicians actually made rationing decisions in their daily practice. Second, the types of interventions that tended to be rationed were not known. Third, the criteria that physicians used in making these decisions had not been explored either. Therefore, these three questions constituted the main focus of our own study.

There are two reasons to look at physician bedside rationing. If we find that it happens, it points to situations where scarcity is identified. But there is a more important reason. If we wonder whether or not physicians should take part in resource allocation, then we may need to know whether, and especially how, rationing takes place in clinical practice (Asch & Ubel, 1997; Ubel, 2001). The key question here is whether physicians *should* participate in allocation decisions. This, however, may very much depend on how they tend to do so. Descriptive data about what physicians withhold, from whom, and how they make these decisions is very important if we are to make normative judgments about the ethical acceptability of bedside rationing. If one takes the normative perspective, as we do, that rationing ought to maximize fairness, data can eventually be used to examine whether physicians withhold in a discriminatory or evenhanded manner and hence whether or not bedside rationing is morally problematic. If physician reasoning is consistent with practice guidelines and cognizant of issues of fairness, then bedside rationing might be an ethically acceptable component of the processes dictating the distribution of medical resources. If not, it may not be.

■ A SURVEY OF EUROPEAN PHYSICIANS

We surveyed general physicians, whom we identified through the 2002 official list of the Norwegian Medical Association, the Swiss Medical Association, published listings of UK general practitioners and general physicians, and regional listings of Italian general practitioners and members of the Italian Society of Internal Medicine. In each country we selected a random sample of 400 individuals in proportions of general practitioners and general internists reflecting that of each national physician population. This sample was chosen to capture similar physician populations, who do the same kind of work in general internal medicine, in both inpatient and outpatient care. We developed a survey to explore their perception of, and attitude toward, scarcity and rationing both at the system-wide level through resource unavailability and in clinical practice through bedside rationing (Hurst, Slowther, et al., 2006). We chose four European countries that offer universal access to health care, with per capita expenditure on health care ranging from $3,322 in Switzerland to $1,989 in the United Kingdom.

We were particularly careful in wording the questions about clinical rationing. The term "rationing" is of course a socially loaded word, and asking physicians something like "do you ration?" would have been very likely to yield false-negative results. Consequently, we made our questions as descriptive and morally neutral as possible. Our main question was worded as follows: "During the last 6 months, how often did you personally refrain, because of cost to the health care system, from using the following interventions when they would have been the best intervention for your patient?" We then listed 10 concrete interventions, chosen to represent the range of interventions across the spectrum of care from prevention to life-sustaining treatment. Thus, we hoped, physicians would feel more free to respond accurately and do so based on specific cases they remembered.

We mailed questionnaires to 1,600 physicians and received responses from 43%. Respondents covered the full range of physicians' ages (from 28 to 82)

TABLE 1.1. *Characteristics of Physicians Who Responded to the Survey*

Physician characteristics	(N = 656)
Age, years	28–82 (mean 51)
Years in practice	1–62 (mean 25)
Male	546 (85%)
Specialty	
Family medicine	195 (30%)
General medicine	188 (29%)
Internal medicine	179 (28%)
Country of practice	
Italy	139 (21%)
Norway	222 (34%)
Switzerland	183 (28%)
UK	112 (17%)
Primary practice site	
Hospital	258 (38%)
Solo practice	182 (28%)
Primary care group practice	164 (25%)
Multispecialty group	23 (4%)
Other	28 (4%)
Admitting hospital	
Public	572 (94%)
Private	21 (3%)
For-profit	81 (17%)
Not-for-profit	406 (82%)
Teaching hospital	264 (46%)

Numbers in parentheses are percentages of the sample shown exclusive of missing data, and rounded to the nearest whole number

and were, with an average length of time in practice of 25 years, a rather experienced group. TABLE 1.1 provides their characteristics. Results from this survey are presented in this chapter and the next.

Clinical Rationing Is Accepted

Most of our respondents (82.3%) showed some degree of agreement with rationing. As shown in *Figure 1.1*, over a third of respondents agreed that they should sometimes deny beneficial but costly services. Half agreed that cost to society was important in their decision to use or not to use an intervention. Two-thirds agreed that physicians should adhere to clinical guidelines that discourage the use of interventions that have a small proven advantage over standard interventions that cost much more. Nevertheless, over half thought that denying costly but beneficial care would interfere with the physician–patient relationship. Physicians in the four countries gave different responses regarding agreement with rationing, agreement with guidelines discouraging the use of expensive treatments, and rationing-related fear for the physician–patient relationship. There were, however, no significant differences in physicians' agreement that they should deny services or that cost to society is important

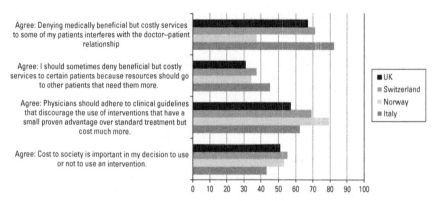

Figure 1.1 *Percentage of respondents who agreed with rationing.*

in clinical decision making. Agreement with rationing was prevalent in our sample but differed according to the sort of limit-setting described. Agreement was, for example, greater with adherence to limit-setting guidelines than with clinical bedside rationing by physicians themselves.

Clinical Rationing Is Practiced

A little over half of our respondents (56.3%) reported that they had practiced rationing in the previous 6 months. The most frequently rationed interventions were magnetic resonance imaging and screening tests. The latter is not so surprising, as the efficacy of screening tests is not always well established before they are made available to physicians. The interventions least frequently rationed were also those least frequently considered or needed: referral to an intensive care unit and dialysis. We assigned clinicians a mean score of bedside rationing related to how often they reported rationing. The identical score could correspond to situations such as rationing each of six interventions less than once a month, or rationing one intervention daily and one intervention monthly. Rationing was reported as often as daily for all interventions. Rationing of time was reported by 61.3% of respondents for the prior 6 months (*Figure 1.2*).

When asked about strategies for rationing, most respondents (82.4%) reported that they explained their reasoning to their patients when avoiding an expensive intervention. However, 36.5% also reported that they sometimes did not let a patient know about an expensive alternative (*Figure 1.3*).

Physicians reported that they tended to withhold interventions more if the expected benefit was small, chances of success were low, if an intervention was intended to prolong life when quality of life is low, or when the patient was over 85 years of age. Some criteria were reported by a number of physicians as a reason to be more likely to use an intervention, while also being reported

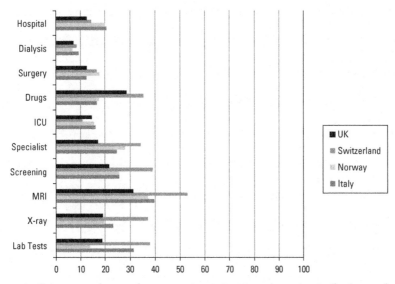

Figure 1.2 Percentage of respondents reporting rationing to any extent in the 6- month period prior to the survey.

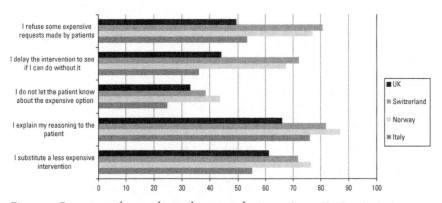

Figure 1.3 Percentage of respondents who reported using various rationing strategies.

by other physicians as a reason to use the intervention less (TABLE 1.2). For example, if an intervention were intended to improve the quality of life of a patient with a short life expectancy respondents were quite evenly divided with a third reporting being more inclined to use it and a third being less inclined to use it.

Our results complement studies that have examined specific examples of clinical rationing such as nonreferral to dialysis. (Mendelssohn, Kua, et al., 1995; Wilson, Godwin, et al., 2001) While it has been suggested that physicians often deny scarcity (Alexander, Werner, et al., 2004), our findings

TABLE 1.2. *Criteria Reported as Influencing the Use of Expensive Interventions*

	Physicians (N = 656)		
	Less likely	No change	More likely
A patient you are treating would benefit from an intervention. This intervention is very expensive. It is paid for by public money, or by a private insurer, or both. Under these circumstances, do the following factors make you **more or less likely to use this intervention?**			
The benefit to the patient is small	82.3%	0.7%	7%
Chances of success for the intervention are low	79.8%	13.8%	6.4%
The aim is to prolong the life of a patient whose quality of life you judge to be low	70.6%	17.7%	11.7%
The patient is over 85	70%	24.1%	5.9%
The patient is frail	63.2%	26.4%	10.4%
While you think the patient would benefit, the evidence base for the intervention is lacking	57.5%	28.5%	14%
The patient is cognitively impaired	49.5%	45.4%	5.1%
The aim is to improve quality of life in a patient whose life expectancy is short	35.3%	29.7%	35%
The condition requires chronic care	30.2%	50.9%	18.9%
The intervention is primary prevention	26.1%	32.8%	41.1%
The condition is attributable to smoking	17.8%	77%	5.2%
The patient will not work again	14.9%	77.7%	7.4%
The condition is attributable to a dangerous sport	14.7%	79%	6.3%
The patient asks for the intervention	12.3%	45.3%	42.4%
The patient is poor	8.4%	82%	9.6%
The condition is attributable to pregnancy	6.6%	67.4%	26%
The patient holds an important position in society	6.6%	81.3%	12.1%

Percentage shown in valid percent

indicate that physicians are aware of personally denying some benefits—or at least potential benefits—to their patients.

Should we be concerned about these results? The prevalence of rationing of nonvital benefits and of interventions for which there are alternatives does suggest that at least some rationing practices are justifiable and could be safely and legitimately entrusted to the physician at the bedside. Perhaps we even should entrust physicians with such decisions: physicians need to be aware of resource contraints and are in a particularly good position to ration in a way that takes individual specificities into account. When rationing is considered within budget constraints, physicians are not merely denying a benefit to someone; they are exercising their best judgment about where the available resources can do the most good. While rationing may be perceived as having negative consequences, it can be practiced in an effort to minimize inconvenience and risk. Indeed, the crucial question seems to be how, rather than if, rationing should be practiced. Discussion is thus needed regarding what an ethically appropriate and practically applicable process for bedside rationing could look like. While it is reassuring to see so few physicians report rationing based on poverty, the fact that some physicians report rationing based on the criterion that a patient has a low likelihood of future employment is worrisome. While rationing criteria such as cognitive impairment may be viewed as representing instances of discrimination, they may, alternatively, reflect concerns for quality of life that are shared by patients and their families. Such a range of more and less acceptable rationales for forgoing medical interventions highlights the need for a more detailed look at what elements should be taken into account to make rationing ethically acceptable. Given the prevalence of rationing, the public may be well served by more explicit discussion of how best to ration care at the bedside in an ethically justifiable manner. Concerns about justice, which have been shown to be relatively absent from physician choices in situations of scarcity (Hurst, Hull, et al., 2005), would surely be among the elements relevant to the acceptability of bedside rationing.

Determinants of Clinical Rationing Are Individual and Systemic

Bedside rationing, then, is practiced by physicians in all European countries studied. Physicians who personally agree with rationing, perceive more pressure to ration, and perceive more scarcity are more likely to report rationing.

Surprisingly for us, physicians from Norway were 2.5 times as likely to report rationing as physicians from the United Kingdom, while physicians in Italy were 3.5 times as likely and Swiss physicians were 5 times as likely as UK physicians to report rationing. While one might expect that physicians in countries that spend more money per capita would report rationing less, this does not appear to be the case. Physicians in Switzerland, where the most money per capita is spent, report the most rationing. This result is difficult to explain based on individual physician characteristics. Are Swiss physicians, who practice in an environment where scarcity is less pressing, more reluctant to act as the agent responsible for denying beneficial care and more self-consciously aware of instances where they do so? We found this explanation unconvincing, as Swiss respondents were as likely as others to agree with the necessity to sometimes deny beneficial care and did not score lower than average on the agreement with rationing scale. Swiss physicians, however, feared for their financial and professional security much more than physicians from the other surveyed countries. This, then, may have been at play in leading them to more frequently limit costly interventions. This is one of the results that requires an examination of the interaction between physician attitudes, reported rationing practices, and the broader environment within their respective health care systems.

■ STRENGTHS AND LIMITS OF THIS STUDY

The Values at the Bedside study was the first empirical report on bedside rationing to show that physicians not only practiced rationing but were also aware of it and agreed to some degree at least that they should. Our study nevertheless had several limitations. Using self-reports may have led to an underestimation of actual rationing by physicians in the countries we studied. First, withholding medically beneficial interventions from patients is controversial and is thus less likely to be reported fully than less sensitive information, even in an anonymous survey. Second, self-reports only capture instances of rationing of which practitioners are aware. This will exclude cases where physicians may have reassessed the medical indications so they were better aligned to match available resources. One of the criteria for rationing was that the expected benefit was small: but when does a small benefit become no benefit at all? Here, too, our study is likely to have underestimated the frequency of rationing due to self-reporting. As we only surveyed general physicians, generalizations to other medical specialties should be cautious, as should generalizations to different health care systems. Finally, although the response rates of physicians to mailed surveys are generally modest (Asch, Jedrziewski, et al., 1997), we would have liked to have a higher response rate. Nonrespondent bias is most likely to be associated either with lack of time or with lack of interest for the topic. In the first instance, we would expect an underestimation of the rationing of time. In the second instance, we may have to expect an overestimation of reported rationing of interventions. However, if we extrapolate our results to a response rate of 100% and if we consider all nonrespondents to report no rationing, that results in a percentage of physicians reporting rationing of interventions of 23%. This would still mean that 1 in 4 physicians was aware of withholding beneficial interventions on the basis of cost.

■ THE INEVITABLE REALITY OF BEDSIDE RATIONING BY PHYSICIANS

Bedside rationing by physicians was reported in all four surveyed countries, with a high prevalence ranging from 43.3% to 64.7%. Some physicians reported that they practiced it daily. A majority of physicians in all four countries agreed that some degree of rationing was part of their role.

Based on our definition of rationing, these results can be understood to mean that physicians are attempting to define a "reasonable limit" to the care they provide and the costs it generates. Whether the decisions they report are "reasonable" and ethically justifiable is, of course, still an open question. It is likely that some of these instances of rationing are not justified. Note, however, that it is also likely that some instances of non-rationing will similarly be unjustified. In some cases, spending resources where very little medical benefit is to be expected is harmful in that it takes away these resources from others who would need them more. Given the importance of limit-setting decisions, it is reassuring that the most frequently rationed interventions were of exactly this kind: interventions with small benefits, unlikely to reflect life or death choices, and for which alternatives are likely to exist. The criteria reported by physicians were, however, highly variable and this could reflect concerning disparities between decisions made by different professionals. While this may reflect a situation that could generate unfair outcomes, it could also reflect the diversity of clinical situations that respondents may have been thinking of in answering our survey. It could also reflect different priorities and processes in making limit-setting decisions and could point to difficulties in the practice of bedside rationing.

Our results, then, predictably do not enable a straightforward answer regarding the ethical acceptability of bedside rationing by physicians. Rather than *whether* physicians ought to ration care, the relevant question seems to be *how* they can feasibly and justifiably do so and whether they can contribute to more fair and justifiable limit setting in society as a whole through their role at the bedside. Thus, the Values at the Bedside study sets the stage for addressing these questions in the remainder of this book.

REFERENCES

Alexander, G. C., Werner, R. M., & Ubel, P. A. (2004). The costs of denying scarcity. *Archives of Internal Medicine*, 164(6), 593–596.

Arnesen, T., & Fredriksen, S. (1995). Coping with obligations towards patient and society: an empirical study of attitudes and practice among Norwegian physicians. *Journal of Medical Ethics*, 21(3), 158–161.

Asch, D. A., Jedrziewski, M. K., & Christakis, N. A. (1997). Response rates to mail surveys published in medical journals. *Journal of Clinical Epidemiology*, 50(10), 1129–1136.

Asch, D. A., & Ubel, P. A. (1997). Rationing by any other name. *New England Journal of Medicine*, 336(23), 1668–1671.

Ayres, P. J. (1996). Rationing health care: views from general practice. *Social Science & Medicine*, 42(7), 1021–1025.

Cooke, L., & Hutchinson, M. (2001). Doctors' professional values: results from a cohort study of United Kingdom medical graduates. *Medical Education*, 35(8), 735–742.

Escher, M., Perneger, T. V., & Chevrolet, J. C. (2004). National questionnaire survey on what influences doctors' decisions about admission to intensive care. *British Medical Journal*, 329(7463), 425.

Hurst, S. A., Forde, R., Reiter-Theil, S., Slowther, A. M., Perrier, A., Pegoraro, R., & Danis, M. (2007). Physicians' views on resource availability and equity in four European health care systems. *BMC Health Services Research*, 7(1), 137.

Hurst, S. A., Hull, S. C., DuVal, G., & Danis, M. (2005). Physicians' responses to resource constraints. *Archives of Internal Medicine*, 165(6), 639–644.

Hurst, S. A., Slowther, M. A., Forde, R., Pegoraro, R., Reiter-Theil, S., Perrier, A., Garrett-Mayer, E., & Danis, M. (2006). Prevalence and determinants of physician bedside rationing: data from Europe. *Journal of General Internal Medicine*, 21(11), 1138–1143.

Mendelssohn, D. C., Kua, B. T., & Singer, P. A. (1995). Referral for dialysis in Ontario. *Archives of Internal Medicine*, 155(22), 2473–2478.

Rosen, P., & Karlberg, I. (2002). Opinions of Swedish citizens, health-care politicians, administrators and doctors on rationing and health-care financing. *Health Expectations*, 5(2), 148–155.

Ryynanen, O. P., Myllykangas, M., Kinnunen, J., & Takala, J. (1997). Doctors' willingness to refer elderly patients for elective surgery. *Family Practice*, 14(3), 216–219.

Ryynanen, O. P., Myllykangas, M., Kinnunen, J., & Takala, J. (1999). Attitudes to health care prioritisation methods and criteria among nurses, doctors, politicians and the general public. *Social Science & Medicine*, 49(11), 1529–1539.

Ubel, P. (2001). *Pricing Life: Why It's Time for Health Care Rationing.* Cambridge, MA: The MIT Press.

Wilson, R., Godwin, M., Seguin, R., Burrows, P., Caulfield, P., Toffelmire, E., et al. (2001). End-stage renal disease: factors affecting referral decisions by family physicians in Canada, the United States, and Britain. *American Journal of Kidney Diseases*, 38(1), 42–48.

2 The Interaction of Bedside Rationing and the Fairness of Health Care Systems

Physicians' Views

■ SAMIA A. HURST, REIDUN FØRDE, ANNE SLOWTHER, AND MARION DANIS

In this chapter, as in chapter 1, we present results from the Values at the Bedside study, a survey of European physicians exploring their reported experience with rationing, their perception of scarcity and fairness in their health care system, and their attitudes toward clinical rationing and various other cost-containment strategies (Hurst et al., 2007). Some of the results from this study have been published and have already been alluded to in the previous chapter. Some of the results pertaining to the interactions between physician bedside rationing and the structure of health systems has, however, not been published before. Here we report results from our study regarding physicians' assessment of their health care systems' resource availability and fairness, and other relevant elements, in order to begin exploring the interactions between macro-level policy decisions and resource allocation decisions by clinicians.

When we started our study, contradictory data existed as to whether physicians were aware of facing scarcity. In *The Painful Prescription: Rationing Hospital Care*, Aaron and Schwartz noted that British physicians rationalized or redefined health care standards to face scarcity more comfortably (Aaron & Schwartz, 1984). Twenty years later, researchers conducting interviews with physicians regarding scarcity reported being struck with the strength with which scarcity was denied (Alexander et al., 2004). In the United States, however, general internists, intensive care specialists, and oncologists did report difficulties explicitly associated with resource scarcity (Hurst et al., 2005). Physicians at the point of care are uniquely situated to observe the impact of priority setting decisions on patients in the form of scarcity and inequity. Their experience may thus yield useful insights and feedback about the impact of priorities on clinical care, which could contribute to evidence-based health policy (van Kammen et al., 2006). Despite this, insufficient attention is usually paid to their experiences.

Gathering such data gains additional importance once we recognize that, as is suggested in our study, complex interactions exist between macro-level policy decisions and clinical rationing decisions at the micro level of patient care. Fair bedside rationing may thus be dependent on the structure of health systems.

■ PHYSICIANS PERCEIVE SCARCITY

The four European countries in our survey all offer universal access to health care, although their health care systems different significantly with per capita expenditure on health care ranging from $3,322 in Switzerland to $1,989 in the United Kingdom. As shown in TABLE 2.1, despite differences in structure and health care expenditure the health care systems of all four countries received similar evaluations regarding fairness of financial contribution to the health system and distribution of responsiveness in the World Health Organization (WHO) world health report of 2000.

Survey respondents of all four countries reported perceiving scarcity in their country. Resources reported as scarce are shown in *Figure 2.1*. There were significant differences between the four countries in the degree of perceived scarcity and in the degree of perceived underinsurance. Respondents working in the four countries also varied on how troubled they were by limited resources in health care (*Figure 2.2*). The resources most frequently reported

TABLE 2.1. *Four Health Care Systems—WHO and OECD Data at the Time of the Study*

Per capita expenditure on health care[a]	Italy	Norway	Switzerland	United Kingdom
Total (US $)	2,166	3,409	3,446	2,160
Public (US $)	1,639	2,845	1,995	1,801
Out of pocket (US$)	440	546	1,085	200
Proportion of expenditure on health care[a]				
Social security	0.1%	0%	40%	0%
Other public	75.5%	83.5%	17.9%	83.4%
Prepaid plan	1%	0%	9.6%	3%
Out of pocket	20.3%	16%	31.4%	9.2%
Other private	3%	0.5%	1.4%	4.3%
Beds, physicians, nurses[b]				
Acute care beds/1,000 pop.	3.7	3.1	3.9	3.7
Nursing home beds/1,000 pop.	2.7	9.1	11.6	3.1
Nurses/1,000 pop.	5.4	10.4	10.7	9.7
Physicians/1000 pop.	4.1	3.4	3.7	2.2
Elements of health policy				
Universal coverage	Yes	Yes	Yes	Yes
Freedom to choose general physician	Yes	Yes	Yes	No
Gatekeeping for specialist consultation	Yes	Yes	No	Yes
WHO assessment of equity[c]				
Fairness of financial contribution to health system	0.961	0.977	0.964	0.977
Distribution of responsiveness	0.995	0.995	0.995	0.995

[a] WHO 2002 country information
[b] OECD 2003 country information
[c] WHO 2000 World health report

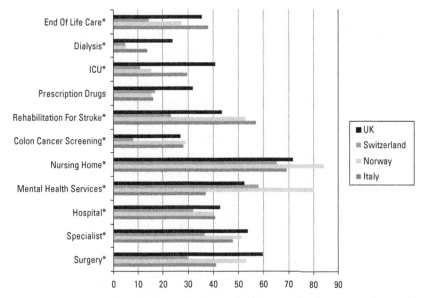

Figure 2.1 Percentage of respondents who reported shortages of various types of resources in their countries.

as scarce were nursing homes and mental health services, with referral to surgery reported as more scarce in the United Kingdom and rehabilitation for stroke in Italy.

Reports of scarcity in all the surveyed health care systems are not surprising. Every system in the world rations health care, some by waiting times and some by availability of services, coverage decisions, or by ability to pay. There are compelling reasons for some resources to be unavailable, as choices will have to be made whenever demands exceed resources. Physicians are in a unique position to observe the impact of these choices, particularly when they may be unexpected. Our respondents' aggregate assessment of how various interventions were more or less sufficiently available differed across interventions and between countries. Health care systems do not allocate their resources in

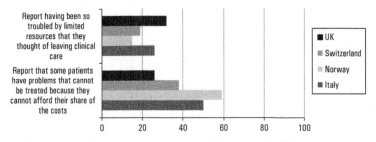

Figure 2.2 Percentage of respondents who reported being troubled about resource scarcity.

identical ways; assessement of how existing services fit with perceived need, however, can be difficult. In our study we assessed unavailability of services based on physicians' assessment of need rather than on a measure derived from utilization (Andersen & Aday, 1978; Penchansky & Thomas, 1981). The location of physicians at the point of care enables them to perceive discrepancies between need and utilization. Their view may also contribute to an understanding of what a reasonable level of resources, or a more appropriate level, ought to be. Mean scores on the scarcity scale were consistent with differences in national health expenditures. Where comparisons are possible, physician reports of scarcity based on our findings are supported by Organisation for Economic Co-operation and Development (OECD) mortality data, which yields identical rankings with regard to colon cancer screening and mental health services and an almost identical ranking regarding rehabilitation for stroke (TABLE 2.2; OECD, 2006).

It would not be appropriate to conclude that scarcity is the major cause of the differences in mortality reported here. An alternative interpretation could be that physicians are more aware of problems related to diseases that are more prevalent. These comparisons, however, give construct validity to differences in the perception of scarcity among the four countries. If physicians were reporting different degrees of scarcity for, say, cultural reasons, we would not expect scarcity and disease-related mortality to be so parallel.

■ PHYSICIANS ARE IN A UNIQUE POSITION TO VIEW FAIRNESS AND DISPARITY

Virtually all respondents thought that everyone in their country should have equal access to needed medical services, but a little less than half thought that health care resources in their country were not distributed fairly, one-quarter

TABLE 2.2. *Differences in Reported Unavailability are Parallel to Health Outcomes*

	Italy	Norway	Switzerland	United Kingdom
% respondents who reported unavailable rehabilitation for stroke[a]	57	53	23	44
Potential years of life lost, cerebrovascular disease/ 100,000 pop. >70 years[b]	89	74	58	121
% respondents who reported unavailable colon cancer screening[a]	28	29	8	27
Potential years of life lost, malignant neoplasia of the colon/ 100,000 pop. >70 years[b]	73	89	56	70
% respondents who reported unavailable mental health services[a]	37	80	58	53
Potential years of life lost, mental disorders/ 100,000 pop. >70 years[b]	33	267	132	113

[a] Survey responses
[b] OECD 2002–3 country information

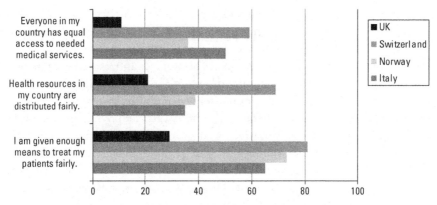

Figure 2.3 Percentage of respondents who agreed with statements about the degree of fairness of distribution of resources.

considered that they were not given enough means to treat their patients fairly, and half did not agree that everyone in their country had equal access to needed medical services (*Figure 2.3*). Respondents working in the four surveyed countries differed on whether they thought they were given enough means to treat their patients fairly. Physicians working in the United Kingdom reported less equity; similarly, physicians who reported more pressure to ration and physicians who reported more adverse events attributed to scarcity reported less equity.

We also asked physicians about their perception of discrimination against some groups of patients. As shown in *Figure 2.4,* eight out of ten respondents reported that at least one group of patients was more likely than others to be

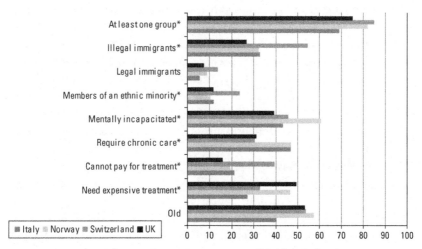

Figure 2.4 Percentage of respondents reporting greater likelihood of treatment denialbased on group identity.

denied beneficial care on the basis of cost in their health care environment. The most frequently identified groups were patients who are mentally incapacitated, patients who require chronic care, illegal immigrants, and patients who are old. There were significant differences between countries in the frequency with which each group was identified, except for legal immigrants and the elderly (*Figure 2.4*). More discrimination was reported by respondents who reported more underinsurance or more scarcity. Italian physicians were only half as likely as other physicians to report discrimination in their environment.

Access to care was often reported as inequitable. More specifically, some patient groups were identified as more likely than others to be denied care on the basis of cost. Although the distribution of responsiveness as reported by WHO was identical in the four study countries, evaluation of the equity as judged by the Perceived Equity scale that we developed (Hurst et al., 2007) and discrimination as judged by the Perceived Discrimination scale that we developed (Hurst et al., 2007) did vary in these countries. Respondents thus perceived that access, viewed as a concern that "health care resources are mobilized to meet the needs of different groups in the population" (Gulliford et al., 2002) was not fully realized. This finding raises the possibility that physicians, who are in a unique position to observe unequal access or discrimination in the health system, may be situated to address it. In saying this we recognize that it is relatively easy for persons in a health care system to express a need for more resources, but it is more difficult to develop an allocation process to ensure equitable distribution and resource allocation in a manner that maximizes benefit in terms of organizational or system objectives. Could physicians contribute to this? At minimum, our results suggest that efforts to measure a health system's equity might incorporate feedback from physicians about adverse events stemming from distributional decisions made at the system level. This feedback loop could be a way to connect the macro and meso levels of priority setting with the micro level. Such feedback loops are often missing. For example, in countries where the length of waiting lists is monitored, we often know little about the patients who wait and about the effects of waiting on treatment effectiveness. Likewise, there is often little information on the frequency of paradoxical results: if waiting lists are required to be short, for example, this could result in pressures to see patients quickly even in situations where there is no urgency, thus possibly taking needed clinical attention away from others who may need it more.

Additional comparisons of our study results with other assessments of equity and utilization in the four countries included in our study show some convergence. An OECD working paper concluded that the distribution of general practitioner care utilization favored the poor in all four countries included in our study, but the distribution of specialist utilization favored the rich in all of them (van Doorslaer et al., 2006). Reports by general physicians in our study, that patients who cannot afford to pay for treatment are more likely to be denied care, fits with those results.

■ COST-CONTAINMENT POLICIES SHOULD NOT BE DETACHED FROM THE BEDSIDE

Most responding physicians agreed that they should help their patients when the health care system was unfair or make sure their patients obtained needed medical services. There were no significant differences among the respondents from the four countries on these points. Older, more experienced physicians were more likely to agree that they ought to provide such help to patients, as were those who perceived more discrimination in their health care system or practiced in a rural area.

Almost all respondents found at least one cost-containment policy acceptable (*Figure 2.3*). Classification of referrals by degree of urgency, emphasis on evidence-based practice, and waiting lists for elective surgery were the policies most frequently found acceptable. Administrative prioritization of patient groups and closing hospital beds were least frequently found acceptable, with the latter found acceptable more frequently (52%) in Italy where the number of beds per capita was much higher than in the other countries. Restriction of expensive treatments and interventions, and direct treatment fees, were found acceptable by over half of respondents only in Norway. Overall agreement with cost-containment policies was greater in Norway and Italy than in the United Kingdom and Switzerland (*Figure 2.5*).

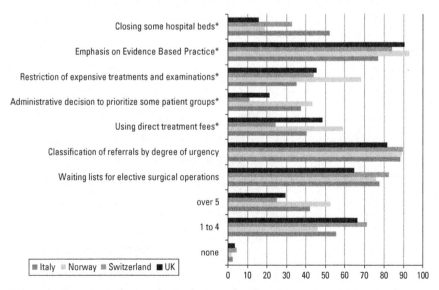

Figure 2.5 Percentage of respondents who agreed with various cost containment policies.

■ FREEDOM AND PRESSURES INFLUENCE BEDSIDE RATIONING

Although a majority of respondents felt free to use resources in their patients' best interest (73.3%), there were significant differences between respondents in the four countries in the perception of freedom to use resources in patients' best interests, pressure to deny interventions, and in agreement that respondents' jobs or financial security were threatened by pressures on health care costs (*Figure 2.6*). This was a striking result, reflecting what could be central differences between the four health care systems. It also highlights how our results on physician perceptions regarding bedside rationing need to be understood in the context of very different health care environments that provide physicians both variable quantities of resources and varying degrees of freedom to use them as they see fit. Physicians from Norway and Switzerland reported greater availability of resources than did physicians from Italy and the United Kingdom. Physicians from Switzerland and Italy, however, reported both more freedom to utilize resources as they saw fit and greater fear for their financial or professional security. This may provide context for the otherwise puzzling finding that physicians working in Switzerland, the richest health care system at the time of our survey, reported the greatest prevalence of physician bedside rationing. In comparing the four countries on this variable, our data suggest a stronger association with perceived pressure rather than with available resources. In other words, the reason Swiss physicians are reporting more bedside rationing may be that although they feel spared from scarcity and free to use resources in their patients' best interests, they nevertheless fear what may happen to them if pressures on health care costs were to continue.

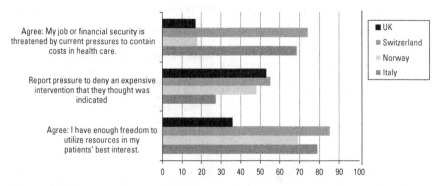

Figure 2.6 Percentage of respondents who perceived pressures to contain costs, pressure to ration, or freedom to use resources as they consider necessary for their patients' interests.

■ PHYSICIANS AND THEIR HEALTH SYSTEMS

While we will explore more extensive details about each of the country contexts in the next several chapters, we draw some preliminary conclusions
regarding the characteristics of their health care systems as perceived by physicians in our study.

Norwegian physicians' responses seem to reflect a situation of deliberative agreement. They seem less concerned than responding physicians in the
other countries that rationing may be a problem for the physician–patient
relationship. One possible reason may be that resource allocation was abun-
dantly discussed in the public sphere, and patients are expected to understand. Norwegian physicians also reported greater trust of guidelines and
administrative allocation decisions.(Hurst et al., 2007) We remain puzzled
by the high underinsurance report in a rich health care system. As different
aspects of health care are covered or not covered in different European countries, this may have a very local explanation. A greater degree of cost-shifting
from health care coverage could lead to such a response: this would not be
mutually exclusive with the previous hypothesis, as rationing questions specifically excluded limits due to cost-shifting.

British physicians' responses seem to reflect a rule-bound system. Financial
coverage is reported as high, but more frequently than elsewhere resources
are reported as not available when indicated. Physicians report less freedom,
suffer less indirect pressure, and make personal rationing decisions less often
than in the other three countries. One of the reasons they seem to agree with
clinical rationing rather less may be that they feel enough strictures are in place
already. That they report themselves as less equipped to treat their patients
fairly, and are more frequently troubled enough to think of leaving clinical
care, would seem to fit with this. They trust guidelines the least.

Swiss physicians' responses reflect a situation of freedom under pressure in
conditions of plenty. They reported a high degree of freedom, a higher availability of resources, but also high direct and indirect pressure to ration. In our
study this was associated with the highest rate of reported rationing. Despite
high pressure, Swiss physicians are the second happiest with the limits in their
system. Despite the lack of effective guidelines regarding resource allocation,
trust in such guidelines was high. Perhaps there is the perception that they
are needed. A Swiss Academy of Medical Sciences report published after our
study seems to indicate this (Swiss Academy of Medical Sciences "Rationing"
working group, 2007). Swiss physicians also have the patients with the highest
copays, and this too may play a role in their more frequent decisions to limit
expensive care.

Italian physicians also seem to practice in a situation of freedom under pressure, but in conditions of scarcity. They simultaneously reported important

limitations in the availability of resources, feeling personally at risk due to pressures on health care costs, and personally deciding to refrain from using interventions with the second highest frequency in our sample. Based on our data, we would predict that physicians in Italy do not feel that there are many explicit limits as to how they can use resources.

It seems clear that the structure of a health care system has an influence on attitudes of health care providers working within it. It also seems clear, though perhaps to a lesser degree, that the attitudes of health care providers would be one of the components shaping a health care system. It would be quite surprising if there were no connection between physicians' attitudes toward rationing and the extent to which they practice it. Ultimately, a valuable goal would be to clarify what system-wide characteristics are most likely to lead to fair distribution of resources among patients. Resources available within a health system, physicians' degree of discretion, and their readiness to assume a role in allocating resources at the micro level are all a part of this interesting mix.

In order to understand the interrelationships between a particular health care system, the attitudes of practitioners within it, and the characteristics that influence fair distribution of resources, in the following chapters we explore the specific health care context of the four countries involved in the Values at the Bedside study. Each country chapter provides an historical overview of the health care system with a particular focus on how it approaches distribution of resources. The authors reflect on how the structure and underlying principles of the system may have affected the responses of that country's physicians to the survey questions. Each chapter concludes with an update of how the system has changed since the Values at the Bedside study and looks forward to consider future challenges.

REFERENCES

Aaron, H. J., & Schwartz. W. B. (1984). *The Painful Prescription; Rationing Hospital Care.* Washington. DC: The Brookings Institution.

Alexander, G. C., Werner, R. M., & Ubel, P. A. (2004). The costs of denying scarcity. *Archives of Internal Medicine, 164*(6). 593–596.

Andersen, R., & Aday. L. A. (1978). Access to medical care in the U.S.: realized and potential. *Medical Care, 16*(7), 533–546.

Gulliford, M., Figueroa-Munoz, J., Morgan, M., Hughes, D., Gibson, B., Beech, R., & Hudson, M. (2002). What does 'access to health care' mean? *Journal of Health Services Research & Policy, 7*(3), 186–188.

Hurst, S. A., Forde, R., Reiter-Theil, S., Slowther, A. M., Perrier, A., Pegoraro, R., & Danis, M. (2007). Physicians' views on resource availability and equity in four European health care systems. *BMC Health Services Research, 7*(1), 137.

Hurst, S. A., Hull, S. C., DuVal, G., & Danis, M. (2005). Physicians' responses to resource constraints. *Archives of Internal Medicine, 165*(6), 639–644.

Organisation for Economic Co-operation and Development [OECD] (2006). OECD Health Data; Statistics and indicators for 30 countries. Paris: Organisation for Economic Co-operation and Development.

Penchansky, R., & Thomas, J. W. (1981). The concept of access: definition and relationship to consumer satisfaction. *Medical Care, 19*(2), 127–140.

Swiss Academy of Medical Sciences 'Rationing' working group. (2007). [Rationing in the Swiss Health-Care System: Analysis and Recommendations.] (Original in French) Retrieved May 2014 from www.samw.ch/dms/fr/Publications/Feuilles-de-route/f_Rationnement.pdf.

van Doorslaer, E., Masseria, C., & Koolman, X. for the OECD Health Equity Research Group (2006). Inequalities in access to medical care by income in developed countries. *Canadian Medical Association Journal, 174*(2), 177–183.

van Kammen, J., de Savigny, D., & Sewankambo, N. (2006). Using knowledge brokering to promote evidence-based policy-making: The need for support structures. *Bulletin of the World Health Organization, 84*(8), 608–612.

PART TWO

The Societal Context

3   The Swiss Context

■ SAMIA A. HURST

Swiss doctors who responded to the Values at the Bedside study reported a high degree of freedom, a high availability of resources, but also high direct and indirect pressure to ration. In our study—and this was a surprising result initially—this was associated with the highest rate of reported rationing (Hurst et al., 2006). What does the health system reflected here look like? This chapter will provide an overview of the Swiss health care system at the time of the Values at the Bedside study, and of discussions regarding priority setting at the time and since then, in order to provide some background for the interpretation of the study results.

Health outcomes in Switzerland are generally excellent, with very low infant mortality and one of the highest life expectancies in the world at 85 years for women and 80 years for men (WHO, 2013). Over eight out of ten Swiss describe their health as good or very good (Swiss Office for Statistics, 2010). The Swiss health care system, like the country, has a complicated governance structure. On the supply side, 26 cantons and half-cantons have the task of overseeing hospital care and conferring rights to practice to individual professionals. On the payment side, the Swiss health care system is based on three funding sources: federally mandated private insurance, taxation, and out-of-pocket payments.

■ HEALTH CARE ORGANIZATION

The structure for health care coverage is a public–private mix for both the funding and delivery of health care. It is built on a private insurance mandate with federal oversight, intended to be a publicly accountable system grounded in values of reciprocity and solidarity but also incorporating the advantages of competition in making the system more efficient. Each resident of Switzerland must buy health insurance from one of over 50 health insurance funds authorized to provide basic insurance under the federal mandate (Swiss Confederation, 2013a). Authorized insurance funds design and price insurance plans within legally prescribed parameters. The federal government oversees the application of these parameters. Cantonal governments are responsible for coordinating the delivery of care, as well as for public subsidies to hospitals and to individuals who meet criteria for premium subsidies.

This makes for a complex system (Reinhardt, 2004; OECD, 2011). It was enacted in 1996 through the adoption of the first federal law on health insurance, which initiated compulsory universal health coverage in Switzerland. Many of the current aspects of the organization of the Swiss health care system have remained in place since the Values at the Bedside study. Where changes have occurred, the description provided here refers to the time of our study.

The main components of the system are as follows.

Insurance plans may provide basic coverage provided they have received the authorization to do so, with this authorization contingent on their respect for four basic rules. First, they must cover all interventions that have not been excluded from basic coverage and all drugs authorized for prescription on the Swiss market. Second, they must accept all candidates for insurance without restrictions. Third, although they may charge different premiums in different cantons, and for adults and children, they may not adjust premiums based on any other factors. Fourth, basic insurance is not-for-profit. The same companies may provide additional voluntary insurance on a for-profit basis and may practice risk-rating in such additional plans, but there can be no transfer of funds from one of these activities to the other.

Adult individuals must purchase insurance from one of the authorized plans, and parents must also purchase insurance for each of their children. They may freely choose which insurance fund they prefer. Once a year, there is a window of time during which each insurance holder may leave his or her insurance plan and contract with a different insurance fund. Anyone who applies to a health insurance fund must be covered, with no restrictions for age or preexisting conditions. Health insurance covers the same basic package throughout the country. Insured individuals can consult any physician they choose and at any hospital of their choice. Although this has recently changed, initially this choice was limited to the canton of residence. Out-of-canton care was covered in case of an emergency or if equivalent care was not available within the canton of residence.

Government is responsible at the federal level for oversight of the system and adaptations of the Swiss health insurance law, and at the cantonal level for the organization of the supply side of health care and for subsidizing individuals and public hospitals. The Swiss government has no ministry of health: instead, health is one of the topics overseen by the minister for home affairs, with many tasks implemented through the Federal Office of Public Health. It is this office which supervises the application of the Swiss health insurance law. The organization of the supply side of the health care system lies mostly within the jurisdiction of the 26 cantons. This results in 26 semi-independent health care systems for the delivery of care, each coordinating supply in hospital care, licensing individual professionals, and covering part of the costs of public hospitals. Cantons also subsidize individual insurance holders. Because premiums are individual, total costs vary with family size. Moreover, as they are fixed, the burden on individuals and households changes with income. For these reasons, cantons subsidize the cost of health insurance premiums, in part or completely, based on a sliding scale according to household size and total income.

■ HEALTH CARE FINANCING

At the time of the Values at the Bedside study, Swiss health care spending was the second highest in the world after the United States at a total of $3,446 per capita annually, slightly ahead of Norway among the study countries. Approximately one third of health insurance costs are covered through health insurance funds for compulsory basic coverage (35%), a second third of costs is covered directly out of pocket by individuals (31%), one-fifth (19%) is financed through (mostly cantonal) government expenditure, and 9% is covered through voluntary private health insurance (OECD, 2011). Government expenditure on health care in 2002 was $1995 per capita.

There are two areas of tension in Swiss health care financing. First, since only one-fifth of Swiss health care costs are covered through redistributive means, most of the financial burden for health care is inequitably distributed. Neither premiums nor outpatient costs are income-sensitive. While it is true that health insurance is supported by subsidies to help families with lower incomes to afford coverage, despite this, health insurance financing remains regressive and places considerable financial stress on some households (OECD, 2011). This is problematic for these households but also for others: pressures on young families have, for example, led older patients to express guilt when they use the healthcare system, although they too have paid for it (Coutaz, 2013). In the decade between 1999 and 2009, the average annual subsidy per household rose from 2187 to 2881 Swiss francs (OFSP, 2011). During the same period, the percentage of individuals receiving such subsidies has remained stable at about 30%, but financing them has placed increasing burdens on cantons as federal input decreased over same the period.

The second source of tension is regional distribution. Premiums can and do vary between cantons. In 2011, the OECD commented on this point as follows: "According to various stakeholders, inter-cantonal inequities are considered an acceptable consequence of a federal system. However, there is a lack of analysis providing evidence on the level of inequity in health financing."(OECD, 2011). The burden represented by the costs of health care also varies substantially between the cantons. In 2001, costs ranged from $1,051 per capita in the canton of Appenzell to $2,781 per capita in the canton of Geneva. In 2002, the share of disposable income spent on health insurance premiums for a family with a gross income of 45,000 euros ranged from 1.5%

in the canton of Valais to 14% in the canton of Geneva. (Crivelli, Filippini, & Mosca, 2006).

■ HEALTH CARE RESOURCES

Switzerland had 3.7 doctors per 1000 inhabitants in 2002, the second highest number after Italy among the Values at the Bedside study countries. It had the highest number of nurses (10.7/1000 inhabitants), acute care beds (3.9/1000 inhabitants), and nursing home beds (11.6/1000 inhabitants) in the study countries.

Among the four study countries, Switzerland is the only one without a gatekeeper system for specialist consultation. Patients are free to choose any providers within the covered geographic area, both in general practice and specialized medicine. Health care professionals are trained in public universities and higher education institutions. Physicians must obtain a license to practice medicine from the canton.

Hospital and nursing home beds are planned at the level of cantons or regions. Tertiary care teaching hospitals are all public, and there is a dense network of public regional hospitals as well as a number of private hospitals. Despite short distances between hospitals, considerable controversy often arises when a local hospital is scheduled for closure or a change in mission.

Health care providers are salaried in the public sector but paid on a fee-for-service basis in the private sector. The fee schedule for physicians is centrally determined, with a stable cost structure and unit prices that vary between cantons. Fee-for-service payment has been criticized as a potential source of provider-driven health care costs. This criticism is based on an association between provider density and health care utilization and costs (Busato et al., 2010). It is possible, of course, that greater physician density simply covers otherwise unmet needs (Carlsen & Grytten, 1998; Swiss Federal Office for Statistics, 2007). In the absence of better outcomes in areas of greater provider density, however, this second hypothesis also remains unproven.

The health insurance benefit package is determined centrally by the ministry of home affairs following advice from the Swiss Federal Office for Public Health, itself advised by specific commissions on drugs, interventions, and devices. The health insurance law requires "effectiveness, appropriateness, and efficiency" for the inclusion of services in the benefit package. The processes testing this have been criticized as lacking a rigorous methodology and a transparent decision-making process (OECD, 2011). Moreover, the costs of covered interventions are rarely negotiated with the provider.

■ COPAYMENT

Drugs and interventions not covered under the basic health care package are paid for out of pocket by patients. Dental care is excluded unless required for a condition associated with another physical disease. Contraception and medically assisted reproduction is excluded as well, with some exceptions. Any professional care not directly linked to the treatment of a disease is also excluded. For example, long-term care in a nursing home is not covered.

Even for covered interventions, out-of-pocket payments are high in the Swiss health care system. All insurance comes with a deductible, a specific amount which the insurance holder must pay before insurance coverage starts, which can be set at different levels and which is one determinant of the price of monthly insurance premiums. Persons who use the health care system must also contribute a copay of 10% of the costs, although this is capped at 700 Swiss francs per year. As a result of these costs, and noncovered interventions, financial contribution from out-of-pocket payments in Switzerland was $1,085 per capita in 2002, almost twice the amount in Norway and over five times the amount paid out of pocket in the United Kingdom for the same year.

One consequence is that despite a system with mandatory health insurance, forgoing care for financial reasons is documented in Switzerland. One study conducted in Geneva showed the prevalence to be 13% to 14% over a 3-year period from 2007 to 2010. Prevalence of forgoing care for financial reasons was higher among the lower income group, with 22.5% and 34.7% reporting this in 2007 and 2010, respectively (Guessous et al., 2012).

■ SETTING PRIORITIES WITHIN THE SWISS HEALTH CARE SYSTEM

The organization of the Swiss health care system is under constant examination (Moresi-Izzo, Bankauskaite, & Gericke, 2010). One of the intentions of the Swiss health insurance law was to reach a balance between market-based competition and the protection of access to health care for all (Reinhardt, 2004). Since 1996, multiple revisions have attempted to fine tune, correct, or even abandon this intention.

The need to set priorities is recognized for two main reasons. One is the constant rise of insurance premiums, which have led to critiques that the current system is unsustainable (von Elm et al., 2005). A second reason is the question of governance. In the highly federalized Swiss health care system, many stakeholders participate in setting priorities. Lack of coordination, which is sometimes valued as part of the federal system, can however also mean a lack of transparency in decision making. It also makes an exhaustive synopsis of discussions almost impossible to achieve. For this reason, this section will outline illustrative aspects of priority setting in Switzerland rather than attempt a systematic overview.

A Dense Network

One of the most important aspects of priority setting in Switzerland is the number and diversity of stakeholders. The Swiss health insurance law gave insurance companies the task of reimbursing care, and with it a key role in controlling provider costs. The Swiss federal office for public health has the mandate to oversee insurance providers and also makes recommendations to the ministry of home affairs on coverage of goods and services. Local resource availability is determined by cantonal governments and hospital authorities, with coordination bodies overseeing regional planning in some circumstances. There are frequent popular votes on matters related to the health care system. In addition, independent bodies such as the Swiss Academy of Medical Sciences have published reports on the Swiss health care system (Swiss Academy of Medical Sciences "Rationing" working group, 2007). Since 2008, the Swiss Medical Board has made recommendations based on technology assessment for the coverage and use of medical technologies, first for the canton of Zurich on a pilot basis and now nationwide.

Setting priorities in such a decentralized and deliberative system, with its strengths (such as inclusiveness and buy-in) and weaknesses (such as delays and conflicts of interest), is difficult. Discussions on priority setting in Switzerland can be described from several different angles: political difficulties, initiatives by stakeholders, recommendations, and structural proposals. Recently, a landmark court decision has also contributed to priority setting in Switzerland.

Limit Setting: A Politically Difficult Exercise

The political difficulty of setting priorities in the Swiss health care system can best be captured by a story. In 1999, a patient was being discussed in a teaching hospital. This 86-year-old man was scheduled for a surgical intervention during which severe bleeding was a possibility. The staff discussed whether a new recombinant clotting factor, which had just been authorized but which could cost up to 1 million Swiss francs for a single patient, might be used in his case. Given the cost, they discussed this eventuality with the minister of health for this canton. The decision was to not provide the drug. The patient was a former Federal councilor and president of Switzerland, who had been one of the architects of the Swiss social safety net. Neither he nor his family requested special treatment, but the media seized the case. Although the intervention went well and would not have made the drug necessary in any case, the local minister of health was not reelected. This led to lasting hesitations to discuss anything that might seem like limit setting within the Swiss health care system.

Although this reluctance was greatly diminished, in part through publications calling for explicit deliberations rather than implicit decisions (DIALOG-ETHIK, 1999; Swiss Academy of Medical Sciences "Rationing" working group, 2007), agreeing to limits that might affect individual patients remains difficult. In 2005, the federal councilor for home affairs decided to remove coverage for five complementary medicine approaches on the grounds that their efficacy was insufficiently demonstrated. Following a popular vote in 2009, coverage for these still-unproven approaches was reintroduced in 2011.

Stakeholder Initiatives

Health insurance providers must apply coverage for the basic health care package and must, in case of doubt, follow the recommendations of physicians hired for this purpose. Attempts to limit expenditure by insurance companies have included increasing the number of requests for justification, which allows better verification that expenditure is justified but also sometimes leads to denials of justified care. Although some cases of denied coverage were later overturned in court, initiating this procedure in such cases is the task of the patient and this is perceived as adding burdens to situations that are already difficult. Insurance providers have also supplied individual physicians in private practice with information regarding their cost-based ranking in comparison with colleagues in the same specialty. This has been perceived by physicians as threatening, especially at times during which the introduction of selective contracting was being discussed. Insurance providers have also discussed the possibility of raising premiums for persons who engage in unhealthy behavior. Another controversial topic taken up by political parties regards a proposal to bill patients for alcohol-related health care costs.

Physicians have been more reluctant and have only more recently started stakeholder initiatives for priority setting. One such attempt is an adaptation to Switzerland of the *Choosing wisely* approach adopted in the United States. In this approach, medical societies develop lists of the "top five" tests, treatments, or services commonly used in their specialty and "for which the use should be reevaluated by patients and clinicians" (Brody, 2010).

Direct democracy allows popular initiatives to bear on the Swiss health care system. There have thus also been direct popular votes on the topics of hospital costs (twice), prescription drug costs, health care costs (twice), the creation of a single state-funded insurance fund, the inclusion of some forms of alternative medicines, and an obligation to create health management networks (Swiss Federal Administration, 2013).

Recommendations

Recommendations to make priority setting and its methodology more explicit and transparent have been made by several bodies. In 1999 Dialog Ethik, a for-profit independent ethics institution, published a "Manifesto for a fair allocation of resources in our Health Care System" recommending explicit decision making on the basis of cost-effectiveness analysis (DIALOG-ETHIK, 1999). In 2007, the Swiss Academy of Medical Sciences published a report on "Rationing in the Swiss health care system: analysis and recommendations," recommending explicit limit-setting based on national priorities, evidence of effectiveness, and the protection of vulnerable persons (Swiss Academy of Medical Sciences "Rationing" working group, 2007). In 2012, the Swiss Academy of Medical Sciences published a report on "sustainable medicine," which recommended that a minimal clinically relevant effect size be demonstrated for new medical technologies and that health technology assessment should be supported for medical technologies (ASSM, 2012). That this second report moved from the language of rationing to the language of sustainability was welcomed during expert consultation as a strategy that might facilitate future discussions on priority setting.

Such recommendations highlight two aspects of the governance of health care in Switzerland. First, they are part of the deliberative structure of decision making. Second, they also highlight the political difficulty of this topic, which is taken up by civil society in part because of the difficulty of the political discussion. Moreover, the effects of these reports has been modest.

The Swiss medical board, the institution for medical health technology assessment, publishes a different type of recommendation as it focuses on specific interventions. Since 2009, it has published ten reports on topics including percutaneous mitral valve repair, prostate-specific antigen screening, and surgical treatment of hepatic metastases of colorectal tumors. These reports are consultative and their effect on the delivery and coverage of care remains to be assessed.[1]

Structural Proposals

Despite the difficulties outlined here, changes have been implemented. As in other areas, decisions regarding health care in Switzerland tend to be slow and require considerable input. However, they are not impossible and the hope is always that they may be improved in the process. Among the principal changes implemented since the Values at the Bedside Study, insurance holders can now choose providers and hospitals across the country regardless of their place of residence. Insurance funds have also introduced lower premiums for individuals who accept health care through a designated provider network. Finally, hospitals are now paid on the basis of diagnosis-related groups rather than on the basis of the length of stay. Several revisions to the legal framework were also discussed and, at least temporarily, rejected (Moresi-Izzo et al., 2010). For example, a right for insurance funds to selectively contract with providers was being discussed around the time of the Values at the Bedside study (Hurst & Mauron, 2004).

Since 2002, the number of new licenses to practice has been capped following a federal decision to limit the number of physicians in an attempt to control health care costs, with attempts at needs-based limits on the number of general practitioners and specialists who are given licenses to practice in each canton. In parallel, discussions have focused on the number of physicians trained in Switzerland. Admissions into the second year of medical school are competitive, with 3.8 candidates for each slot in 2009 (Kraft, 2009). Switzerland is a destination country for the migration of health professionals. In 2007, 19% of doctors practicing in Switzerland were foreign-trained (Garcia-Perez, Amaya, & Otero, 2007). Calls to decrease this reliance on physicians imported from poorer countries have repeatedly been made (ASSM, 2012), and this has resulted in some increase in medical school capacity and some limits on the rights granted to foreign physicians to practice in Switzerland.

Highly controversial discussions have also focused on regional hospital concentration, which implies the closure of wards and sometimes entire institutions, as well as the designation of national or "language-regional" centers for highly specialized medicine in the case of technical interventions for which greater volumes tend to be correlated with better outcomes. Both illustrate a tension between the quality of care and the proximity at which it is available. Switzerland has a highly decentralized system and, at the same time, a rich one that places a premium on high-quality care. When these dimensions conflict, enduring controversy is inevitable.

The "Myozyme Case": A Landmark Court Decision

In November 2011, the Swiss supreme court ruled in the case of a 70-year-old woman who was diagnosed 3 years earlier with late-onset Pompe' disease, the adult-onset form of an rare disease of muscular tissue that causes patients to lose muscular function including the heart and breathing muscles, leading to early death. Enzyme replacement therapy was available but not approved for use in Switzerland at the time (Hurst, 2011). This patient's doctors obtained approval for off-label use and coverage of the drug for the first 6 months. The patient's condition improved, but the required dosage was greater than anticipated, as was the expense. After the first 6 months, the insurer denied continued coverage. The drug was discontinued, following which the patient's symptoms worsened. The patient sued the insurer for coverage and won in the first instance. The insurer appealed the decision to the Swiss Supreme Court, which ruled that coverage in this case could be denied. The reasons were that off-label coverage requires that a "high therapeutic value" be demonstrated, which was not the case here. The Court further argued that even if a "high therapeutic value" had been present, coverage could still have been denied on the grounds of an insufficient cost effectiveness ratio.

This "Myozyme" ruling contains a number of important points. First, it again underlines the difficulty of the political discussion by stating that "Case law has attempted in several cases to decide on the relationship between cost and utility, in the absence of criteria which the political level has until now not set down"(Swiss Supreme Court, 2011). Second, it defines the required benefits as those effects which are not only statistically significant but also clinically relevant. It further makes a distinction between life-extending treatment and treatments that do not extend life. Third, it set a precedent by determining the cost effectiveness of the drug as part of the ruling. Fourth, this ruling took an explicit stand on fairness by stating that equality before the law required that for the same impact of disease on the quality of life, everyone should have the same resources when these resources have a similar effect.

■ IMPLICATIONS FOR THE VALUES AT THE BEDSIDE STUDY

The political difficulty of priority setting made the topic of the Values at the Bedside a particularly sensitive one. Swiss respondents were reporting behavior that was at the time largely taboo. The results are thus all the more striking, as this effect may have led them to underreport bedside rationing.

Swiss respondents reported considerable pressure to ration care. This could be linked to at least two aspects of the Swiss context. First, increasing requests for justification by insurance providers could have played a role. Second, the possibility of selective contracting was certainly viewed as a threat at the time. Both of these factors could have contributed to Swiss physicians practicing bedside rationing as a form of defensive medicine, against what might happen to them should health care costs continue to rise uncontrollably. This situation might be described as *freedom under pressure*—one in which incentives were in place for physicians to limit care in the absence of guidance. This may explain the extent to which Swiss respondents in the Values at the Bedside study expressed agreement with the value of guidelines. Under the circumstances, more guidelines were viewed as potentially helpful to clinicians. The 2007 Swiss Academy of Medical Sciences report also offers this interpretation, in part on the basis of the Values at the Bedside study (Swiss Academy of Medical Sciences "Rationing" working group, 2007).

The court hearing the Myozyme case cited the Values at the Bedside study among its references. The point this reference supported was that physicians were already engaged in limit setting, but that in the absence of official guidance this represented a legal risk for them. This situation, where physicians were participating in rationing decisions in the absence of guidance, lent importance to the court ruling and the political discussion it hoped to encourage.

■ CONCLUSIONS AND FUTURE TRENDS

That Switzerland, with its decentralized, multipiloted health care system, reported the highest rate of physician bedside rationing among the four study countries contradicts the hypothesis that physician bedside rationing is the result of centralized rules. The Swiss context highlights the fact that a market-based and well financed health care system will also generate physician rationing. It will, however, be of a different kind: more individualized but also more implicit; a reflection, perhaps, of a health care system that values regional diversity but also seems to function with some rather opaque decision-making processes.

Future trends in priority setting in Switzerland are likely to include a greater focus on health technology assessment, as the Swiss medical board gains support and begins to function nationwide. Regional concentration of hospitals and highly specialized medicine are likely to continue and to continually raise controversy. Although frequently discussed, tougher negotiations of the cost of drugs and services are not likely to take place. This could, however, change: one current controversy as of this writing is the tenfold difference in price of two drugs proven effective in the treatment of age-linked macular degeneration. Only the more expensive one is currently registered for use in Switzerland. Redistributive aspects of healthcare funding, both between individuals and between regions, are likely to remain a difficult point. In 2012, considerable tensions arose when it was discovered that health insurance premiums had been systematically overestimated, and thus overcharged, in five cantons from 1996 until 2011. The resulting agreement, which provides for partial reimbursement, was mostly deemed to represent a politically expedient compromise rather than a full-scale solution.

The development most likely to make a mark on priority setting is a recent decision by the ministry of home affairs to launch an extensive campaign for reform in the Swiss health care system (Swiss Confederation, 2013b). The objectives of this reform include promoting integrated care and prevention, increasing equity in health care financing, limiting the possibility of risk selection by insurance providers, reforming the determination of drug costs, promoting patients' rights including in the elaboration of health policy, promoting e-health, increasing the number of health professionals trained in Switzerland, increasing the oversight of insurance providers by the federal government, and increasing the coordination between the different levels of government.

Objectives such as continuing the concentration of highly specialized medicine and the development of health technology assessment are also included. This is an ambitious agenda to say the least, but if even some of these objectives succeed the resulting health care system could become very different from the one described in this chapter.

Note

1. An updated list of Swiss Medical Board reports, some with English summaries, can be found at http://www.medical-board.ch/index.php?id=809&L=1.

REFERENCES

Swiss Academy of Medical Sciences (SAMS) (2012). Médecine durable. Basel: Schwabe.

Brody, H. (2010). Medicine's ethical responsibility for health care reform—the Top Five list. *New England Journal of Medicine, 362*(4), 283–285.

Busato, A., Matter, P., Kunzi B., & Goodman, D. C. (2010). Supply sensitive services in Swiss ambulatory care: an analysis of basic health insurance records for 2003–2007. *BMC Health Services Research, 10,* 315.

Carlsen, F., & Grytten, J. (1998). More physicians: improved availability or induced demand? *Health Economics, 7*(6), 495–508.

Coutaz, M. (2014). Too old, too expensive? The impact of health costs on senior citizens in Switzerland. *European Geriatric Medicine, 5,* 39–42.

Crivelli, L., Filippini, M., & Mosca, I. (2006). Federalism and regional health care expenditures: an empirical analysis for the Swiss cantons. *Health Economics, 15*(5), 535–541.

DIALOG-ETHIK. (1999). Manifest for a fair allocation of resouces in our health care system. *Bulletin of the Swiss Medical Association, 80*(45), 1–9.

Garcia-Perez, M. A., Amaya, C., & Otero, A. (2007). Physicians' migration in Europe: an overview of the current situation. *BMC Health Services Research, 7,* 201.

Guessous, I., Gaspoz, J. M., Theler, J. M., & Wolff, H. (2012). High prevalence of forgoing healthcare for economic reasons in Switzerland: a population-based study in a region with universal health insurance coverage. *Preventive Medicine, 55*(5), 521–527.

Hurst, S. A. (2011). Important discussion. *Bioethica Forum, 4*(2), 79–80.

Hurst, S. A., & Mauron, A. (2004). Selective contracting of Swiss physicians: ethical issues and open questions. *Swiss Medicine Weekly, 134*(43–44), 632–639.

Hurst, S. A., Slowther, A. M., Forde, R. Pegoraro, R., Reiter-Theil, S., Perrier, A., et al. (2006). Prevalence and determinants of physician bedside rationing: data from Europe. *Journal of General Internal Medicine, 21*(11), 1138–1143.

Kraft, E. (2009) "[Swiss medical professionals : pre- and postgraduate training]" (Original in French) *Bulletin des Médecins Suisses, 90*(45), 1733–1735

Moresi-Izzo, S., Bankauskaite, V., & Gericke, C. A. (2010). The effect of market reforms and new public management mechanisms on the Swiss health care system. *International Journal of Health Planning Management, 25*(4), 368–385.

OECD [Organisation for Economic Co-operation and Development]. (2011). "OECD Reviews of Health Systems—Switzerland" OECD & WHO. Retrieved May 2014 from http://www.oecd.org/switzerland/oecdreviewsofhealthsystems-switzerland.htm

Federal Office of Public Health. (2011). [Statistics for mandatory health insurance in 2009] (Original in German). Retrieved May 2014 from http://www.bag.admin.ch/shop/00102/00559/index.html?lang=en.

Reinhardt, U. E. (2004). The Swiss health system: regulated competition without managed care. *Journal of the American Medical Association*, 292(10), 1227–1231.

Swiss Academy of Medical Sciences 'Rationing' working group. (2007). [Rationing in the Swiss health-care system: analysis and recommendations.] (Original in French) Retrieved May 2014 from www.samw.ch/dms/fr/Publications/Feuilles-de-route/f_Rationnement.pdf.

Swiss Confederation. (2013a). List of accepted health insurance companies. Retrieved May 2014 from http://www.bag.admin.ch/themen/krankenversicherung/00295/11274/index.html?lang=fr

Swiss Confederation. (2013b). Health2020—A comprehensive health care strategy. Retrieved May 2014 from http://www.bag.admin.ch/gesundheit2020/index.html?lang=en

Swiss Federal Administration. (2013). Results of topics submitted to federal votes. Retrieved September 2013 from http://www.admin.ch/ch/f//pore/va/vab_2_2_4_1_gesamt.html.

Swiss Federal Office for Statistics. (2007). Determinants and evolution of costs of the Swiss healthcare system: a review of the literature and projections to the horizon of 2030. Neuchatel: Swiss Federal Office for Statistics.

Swiss Office for Statistics. (2010). [Health and health behavior in Switzerland 2007] Santé et comportements vis-à-vis de la santé en Suisse 2007. *Swiss statistics*. Neuchatel: Swiss Office for Statistics.

Swiss Supreme Court. (2011). Decision 9C_334/2010. Lausanne.

von Elm, E., Egger, M., Pewsner, D., & Bisig, B. (2005). Holes in the Swiss health care system. *Journal of the American Medical Association*, 293(19), 2337–2338; author reply 2339–2340.

WHO [World Health Organization]. (2013). Countries: selected indicators. Retrieved September 2013 from http://www.who.int/countries/en/.

4   The United Kingdom Context

■ ANNE SLOWTHER

■ THE UK HEALTH CARE SYSTEM

Health care in the United Kingdom is primarily delivered through a publicly funded, nationally delivered, comprehensive service that includes public health, primary care and community care, hospital-based services, and national services such as blood and tissue donation. The National Health Service (NHS) was founded in 1948 with the enactment of the NHS Act (1946) and the NHS Scotland Act (1947), and its founding principles were the provision of a comprehensive system of health care for all citizens, free at the point of delivery and based on clinical need rather than ability to pay (NHS Choices, 2011; Bevan, 1948a). These principles were restated in the NHS Constitution (England), first published in 2010 Department of Health, 2012). Although each country is responsible for its own health service, the fundamental principal of a universal publicly funded service applies to all four health services (England, Scotland, Wales, and Northern Ireland). A key feature of the NHS system is the gatekeeping role of the general practitioner (GP). All NHS secondary medical care (except for emergency care), together with a significant proportion of private health care, is accessed through a referral from a GP. Thus, GPs facilitate appropriate use of NHS services on behalf of both the patient and the health care system.

■ UK HEALTH CARE FUNDING

Funding for the NHS comes from general taxation, and its budget is set by the Department of Health (England) and the devolved administrations (Scotland, Wales, and Northern Ireland). The budget for 2011/2012 for England was £106 billion and for Scotland £11.3 billion (Department of Health, 2011; Scottish Government, 2011). As public health care provision is universal, there is a correspondingly small but significant private health care sector. In 2009 total UK health care expenditure was 9.8% of gross domestic product (GDP) compared to 6.9% in 1999, with private health care expenditure accounting for 1.6% (Office for National Statistics, 2011). Private health care expenditure includes health insurance schemes funded either through an employer or by an individual, as well as direct out-of-pocket expenses for over-the-counter medication and services not funded by the NHS (for example, many complementary therapies and most cosmetic procedures are not funded). Not all treatment provided by the NHS is entirely free. In England a flat-rate charge for prescriptions for drugs is made (currently £7.65 per item prescribed (2012), although there are a number of exemption criteria including age (under 16 and 60 or over), pregnancy, receiving income support, inpatient treatment, and suffering from certain specific conditions such as diabetes (NHS Choices, 2012)). Similarly, there are standard charges for dental care and optometry with corresponding exemptions. Specific regulations differ between the administrations; for example, in Wales there are no prescription charges. Beyond these clearly demarcated areas the issue of copayment within the NHS is a controversial one. In 2002, at the time of the Values at the Bedside study, copayment for other treatments and services was not officially permitted in the NHS, but in 2009 the Department of Health published guidance on copayment which set out the circumstances in which this was permissible within the NHS (Department of Health, 2009a).

The funding for long-term care for older people and people with chronic disabilities who cannot care for themselves is more complex. The medical and nursing aspect of such care has been funded by the NHS since its inception and is part of the publicly funded health care system. Social care is also funded through general taxation, but social care is means-tested so, depending on a person's financial situation, there will be an element of copayment for social care (e.g., accommodation, help with personal care, etc.). People requiring long-term care often have both health and social care needs, and the difficulty of addressing responsibility for funding complex long-term care has thus been a source of public and political debate over recent decades. In the 1990s there was increasing public dissatisfaction with the existing system of funding long-term care, which placed the main burden on the individual rather than the state. In 1999 the report of the Royal Commission on Long Term Care and Older People recommended that long-term care should be split between living costs, housing costs, and personal care, and that personal care (wherever delivered) should be funded from general taxation (Royal Commission, 1999). Personal care includes assistance with washing, dressing, feeding, and the like. The report's conclusions specifically addressed the difficulty of separating "health care" and personal care, finding that such a distinction was unhelpful and discriminatory. In doing so, they echoed the founding principles of the NHS as a system based on need rather than ability to pay.

> "The most efficient way of pooling risk, giving the best value to the nation as a whole, across all generations, is through services underwritten by general taxation, based on need rather than wealth. This will ensure that the care needs of those who, for example, suffer from Alzheimer's disease—which might be therapeutic or personal care—are recognised and met just as much as of those who suffer from cancer" (Royal Commission, 1999, executive summary).

The devolved administrations responded differently to the Commission's rec-
ommendations. In England free nursing care was introduced in 2001, while in
Scotland both personal and nursing care is free (Department of Health, 2001a;
Scottish Parliament, 2002). The NHS Act (2006) and subsequent court cases
led to a clarification of the level of care that was to be funded by the NHS
in England (and therefore not subject to potential copayment by the patient).
Two types of care were identified: NHS continuing care (wholly funded by the
NHS); and NHS-funded nursing care, funded by the NHS as part of a package of care where non-nursing care (i.e., personal care that does not require
medical or nursing input) is funded by either the local authority or the person requiring care depending on their financial status. The "National Service
Framework for NHS continuing health care and NHS funded nursing care"
(2007, revised 2009) sets out the separate responsibilities for health care organizations and local authorities in assessing a person for these different types
of care (Department of Health, 2009b). A person is eligible for NHS continuing care if his/her primary need is assessed as a health need. In this case the
NHS is responsible for providing all of that person's assessed needs, including
accommodation if that is part of the overall need. If the primary need is not a
health need but there are ancillary health needs, the person may be eligible for
NHS-funded nursing care but not for free personal care. A primary health care
need is not related to a specific diagnosis but rather to the complexity, intensity, and unpredictability of the needs of the patient across a range of specified
areas including cognition, mobility, feeding, communication, breathing, and
psychological and emotional needs. Thus someone with a severe neurological
disability with complex and fluctuating needs involving medical treatment,
feeding, and assistance with breathing and mobility might be identified as
having a primary health need such that all care is funded by the NHS, whereas
someone with a stable condition requiring some medical care but where the
main caring requirement relates to personal care might only have their medical and nursing treatment funded by the NHS.

■ ORGANIZATIONAL STRUCTURE OF HEALTH CARE PRIOR TO 2002

Since its inception in 1948, the NHS has undergone several major structural
reorganizations in 1974 1984, 1990, 2001, and 2012. While these reforms have
had profound effects on management and resourcing within the NHS, the
experience of patients in terms of accessing services has remained, in broad
terms, the same. Everyone is entitled to and is expected to be registered with
a GP, who provides first point of contact with the health care system in most
situations. Hospitals provide inpatient and specialist outpatient care as well
as emergency care, and these are supported by a range of community services

such as community nursing, midwifery, and community child health. GPs do not usually have admitting rights to hospitals but are the main primary care physicians and often coordinate care between agencies. GPs are not directly employed by the NHS but are independent contractors with the NHS. A GP's payment in 2002 was based on a complex formula that includes a capitation fee for every patient registered with the GP, a weighting payment based on a calculation of the deprivation level in the community in which they practiced, and a fee-for-service payment for certain specified services outside normal general medical services. In 2002 these included maternity services and contraceptive services. In addition, an element of performance payment had been introduced in 1990 with GPs receiving extra payment for reaching targets in relation to public health activities such as childhood immunizations and cervical screening. Despite GPs not being directly employed by the NHS, the structural reorganizations of 1990 and 2001 marked paradigm shifts in how health care was managed in the United Kingdom and as such had a major impact on GPs as primary care physicians.

The reorganization linked to the NHS and Community Care Act (1990) introduced for the first time into the NHS the concept of a market, by splitting the functions of purchaser and provider. Contracts were set between purchasers (local health authorities or GP fund holders (see below) and providers (hospitals or community services) (NHS and Community Care Act, section 4). This placed a responsibility on providers to accurately cost their services and provide them at competitive rates (purchasers could choose which provider from whom to buy services for their patient population), and on purchasers to accurately assess the needs of their population and allocate their budget accordingly. GP practices with 9,000 or more patients could apply to be fund holders with their own NHS budgets. Fund holders were responsible for purchasing a range of services including specialist outpatient care and a range of defined inpatient services (Audit Commission, 1995). Savings made on the budget could be used to enhance GP practice services and infrastructure, thus providing an incentive for GPs to manage their budgets efficiently. Evaluation studies did not show the expected benefits from fundholding (Coulter, 1995), and by the end of the decade GP fundholding had been discontinued. The internal market more generally also had its critics, who pointed out that while the system might work well for discrete health care episodes such as elective surgery, it would not easily accommodate more complex health care services such as mental health or elderly care. However, the development of an internal market within the NHS brought into sharp relief the need to manage limited health care resources and introduced the idea that GPs should be integrally involved in decisions about how these resources were allocated.

In 2002 another piece of legislation, the National Health Service Reform and Health Care Professions Act, provided the legal framework for yet another major organizational change, which had been outlined in the government white paper, "The NHS Plan: A plan for investment, A plan for reform" (Department of Health, 2000b) and in the supplementary document, "Shifting the balance of power in the NHS" (Department of Health, 2001b). The Act conferred a duty on the Secretary of State for Health to establish Primary Care Trusts (PCTs) for the whole of England. These Trusts covered a population of between 100,000 and 250,000 and had responsibility for managing the budget and commissioning health care services for their populations. By 2004 they controlled approximately 75% of the total NHS budget. Similar changes occurred in Scotland, Wales, and Northern Ireland, although the specific organizational structures were different. Each PCT in England was governed by a Trust Board with a lay Chair and had a Professional Executive Committee that included local health professionals and a social care representative and was chaired by a GP. Thus, local primary care clinicians were actively involved in making decisions about allocation of resources for the delivery of health care to their local population, which would include their own patients. The reforms also further developed the concept of a market in the NHS by a move to allow private health care companies to bid for contracts to deliver health care services paid for by the NHS (Department of Health, 2000b). Health care was still free at the point of delivery, but the provider was now not necessarily an NHS organization. The aim of the 1990 and 2001 reforms was to move resource-allocation decision making away from central government to local decision-making bodies (or, in the case of GP fundholding, to individual clinicians). The belief was that services would thus be more responsive to patients' needs and choices rather than imposed by health service bureaucrats. Primary Care Trusts had a dual function of commissioning services for their community and also providing community-based services.

The provision of long-term care for people with complex health and social care needs also experienced organizational change in the decades leading up to 2002. Throughout the 1990s there was a steady decline in the number of long-stay geriatric and psychogeriatric beds in NHS hospitals with a corresponding increase in the number of nursing home beds in the private and voluntary sector (with individual residents funded through a combination of state and personal finance). Medical care in nursing homes is provided primarily by GPs. As has been noted above, the funding of long-term care in nursing homes was more complex than straightforward NHS care so this structural shift in long-term care provision created challenges for primary care physicians seeking to admit patients for long-term care. Admission needed to be negotiated through social service departments and included an assessment of the patient's ability to contribute to the cost of care. Furthermore, during the 1990s there was a shift in emphasis from institutional long-term care to community-based care, with the aim of supporting people to continue living independently in their own homes. Between 1998 and 2001, the number of nursing home places in the United Kingdom fell from 221,400 to 196,000 (Peace, 2003, p. 24).

■ HEALTH CARE PRIORITIES AND RESOURCE ALLOCATION STRATEGIES PRIOR TO 2002

The challenge of providing universal and comprehensive health care within a limited budget drawn from central taxation has been present since the inception of the NHS. In 1948, at a Royal College of Nurses conference, Aneurin Bevan, the architect of the NHS and Minister for Health at the time commented that expectation would always exceed capacity within the NHS, and that the fact that resources were scarce was all the more reason for ensuring that they were allocated in a well-balanced way.

> *"If there is a shortage of doctors on July 5, when the cash relationship between doctor and patient will disappear, it is very much more important that the doctors who are in short supply should spend their time looking after patients who really need to be looked after than that they should be looking after a lot of hypochondriacs who can afford to pay." (Bevan, 1948b[2])*

The main concern regarding fair allocation of resources in the early days of the NHS centered on the disparity in services between London, where pre-NHS there was a disproportionate number of hospitals and doctors, and the rest of the country. In 1976 the government set up a Resource Allocation Working Party (RAWP) to consider this disparity and make recommendations for a fairer system of allocating health care resources. Its recommendations focused on allocating resources to district health authorities in proportion to the health care needs of their populations, weighted for factors such as age, sex, mortality, and marital status (Department of Health, 1976). In the 1990s, with the development of a purchasing/commissioning role for local health authorities, a more sophisticated model of distributing resources based on a set of needs variables including health and socioeconomic factors was developed (the York model; see Carr-Hill et al., 1994). During this period some health authorities, recognizing their ethical obligation to provide a fair distribution of health care services across their population, set up specific committees (sometimes called *priorities forums*) to develop transparent processes for allocation of resources to provide these services (Hope et al., 1998). One function of these committees was to consider requests from individual patients and their doctors for funding for a treatment or service that the health authority did not normally purchase. Thus these committees had responsibility for making individual patient–level resource-allocation decisions as well as population-level priority setting. As health authorities gave way to PCTs in 2002, the priorities forums continued in the new organizations, with some explicitly developing ethical/values frameworks to support their funding decisions (NHS Oxfordshire, 2012).

In addition to the creation of PCTs, the set of reforms encapsulated in the NHS Plan introduced two further innovations that were likely to have an impact on clinicians' views on allocation of health care resources. The development of a set of National Service Frameworks which set standards for management of care for specific conditions and/or patient groups began in 1999, initially covering mental health, coronary heart disease, cancer, older people, and diabetes services (Department of Health, 2000b, p. 58). To support implementation of the NSFs, specific extra funding was allocated to these areas; for example, in 2002 the Department of Health announced that by 2003/2004 there would be an extra £230 million a year for heart disease services, an extra £570 million for cancer services, an extra annual investment of over £300 million for mental health services, and an extra £1.4 billion each year for better health and social care services for older people (Department of Health, 2002). The development of a set of specific standards against which clinical services could be measured, together with additional funding to support implementation of improved services, sent a particular message to health care commissioners and providers, and also to patients, that the areas covered by a NSF were to be in some way prioritized.

Perhaps the most important innovation with respect to making health care rationing explicit and to some extent transparent was the establishment of the National Institute of Health and Clinical Excellence (NICE) in 1999, an "arm's length" body that is one of the national "Special Health Authorities." The aim of NICE was (and is) to reduce variation in the availability and quality of NHS treatment and care. This could be seen as providing a counterbalance to the decentralization of health care funding to Primary Care Trusts and the ensuing concern about access to treatment being dependent on where you lived (post code lottery). The primary mechanism for achieving this aim is a combination of clinical guidelines (evidence-based guidelines on management of specific clinical conditions) and health technology appraisals (recommendations on whether to fund new and existing treatments based on evidence of clinical and cost effectiveness). The technology appraisal recommendations are in fact mandatory requirements, and commissioning organizations (Now Primary Care Commissioning Groups) must implement the recommendation within 3 months of the recommendation being published (NICE, 2010). The primary focus of the technology appraisal process underpinning recommendations for funding of specific treatments is a cost utility assessment based on Quality Adjusted Life Years (QALYs; NICE, 2010). By 2002 NICE had begun to publish treatment recommendations that would have a significant impact on the newly formed PCTs as they struggled to respond to their particular population's health care needs.

■ THE CONTEXT FOR THE VALUES AT THE BEDSIDE STUDY

In 2002 primary care physicians in the United Kingdom were working in a climate of change with regard to their role in patient care. The core NHS values of universal health care free at the point of delivery still defined their work, so most clinicians would not be faced with denying a patient treatment because of the patient's inability to pay unless the particular service or treatment was not funded by the NHS. This is reflected in the responses of UK physicians in the survey who were less likely than their colleagues in the other three countries to identify a patient's inability to pay as a reason for rationing treatment. However, while UK physicians may have had less worries about whether their patients could pay for treatment, they clearly felt that the resources available to them to treat their patients overall were insufficient, with UK physicians scoring highest on the perceived scarcity scale and only 29% considering that they were given enough resources to treat their patients fairly. This is not unexpected considering that in 2002 the UK per capita expenditure on health care was the lowest of all four countries in the survey, and total health care expenditure was 7.6% of GDP compared to 8.3% in Italy, 9.8% in Norway and 10.9% in Switzerland (World Bank, 2012) Most health care was publicly funded, but the public health care purse was thought to be too small; hence a general feeling of resource scarcity prevailed. In 2002, 2,100 patients were waiting over 13 weeks for an outpatient appointment with a hospital consultant (King's Fund, 2007).

What is perhaps more surprising, given the NHS principle of equal access to treatment, is that UK physicians also scored low on the perceived equity scale with only 11% of respondents agreeing that everyone in their country had equal access to needed medical services. This could in part reflect the overall scarcity of resources as evidenced by the expenditure figures and waiting times. If physicians think that in general needed services are not available or in short supply within the NHS, then the small minority of patients who access private health care will be able to purchase these treatments leading to inequality of access to needed care. However, the move to localized commissioning of services in the 1990s, and the creation of PCTs in 2001, had been accompanied by increasing concerns about regional inequalities or "post code rationing." Different PCTs, commissioning services on the basis of their population needs, would differ in their priorities for funding services, which could result in patients with the same condition but living in different areas having different access to certain services. At an individual clinician level this was perceived as inequitable and for many, unacceptable. The debate on post code rationing, and the publicity given to the emerging activities of NICE, would mean that rationing and priority setting were current topics of debate for physicians at the time of the study. UK GPs were less enthusiastic about suggested cost-containment policies than their European colleagues with the exception of using evidence-based medicine as a resource allocation method. The evidence-based medicine movement has been a strong factor in UK health care since the early 1990s (Davidoff et al., 1996), so GPs in 2002 would be familiar with working in this model. Restriction of expensive treatments was less popular with UK doctors, which would fit with their overall perception of underfunding in the NHS.

However, although UK physicians identified inequity and scored highly on perceived rationing across all modalities of care, they did not identify inequity for specific groups of patients as much as their colleagues in other countries, with the exception of patients who need expensive treatment, which could be a reflection of the overall perceived lack of funding for the NHS. In common with their international colleagues the UK doctors did identify the elderly as a disadvantaged group in relation to resources and also identified nursing home care as a specific area where rationing was frequent. Given the fall in the number of nursing home places between 1998 and 2001, and the complex funding arrangements for nursing and social care for the elderly, this is not entirely surprising.

■ DEVELOPMENTS SINCE 2002

One striking development since 2002 is the increase in UK expenditure on health care, rising from a total of £81.3 billion in 2002 to £136.4 billion in 2009 with health care spending as a percentage of GDP also rising from 7.6% in 2002 to 9.8% in 2009 (Quaiser, 2011). The most recent OECD figure is 9.4%. During this period private health expenditure has remained constant at 1.5%–1.6% of GDP, the rise in total expenditure reflecting a government commitment to increase the health care budget. In parallel with the increased expenditure on health care, and as part of the organizational reforms set out in the NHS plan (Department of Health, 2000b) a series of national targets were set for waiting times for NHS care, including first hospital clinic appointments, elective surgery, GP consultations, and investigation and treatment for cancer. Failure to meet these targets resulted in financial penalties for commissioning organizations (PCTs) and hospitals. In 2004 the government introduced a target of 18 weeks as the maximum time from referral to a hospital consultant to initiation of treatment for any patient (Department of Health, 2004). Waiting time figures from 2006 showed only 35% of inpatients were treated within the 18-week target (King's Fund, 2007), but this had risen to 87% in 2008 and 91.2% in 2012 (Department of Health, 2012). A different set of targets was introduced in 2004 as part of a new NHS contract for GPs. The Quality and Outcomes Framework (QOF) is a set of evidence-based performance indicators against which GPs' performance is measured by awarding points, with payment linked to achieving target percentages of points available for specified sets of indicators. Indicators cover a range of clinical areas such as diabetes, coronary heart disease, and epilepsy, as well as organizational, patient experience, and additional services domains. While there has been general acknowledgement that these targets have improved access and quality of care in some areas, concern has also been expressed that the focus on easily measurable parameters does not necessarily capture overall quality of care and that some patients with less easily measured health care needs will lose out.

While a focus on improving quality and access to health care, with increased funding to support this, has been a feature of the last decade in the NHS, there has nevertheless also been a consistent pressure on health care providers and commissioners to improve efficiency and cut costs. Primary Care Trusts were expected to deliver care to their populations within a specified budget, and failure to do so incurred penalties including financial penalties. The 2011/2012 QOF includes a series of indicators related to reducing outpatient and emergency referrals from primary care (BMA, 2011). A stated aim of these new indicators was to secure "a more effective use of NHS resources through improvements in the quality of primary care," and continuation of these indicators beyond 2012 will occur "if significant progress ha(s) been made in achieving productivity savings at the mid-year point" (NHS Employers, 2011). Overall the NHS is expected to make efficiency savings of £20 billion by 2014. This emphasis on efficiency, while linked to improvement in patient care, makes explicit that there is a limit on NHS resources and that within this limit choices must be made.

Since 2002 the National Institute of Clinical Excellence has become an integral part of the health care system with significant influence on clinical practice and health care commissioning. In December 2011 it had 147 published clinical guidelines available on its website on a wide range of conditions and 254 technology appraisals. NICE's stated aim is to produce evidence-based advice on which interventions provide best quality care and which offer best value for money for the NHS, and it has probably been the most influential agent for raising public awareness of the need to ration health care services in the United Kingdom. Several of its technology appraisal recommendations have been subject to judicial review when patient organizations or pharmaceutical companies have challenged their decision not to recommend a particular treatment for NHS funding. For example, in 2007 the decision of NICE to recommend the use of the drugs donepezil, galantamine, and rivastigmine for moderate Alzheimer disease only was subject to a judicial review brought by the pharmaceutical companies Eisai Limited and Pfizer (NICE, 2007). These high-profile cases not only subject NICE to public scrutiny but increase public debate about the reality of allocating scarce resources in response to increasing heath care need. The voice of the public is included in the work of NICE by representatives of patient and carer organizations on the relevant technology appraisal and clinical guideline committees, and by the formation of a citizen's council whose role is to evaluate the social and moral issues raised by NICE guidelines (NICE, 2008).

The latest organizational change in the NHS took place in 2012 with the passing of the Health and Social Care Act (2102) by parliament. This controversial piece of legislation created Clinical Commissioning Groups, which have now replaced Primary Care Trusts as the main commissioning bodies for health care in England. These groups are led by GPs and include other health professionals and lay members on their governing bodies. All GPs will be members of a CCG (NHS Commissioning Board 2012). The aim of this reorganization is to bring responsibility for commissioning of services as close to the front line of patient care as possible, the argument being that GPs are best placed to understand the needs of their patients and to negotiate appropriate services with their local providers. In the history of NHS reorganization this can be viewed as the latest and most radical step in decentralizing decisions regarding allocation of resources, albeit within a national framework set by NICE. The response of GPs to this development has been mixed, and it is difficult to disentangle reactions to the specific issue of GPs taking responsibility for commissioning from the other wide-ranging changes that will have an impact on patient care. The Royal College of General Practitioners opposed the proposed changes overall but welcomed GP involvement in commissioning in principle and has worked to support and train GP commissioners, including consideration of the ethical challenges that they will face (Oswald & Cox, 2011). At the British Medical Association conference in 2012, a motion for GPs to boycott clinical commissioning groups in protest at the way in which they were organized was defeated. Members argued that "all-out opposition" would remove any GP influence and hasten the privatization of UK health care (Jaques, 2012). The intense debate on clinical commissioning groups is too wide-ranging and complex to discuss in this chapter, but one thing is certain: with their development, GPs will be compelled to confront questions of priority setting and rationing of services for their patients, if not at the bedside then only one step removed.

Increasing awareness of the need to manage and appropriately allocate resources, both at a population level and at the bedside, is also reflected in professional guidance. The General Medical Council (GMC), which is the professional regulatory body for all doctors working in the United Kingdom, updated its guidance on leadership and management for doctors in 2012. In a section entitled "allocating resources" there is specific acknowledgment of the effect of limited resources on treatment options that a doctor can offer to a patient. (GMC, 2012) The guidance reiterates the core GMC principle of making the care of their patients a doctor's first concern, but it points out that a doctor also has responsibilities to the wider population. Acknowledgment of the need to allocate finite resources fairly within the NHS was also made explicit in the NHS constitution (Department of Health, 2011) which, while reiterating the core principles of the NHS as set out in 1948, also included as one of its seven principles a commitment to "providing best value for taxpayers' money and the most effective, fair and sustainable use of finite resources."

■ REFLECTIONS FOR THE FUTURE

In reviewing the development of the NHS in the last decade, one can detect an increasing emphasis on evidence-based treatment decisions informed by national policy and guidance on the delivery of effective and cost-effective care. The discussion of health care rationing or priority setting within limited available resources is now more explicit, although usually conducted at a population rather than an individual patient level. Despite increasing overall funding for the NHS in the last 10 years, clinicians today, like those who took part in the Values at the Bedside study, are likely to experience pressures to limit treatment options because of cost but will tend to perceive these pressures as externally constructed by bodies such as NICE and clinical commissioning groups. However, for GPs the recent organizational changes will shift the responsibility for setting health care priorities to them, making it more difficult to externalize accountability. Critics of clinical commissioning highlighted the potential conflict of interest for GP commissioners between their obligations to manage resources efficiently and their duty of care to their individual patients. Given that another equally significant development in UK health care over the last decade has been an emphasis on patient choice and empowerment, a key challenge for clinicians and commissioners of care, whoever they are in the future, will be to engage patients in an honest and transparent debate about health care rationing.

REFERENCES

Audit Commission. (1995). Briefing on GP fundholding. Available at: http://www.audit-commission.gov.uk/SiteCollectionDocuments/Downloads/BriefingGPFundholding.pdf.

Appleby J. (2005). Cutting NHS waiting times: Identifying strategies for sustainable reductions.London. King's Fund Available at http://www.kingsfund.org.uk/publications/cutting-nhs-waiting-times

Bevan, A. (1948a). A message to the medical profession from the Minister of Health. *Lancet*, 252(6514), 24.

Bevan, A. (1948b). In RCN conference review: hospital planning and method. British Medical Journal, 1, 1197–1198.

British Medical Association and NHS Employers Organization. (2012). Quality and Outcomes Framework for 2012/3 Guidance for PCOs and practices. http://www.nhsemployers.org/~/media/Employers/Documents/Primary%20care%20contracts/QOF/2012-13/Quality%20and%20Outcomes%20Framework%20for%202012-13%20-%20Guidance%20for%20PCOs%20and%20Practices.pdf

Carr-Hill, R. A., Sheldon, T. A., Smith, P., Martin, S., Peacock, S., & Hardman, G. (1994). Allocating resources to health authorities: development of method for small area analysis of use of inpatient services. *British Medical Journal, 309,* 1046–1049.

Coulter, A. (1995). Evaluating general practice fundholding in the United Kingdom. *European Journal of Public Health, 5*(4), 233–239.

Davidoff, F., Haynes, B., Sackett, D., & Smith, R. (1996). Evidence based medicine: what it is and what it isn't. *British Medical Journal, 312,* 71.

Department of Health. (1976). Sharing resources for England: Report of the Resource Allocation Working Party. Available at: http://www.dh.gov.uk/prod_consum_dh/groups/dh_digitalassets/@dh/@en/documents/digitalasset/dh_4122318.pdf.

Department of Health. (2001a). The NHS Plan: the government's response to the Royal Commission on long term care.

Department of Health. (2000b). The NHS Plan: a plan for investment, a plan for reform. 2000.b.

Department of Health. (2001b). Shifting the balance of power in the NHS: securing delivery. Available at http://webarchive.nationalarchives.gov.uk/20130107105354/http://www.dh.gov.uk/prod_consum_dh/groups/dh_digitalassets/@dh/@en/documents/digitalasset/dh_4076522.pdf

Department of Health. (2002). Funding streams: National Service Frameworks: a practical aid to implementation in primary care. Available at http://www.dh.gov.uk/prod_consum_dh/groups/dh_digitalassets/@dh/@en/documents/digitalasset/dh_4050860.pdf.

Department of Health. (2004). The NHS improvement plan, putting people at the heart of public services. Available at: http://www.dh.gov.uk/prod_consum_dh/groups/dh_digitalassets/@dh/@en/@ps/documents/digitalasset/dh_118572.pdf.

Department of Health. (2009a). Guidance on NHS patients who wish to pay for additional private care. Available at: http://www.dh.gov.uk/prod_consum_dh/groups/dh_digitalassets/documents/digitalasset/dh_096576.pdf.

Department of Health. (2009b). The national framework for NHS continuing health care and NHS funded nursing care (revised). Available at: http://www.dh.gov.uk/prod_consum_dh/groups/dh_digitalassets/documents/digitalasset/dh_103161.pdf.

Department of Health. (2011). Spending review. Available at: http://www.dh.gov.uk/en/MediaCentre/Pressreleases/DH_120676

Department of Health. (2012). The NHS Constitution. 2nd edition. Available at: http://www.dh.gov.uk/prod_consum_dh/groups/dh_digitalassets/@dh/@en/documents/digitalasset/dh_132958.pdf.

Department of Health. (2012). Referral to treat time series (England). Available at: http://www.dh.gov.uk/en/Publicationsandstatistics/Statistics/Performancedataandstatistics/ReferraltoTreatmentstatistics/index.htm.

General Medical Council. (2012). *Leadership and management for all doctors.* London: General Medical Council.

Hope, T., Hicks, N., Reynolds, D. J., Crisp, R., & Griffiths, S. (1998). Rationing and the Health Authority. *British Medical Journal*, 307, 1067–1069.

Jaques, H. (2012). BMA meeting: Doctors reject calls to boycott clinical commissioning groups. *British Medical Journal*, 344, 4393

National Commissioning Board. (2012). Towards establishment: creating responsive and accountable clinical commissioning groups. Available at: http://www.commissioningboard.nhs.uk/files/2012/01/NHSCBA-02-2012-6-Guidance-Towards-establishment-Final.pdf.

National Health Service and Community Care Act 1990. National Archives, United Kingdom. Available at: http://www.legislation.gov.uk/ukpga/1990/19/section/2/enacted.

National Institute for Health and Clinical Excellence. (2010). About technology appraisals. Available at: http://www.nice.org.uk/aboutnice/whatwedo/abouttechnologyappraisals/about_technology_appraisals.jsp.

National Institute for Health and Clinical Excellence. (2010). Measuring effectiveness and cost effectiveness: the QALY. Available at: http://www.nice.org.uk/newsroom/features/measuringeffectivenessandcosteffectivenesstheqaly.jsp.

National Institute for Health and Clinical Excellence (2007). Outcome of judicial review for NICE guidance on drugs for Alzheimer's disease. Available at: http://www.nice.org.uk/newsroom/features/outcomeofjr.jsp.

National Institute for Health and Clinical Excellence (2008). Social value judgements: principles for the development of NICE guidance (second edition).Available at http://www.nice.org.uk/media/C18/30/SVJ2PUBLICATION2008.pdf

NHS Choices. (2011). NHS core principles. Available at: http://www.nhs.uk/NHSEngland/thenhs/about/Pages/nhscoreprinciples.aspx.

NHS Choices. (2012). Help with NHS costs. Available at: http://www.nhs.uk/nhsengland/healthcosts/pages/prescriptioncosts.aspx.

NHS Employers. (2011). Available at: http://www.nhsemployers.org/PayAndContracts/GeneralMedicalServicesContract/QOF/Pages/ChangestoQOF2011-12.aspx.

NHS Oxfordshire Priorities Forum. (2012). Available at: http://www.oxfordshirepct.nhs.uk/about-us/how-the-pct-works/priorities-forum.aspx.

Office for National Statistics. (2011). Expenditure on health care in the UK. Available at http://www.ons.gov.uk/ons/dcp171766_308689.pdf

Oswald, M., & Cox, D.; the RCGP ethics committee. (2011). Making difficult choices: ethical commissioning guidance to general practitioners.

Peace, S. M. (2003). The development of residential and nursing home care in the United Kingdom. In Samson Katz, J., & Peace, S. M., eds. *End of Life in Care Homes: A palliative care approach*. Pp. 15–42.Oxford: Oxford University Press

Quaiser, U. (2011). Expenditure on health care in the UK. United Kingdom: Office for National Statistics. Available at: http://www.nhs.uk/nhsengland/healthcosts/pages/prescriptioncosts.aspx.

Royal Commission. (1999). *With respect to old age: Long term care, rights and responsibilities*. London: Her Majesty's Stationery Office. Available at: http://www.archive.official-documents.co.uk/document/cm41/4192/4192.htm.

Scottish Government. (2010). Scotland's spending plans and draft budget 2011/12. Available at: http://www.scotland.gov.uk/Publications/2010/11/17091127/18.

Scottish Parliament. (2002). Community Care and Health (Scotland) Act. Available at: http://www.legislation.gov.uk/asp/2002/5/section/1.

The Stationery Office. (1999). With respect to old age: Long term care, rights and responsibilities: A report by The Royal Commission on long term care (executive summary). Available at: http://www.archive.official-documents.co.uk/document/cm41/4192/4192-sum.htm accessed 1.5.2012/

United Kingdom Parliament. Health and Social Care Act. (2012). Available at http://www.legislation.gov.uk/ukpga/2012/7/contents/enacted

United Kingdom Parliament. (2002). National Health Service Reform and Health Care Professions Act 2002. Available at http://www.legislation.gov.uk/ukpga/2002/17/section/6

United Kingdom Parliament. National Health Service and Community Care Act. (1990). Available at http://www.legislation.gov.uk/ukpga/1990/19/section/47

United Kingdom Parliament National Health Service Act. (2006). Available at http://www.legislation.gov.uk/ukpga/2006/41/contents

World Bank. (2002). Data, Health expenditure. Available at: http://data.worldbank.org/indicator/SH.XPD.TOTL.ZS?page=2.

5   The Norwegian Context

■ REIDUN FØRDE

The Norwegian population is quite privileged. Norway has one of the world's highest employment rates, highest incomes per capita, and relatively small differences in social class. Infant mortality is low, and the average expected life span is 78.7 years for men and 83.2 years for women (2009 OECD data). Eight out of ten Norwegians describe their health as good. Musculoskeletal illness, cancer, and psychiatric illness (especially among the young) are increasing (Statistics Norway, 2012).

Health and care services for the 5 million Norwegians are by and large financed through taxation. Eighty-four percent of health spending was funded by public sources in 2008, compared to the Organisation for Economic Co-operation and Development (OECD) average of 73%. The public share of health care financing has been relatively stable since 2002. Although the number of Norwegians who buy extra health care insurance has increased during the last decade (Berge & Hyggen, 2010), this is still a minor part of the total health care budget.

■ HEALTH CARE ORGANIZATION

In 2001 Norwegian health care was organized in three levels. The first level, the municipal level (430 municipalities) was (and still is) responsible for primary health care, nursing homes, and home-based nursing care. The second level, the county level, was responsible for hospitals and private specialists. Finally the third level, the national, the Ministry of Health and Care Services had overall responsibility for all health and care services.

In 2002 a major health-service reform took place in which the responsibility for hospitals was transferred from the 19 counties (regional political level) to the central government. The purpose of the reform was "to deliver specialized health care services of high quality and equity to anyone in need, independent of age, gender, place of living, economy, or ethnic origin, as well as facilitating research and innovation." (*Lov om spesialisthelsetjenesten m.m. av 2.7.1999 nr. 61*). The hospitals became organized as health enterprises, 100 % owned by the state, specifically the Ministry of Health and Care Services. Every health enterprise forms a separate legal entity. Five (later four) regional health care trusts were established and given responsibility for all specialist health care, including psychiatric treatment and specialist treatment of alcoholism and substance abuse. The regional health care trusts own the hospital trusts in their region. Forty percent of specialist health care is financed by capitation, 60 % by fixed budgets.

As part of the 2002 reform, a Directorate for Health and Care Services was established (later the Norwegian Directorate of Health) responsible for professional guidance to health care, health care cost-analysis, and to represent a bridge between central health care authorities and the health care providers in professional matters.

The last and most recent major reform was launched in 2012 to secure better cooperation between specialist and primary health care services. The aim is to ensure that more treatment is given in primary health care outside the hospitals provided that this treatment is of acceptable quality. Whether this extensive reform will increase quality and reduce spending in the Norwegian health care remains to be seen.

■ HEALTH CARE SPENDING

Total health spending accounted for 9.6 % of GDP in Norway in 2009, and this has been stable since 2002 (OECD, 2011, p. 149). Although Norway's health care spending relative to GDP is on par with many European countries, the spending per capita is much higher. In 2002 Norway spent more money on health care than most European countries. In 2009 per capita spending amounted to $5,352 (adjusted for purchasing power parity), more than all other Nordic neighbors and 30% more than its neighboring country, Sweden, which has a similar health care system (OECD, 2011). One reason for the high spending per capita is that Norway has a decentralized hospital system. Another reason is the high wages in Norway.

■ HEALTH CARE RESOURCES

In 2002 Norway had 3.2 physicians per 1,000 inhabitants, which had increased to 4 physicians per 1,000 inhabitants in 2009—more than the other Nordic countries and more than any of the countries in the Values at the Bedside study (OECD, 2011, p. 63). In 2002 the municipalities with responsibility for primary health care, and health and care for the elderly in nursing homes, had 0.91 physician man-years per 1,000 inhabitants, and this has increased to 0.96 in 2010 (Statistics Norway, 2012). Since 1990 the number of physician man-years has increased by 42 % in primary health care and by 93% in specialist health care (Norwegian Directorate of Health, 2008).

Since 2002 all Norwegians have, through a patient-list system, their own general practitioner / family physician that they are free to choose. This was more or less the situation before 2002, but now it has been formalized. Family physicians receive their income partly from the state, partly from the municipalities (based on the number of patients on their list, independent of patient contacts), and partly from patient copayment for contacts with the doctor.

In principle, access to specialist health care goes through a primary care physician. In addition, primary care physicians are the most important group for certification of sick leave and disability applications. Thus Norwegian primary care physicians have an important gatekeeping function, a function that may be experienced as challenging (Gulbrandsen et al., 2002; Carlsen & Norheim, 2005). The primary care doctor's gatekeeping activity can be challenged as a result of the right to free choice of a family doctor. Competition among doctors may decrease the physician's willingness to risk a conflict with the patient. The gatekeeping function may therefore be in conflict with the doctor's private economic interests. A recent study shows that referrals to specialist health care vary substantially among primary care physicians within the same geographical area (Førde et al., 2011).

■ COPAYMENT

Although Norway's per capita spending is high and largely funded publicly, not all health care is covered through taxation Public financing of drugs is decided by a public board (Norwegian Medicines Agency). This board administers a list of drugs, a "blue label list." The majority of expenses for the drugs on this list is paid for through taxation. In order to obtain a place on the blue label list, certain characteristics of a drug must be met. Effectiveness and cost-effectiveness of a drug are important criteria to win a place on the list. Drugs with expired patents are reimbursed at the price of corresponding cheaper generic drugs. Only treatment for chronic diseases and conditions assessed to be of a certain severity obtain a place on the blue label list. Thus, expenses for drugs for minor ailments and expensive drugs for acute conditions may represent a substantial burden on the personal finances of patients.

Dental health status is closely linked to socioeconomic status. The inclusion of dental health care in public health care is a recurring theme in the public debate.

Maximal copayment for physiotherapy is 30% higher than copayment for other medical interventions (see BOX 1). After this sum of copayment is reached, physiotherapy is covered through taxation for the rest of year. People with particularly low incomes may apply to have their costs covered through the social security system.

The following section describes two areas of health care that have been highlighted in the responses of the Norwegian doctors in the Values at the Bedside study.

BOX 5.1 ■ Patient Copayment in the Norwegian Health Care System

I. **Fully paid for by patient**
   A. Specialist treatment without referral from primary care physician/ without appointment with the health care trust
   B. Drugs not on the blue label list
   C. Most dental care for people over 21

II. **Partly paid for by patients**
   A. Contacts in primary health care
   B. Day treatment, ambulatory treatment in specialist health care
   C. Drugs on the blue label list
   D. Most physiotherapy
   E. A permanent place in nursing homes
      (When the sum of II A, B, C exceeds USD 350 (2011), expenses are fully covered through taxation for the rest of the year.)

III. **All expenses covered through taxation**
   A. In-patient treatment in hospitals
   B. Home based nursing care
   C. Medical treatment for children up to the age of 16
   D. Antenatal care
   E. Treatment of certain infectious diseases
   F. Dental care for patients before age 21 and dental care in nursing homes
   G. Some surgical dental care
   H. Physiotherapy following surgery, and for a few chronic conditions.

■ HEALTH CARE TO PSYCHIATRIC PATIENTS

In 2002, 7.2% of Norwegian doctors were psychiatrists. This has increased to 8.6% in 2011, giving 0.38 psychiatrists per 1,000 inhabitants (Norwegian Medical Association statistics). During this time there has been a shift from inpatient treatment to more ambulatory treatment. The number of beds in psychiatric hospitals has been reduced since 2002, and the number of psychiatrists and psychologists working outside psychiatric hospitals has increased. Waiting lists for patients in need of psychiatric treatment have been long for several decades in spite of national resource allocation guidelines, which since 1987 have recommended that treatment of psychiatric patients should be prioritized (see below). In 1999–2008 a national plan consisting of increased resources to the sector was launched to increase capacity and quality in the field of psychiatry.

▨ HEALTH CARE FOR THE ELDERLY

According to official policy age alone is not considered to be a valid exclusion criterion in resource allocation, and people well over 80 are offered active treatment such as kidney, hip, and knee replacement and advanced cardiac surgery.

In 2010, 2.1 % of the GDP was spent (by the municipalities) on nursing and care services, which represented 34% of the municipalities' net expenses (Hagen et al., 2011). Taking care of old and frail family members is no longer considered the duty of female family members but is seen as a public responsibility. Compared to other European countries, the number of Norwegian women working outside the home is high (Statistics Norway, 2009) so there is greater demand for nursing home facilities. In 2003 Norway had, together with Switzerland, more long-term beds for populations 65 years and over (66.1 and 74.2 /1,000 inhabitants respectively) than Italy and the United Kingdom (14.0 and 54.4 /1,000 inhabitants respectively (OECD, 2013). More Norwegian citizens spend their last days in nursing homes than the OECD average, and 45% die there (Statistics Norway, 2011). Thus, 15 % of the population 65 years and older receive long-term care (nursing home and home-based nursing care).

Home-based nursing care is in most instances considered the best model of care for the elderly, who thereby can continue to live in their own homes in spite of a reduced level of functioning. Home-based nursing care can be given six times a day if necessary. As a consequence, when patients finally are granted a place in a nursing home they have major needs for care and medical treatment. Patients in nursing homes have on average five to seven serious chronic diseases, and 80% suffer from dementia (Husebø & Husebø, 2005). In nursing homes there is one doctor for 167 patients compared to 2 patients per doctor in acute care hospitals (Husebø & Husebø, 2005). In most municipalities there are waiting lists for a place in a nursing home, and home-based nursing care is rationed (Tønnesen, 2011). Medical treatment and care for patients in nursing homes is paid for through taxation, but patients contribute an average of 77% of their income/pension (Hagen et al., 2011). Beyond this, housing, accommodation, nursing care, medical treatment, and dental treatment are covered for nursing home patients.

Most patients in nursing homes have a variety of needs that are expected to be met by the institutions. In addition to medical and nursing needs, they have additional psychosocial and existential needs. They require social stimulation, fresh air, exercise, and emotional support. This represents a huge challenge for the municipalities responsible for the nursing homes. A study indicates that somatic and acute health care to the elderly is prioritized, while psychosocial and existential care are rationed (Førde et al., 2006). To phrase it differently: old, frail people's lives are saved, but what may make life worth living is rationed.

■ SETTING PRIORITIES IN NORWAY

Due to her oil and gas resources, Norway has a very well endowed economy; still, resource allocation in health care and the need to set priorities fairly have been on the public agenda for several decades. Notably, in Norway *setting priorities, resource allocation,* and *prioritization* are the most frequently used words for dealing with limited health care resources. The term *health care rationing* is more rarely used. The first governmental commission on resource allocation issues finished its work in 1987 (Official Norwegian Reports, NOU 1987:23). Through this, Norway was among the first countries to bring resource allocation to public attention. The first commission was followed by a second commission ten years later (Official Norwegian Reports, NOU 1997:18). Both commissions were composed of members of the public, patient organizations, and members from several levels of health care, and both were led by a professor and subsequent parliament member, Inge Lønning. Accordingly, the commissions and their reports are called Lønning I and II.

The first commission concluded in its report "Guidelines for prioritizations in the Norwegian health service" that the most important criterion for resource allocation in health care is the severity of the health condition. The commission defined five priority levels, with acute needs for health care being level 1 and not-prioritized needs being level 5. Psychiatry, care and treatment for the elderly, and rehabilitation services were underscored as areas of special priority that should receive relatively more resources. The report was later criticized for ignoring effectiveness of interventions as well as costs. It was also considered to be too focused on the theoretical level and too little on how prioritizations should take place in clinical practice.

One important effect of the first priority-setting report was, however, that the need to set priorities in health care was communicated to the public; it created a public debate. Thereby, it probably also had some influence on the values and thinking of the nation's health personnel. One indication of this may be that when the ethical guidelines of The Norwegian Medical Association were revised in 1994, a new paragraph (Chapter 1, § 12) was added, stating: *"A doctor shall in his or her practice have due regard for the national economy. Unnecessary or excessively costly methods must not be employed. A doctor must contribute to the distribution of medical resources in accordance with generally accepted ethical norms. A doctor must in no way seek to provide individual patients or groups with unjustified advantages, whether financial, in respect to priorities, or otherwise. A doctor must give notice of insufficient resources in his or her area of responsibility."*

Through this, a doctor's obligation to secure fair priority decisions became not only a practical but also an ethical duty.

In the aftermath of Lønning I, but not a direct consequence of the report, a "waiting time guarantee" was established, organizing the patients waiting for hospitalization based on the need for intervention. According to this "waiting time guarantee" a maximum time for treatment, assessed by a medical specialist, should be set in each individual case. As a result there has been an increased emphasis and focus on the waiting period for treatment both as a measure of the quality and efficiency of the health care delivered and as a measure of the success of the health care's resource-allocation work. There has been much less focus on the quality of the actual health care provided or whether the right patients receive care.

The second public commission (Lønning II) delivered its report in 1997 (Official Norwegian Reports, NOU 1997:18). Part of its mandate was to assess the progress of resource allocation efforts since the first resource allocation guidelines had been launched. The commission concluded that the effect of the 1987 guidelines on resource allocation processes in Norwegian health care was less than expected. The "prioritized" areas such as psychiatry, medical care to the chronically ill, to patients with major care needs, and rehabilitation had lagged behind the already prioritized somatic and especially acute health care. One explanation for this, according to the commission's report, was that health care is a modern, complex system in which most decisions related to distribution are made at a decentralized level by local health authorities and doctors who may not agree with public recommendations. It was emphasized that in order to have an effect on the priorities of the actual health care given, new strategies had to be found.

The Lønning II commission recommended that health care be divided into four priority groups: basic health care, supplementary health care, low-priority care, and care not financed within the public system. Health care interventions were to be assigned to the four priority groups according to three criteria that must be assessed:

1. Health state (for example, poor prognosis, diminished mental or physical function, and pain without treatment).
2. Expected benefit (for example, survival time, reduction of ailment, improvement of function). The assessment of effect should be based on good quality data.
3. Cost-efficiency ("reasonable proportion between costs and benefit of treatment").

As already mentioned, these three criteria were implemented at an early stage in the assessment of drugs considered for the blue label list.

The commission emphasized the importance of a fair and open priority-setting process. To secure this, and to obtain an increased impact of priority-setting work on the everyday level of health care, the commission recommended two additional strategies. The first was to establish expert groups to propose clinical priority recommendations within their fields of expertise. The recommendations were required to be based on the three conditions above: disease severity, benefit of intervention, and cost- efficiency. Besides ensuring that resource allocation was based on expert knowledge of patient needs and effects of intervention, the work was considered by the commission to be important in increasing doctors' acceptance of the need for open and consensus-based resource allocation work.

The second new strategy recommended by the 1997 commission was to establish a national priority council responsible for giving advice about prioritization and to see the conclusions of the different expert groups in relation to each other and in relation to national recommendations. In order to obtain public acceptance of the resource allocation work, the commission recommended that the council should be composed of representatives from the general public, patient organizations, health care personnel, experts on law and ethics, and political-administrative decision makers. Further, the council members had a special obligation to engage in the public debate on resource allocation issues. Raising the public's awareness of the need to prioritize health care was seen as an important pedagogical challenge.

■ ADOPTION OF THE 1997 COMMISSION'S RECOMMENDATIONS

The three priority criteria— severity of the condition, effect of the intervention, and cost efficiency—became the basis of a Patient- and User's Rights Act Act in 1999 (*Lov om pasient- og brukerrettigheter*) and accompanying Regulations Concerning the Prioritization of Health Services (FOR 2000-12-01 nr 1208). These legal regulations give patients the right to receive interventions according to their needs, divided in three categories: needs for emergency intervention, needs that are prioritized and which should receive treatment within an individually defined upper time limit and nonprioritized needs. The aim of the legal regulations was to secure patients' equal rights to good quality health care, including the right to file complaints. For a more detailed review of the Norwegian Health Care laws related to setting priorities, see Søreide et al., chapter 18. If the health care trust does not offer treatment within the guaranteed time span, the patient is given the right to receive immediate care at an alternative hospital (*Lov om pasient- og brukerrettigheter av 2.7.1999 nr. 63*). The trust must then pay for treatment in another health care trust, within the private sector, or for treatment abroad.

■ THE VALUES AT THE BEDSIDE STUDY IN LIGHT OF NORWEGIAN HEALTH CARE AT THE TIME OF THE STUDY

In 2002 Norway had one of the world's highest employment rates, highest incomes, and, in addition, good population health. Most health and care services were financed through taxation, and Norway's total expenditure on health care per capita was, in 2002, on the same level as Switzerland and substantially more than Italy and the United Kingdom. Very little health care was privately funded. Norway had more doctors than any of the other three countries, and the number of psychiatric beds was high.

In spite of this very privileged situation, Norwegian doctors describe some of their health and care services quite critically. One possible explanation for this may be that Norwegian health care is run ineffectively compared to the other three countries. Alternatively, it may be, in line with Wennberg's claim, that with more doctors and more health care offered, more needs for health care are created (Wennberg, 2010). However, there are several other explanations for the study results.

The experience of scarcity of resources is a matter of relative expectations. Thus, when the results of the study are to be interpreted, the population's as well as doctors' values and ideals must be taken into consideration. Most Norwegian doctors hold high ideals regarding the quality of health and care services. Solidarity with the worst off and fairness are deeply founded values in the nation as well as in the doctors' ethical guidelines. When the nation's economy is among the world's most privileged, less than optimal quality of health services may be hard to accept. A standard of care that might be accepted as adequate in another country might not be tolerated by Norwegian doctors, who have high expectations of their health care system.

Rationing may be particularly difficult to accept for the most vulnerable patient groups. Patients with mental health problems and the frail elderly are examples of vulnerable patient groups, and health care for these patient groups was described most critically by Norwegian doctors— indeed, more critically than doctors in the other three study countries. As described above, both these fields have struggled with lack of resources for several decades, and suboptimal care and medical treatment in nursing homes have been highlighted in the media repeatedly. Perhaps the Values at the Bedside findings reflect the fact that Norwegian physicians share the perspective of the two public resource allocation commissions, which highlighted the need to increase resources to these two fields. More recent studies indicate that the quality of the treatment and care to the elderly still is perceived by doctors and nurses as far from optimal (Førde et al., 2006; Tønnesen et al., 2011; Gjerberg et al., 2010), and it was not until 2006–2009 that the increase of resources to psychiatry exceeded resources to somatic health care (Norwegian Directorate of Health, 2012).

Patients' expenses for drugs may represent a substantial imposition on patient finances, and chronically ill patients with complex conditions, who often have relatively low income, may have difficulties paying for some of their treatment. As patient copayments are required for most drug treatments, this may explain why so many Norwegian doctors claim that patients do not receive treatment due to lack of ability to pay.

The need for resource allocation has been on the public agenda in Norway since 1987 and, as described above, the Norwegian Medical Association has actively endorsed efforts to create fair rationing processes, such as guideline development, since 1994 (Norwegian Medical Association, 2007a). The Values at the Bedside study indicates that Norwegian doctors, to a greater extent than their European colleagues, seem to accept rationing, and still do not fear that denial of expensive therapy is a threat to the patient–physician relationship. This may be taken as an indication that the work of setting priorities fairly in Norway has had some effect. A substantial proportion of Norwegian doctors in the study accepted guidelines as a tool for making good resource allocation decisions, which may reflect that such guidelines have been recommended in the national public resource allocation documents (Official Norwegian Reports, NOU 1997:17). However, it is also possible that the doctors, when asked about guidelines in the study, gave what they thought was the expected answer: resources are limited and should be distributed fairly in open processes and, in order to adhere to the principle of fairness allocation, practice should follow guidelines. The high acceptance of the need to ration may explain why a high proportion of Norwegian doctors are aware of and openly admit that they actually do ration. However, acceptance of a theoretical and political ideal does not necessarily translate into acceptance by clinicians of the results of limited resources when confronted with individual patients' needs in their own field/specialty.

■ DEVELOPMENTS SINCE 2002

The Patient- and User's Rights Act in 2004 granted prioritized patients a "waiting time guarantee." A quickly recognized problem was that clinicians' assessments of need for prioritized health care varied substantially. The Lønning II report emphasized that the doctor's clinical assessment should be fundamental in individual priority decisions, but the geographical variation in priorities was violating the principle of fairness. Accordingly, the health authorities could no longer ignore how priority decisions were dealt with at the clinical level; national priority guidelines were needed which also would make resource allocation decisions on a clinical level more explicit.

■ MOVING PRIORITY WORK CLOSER TO CLINICAL PRACTICE

The Lønning II commission emphasized the importance of basing good resource allocation decisions on valid scientific knowledge. An important step in the right direction was the establishment of the first national health technology assessment institution in 1998. This organization was continued through the establishment of the Norwegian Knowledge Centre for the Health Services (NOKC) in 2004, which was intended to ensure that health care services are based upon the best possible scientific evidence and with a national responsibility to communicate knowledge of evidence-based medicine to health care decision makers.

The recommendation to establish experts groups to elaborate allocation guidelines was not followed up until 2007, 10 years after Lønning II. An important reason for this was, in my opinion, that the health authorities considered that this work was in itself a huge resource commitment. However, the substantial variation in priority assessments made it obvious that resource allocation guidelines were necessary. In addition, in 2007 the Ministry of Health and Care Services issued a national health plan that emphasized the need for a comprehensive approach to priority setting and quality improvement work. Accordingly, the Directorate for Health initiated the endeavor to make priority guidelines based on best possible scientific knowledge. Since 2007 more than 33 guidelines have been launched (The Norwegian Electronic Health Library, 2011).

The Norwegian Medical Association took an active role in the development of the guidelines. The association also elaborated their own "white paper" on resource allocation in 2007 (Norwegian Medical Association, 2007b).

The work with priority guidelines was a substantial step forward in securing fair resource allocation in health care but was still no quick fix. Responsibility for interpretation and implementation of the guidelines falls to individual clinicians. Soreide and colleagues' chapter is a demonstration of how guidelines were put into clinical practice by one of Norway's biggest health care trusts. Although not without challenges, this health care trust has managed to control costs and to create a system with open and transparent priority setting.

The next step was to secure a fair balance between the different fields within health care, for example, somatic health care versus psychiatric health care. To secure this, and to give specific and effective advice in resource allocation issues, the National Council for Priority Setting established in 2000 was replaced by the National Council for Quality Improvement and Priority Setting in Health Care in 2007 (Mørland et al., 2010). The members of the latest "priority council" include a strong percentage of managers from different levels of health care in addition to lay members. This is in contrast to the first council, which was criticized for its lack of ability to implement its recommendations in actual health care services. The director of the the Norwegian Directorate of Health is chair of the new council. Accordingly, its work is more closely linked to actual decision making in health care. The Norwegian Ministry of Health has established the Norwegian Council for Quality Improvement and Priority Setting in Health Care for several purposes. First and foremost, the council will secure a comprehensive national approach to the work on quality and prioritization.

The council's aim is to help coordinate efforts on important topics across different positions of responsibility. They do not have the mandate to issue instructions, but to create transparency and legitimacy around difficult quality and prioritization issues (National Council for Quality Improvement and Priority Setting in Health Care, 2012).

The Norwegian Knowledge Centre for the Health Services has become a secretariat for "The Priority Council." One of its aims is to ensure that new medical technology is introduced into clinical care after a thorough assessment of its benefits as well as its cost-effectiveness.

▪ HAS SYSTEMATIC RESOURCE ALLOCATION WORK IN NORWAY BEEN WORTHWHILE?

The National Council for Quality Improvement and Priority Setting in Health Care has managed to set some limits, such as recommending only one cochlear implant for hearing impairment, reducing surgical intervention for sleep apnea, and a recommendation to ration extremely expensive drugs with uncertain effects. The Council is, however, being criticized for being too conservative, since the process of documenting utility and cost-effectiveness of new treatments takes time with the result that the Norwegian population may not receive the newest and the best interventions.

During recent years the field of psychiatry, including child and adolescent psychiatry and treatment for addiction problems, has, through efforts at priority setting on the political level, received substantially more resources than somatic health care (Norwegian Directorate of Health, 2012).

The health care sector is extremely complex. Development, and thereby resource allocation, is influenced by a number of factors of which new technology, scientific knowledge, and financial interests are but a few. Politicians pass laws with good intentions, but laws may influence resource allocation in unintended ways. One example of this may be the right to free choice of hospital, with the result that hospital expenses are difficult to predict since the number of guest patients is unpredictable and the more expensive "guest patients", treatment must be paid for by the local health care trust. Guest patients pose difficulty mainly in several hospitals in the most heavy populated areas of the country.

Relatively few patients who are entitled to prioritized health care, or health care within a certain time limit, choose treatment at locations other than their local hospital even when the guaranteed time limit is exceeded. One explanation for this may be that delayed treatment is tolerable for the patient, and that the predicted "urgency" is less than assessed. Another explanation is that patients who are chronically ill or have psychiatric illnesses may find it difficult to exercise their right to choose. Thus, strengthened patients' rights may favor the strong patient groups who can voice their interests. A national survey published in 2008 indicated that when the strongest patients who can voice their interests receive better care, this caused moral distress for physicians (Førde & Aasland, 2008). When this survey was repeated in 2010, fewer doctors working within specialist health care claimed that this was distressing, indicating that the prioritization guidelines may have begun to function as useful tools in clinical practice (Førde & Aasland, 2013).

Setting priorities in an affluent society has some unique challenges. One particular challenge involves gaining public acceptance of the need to ration. The Priority Council consists of members with different backgrounds who hold different values, some of which may be in conflict with priority guidelines. An example of this is a recent recommendation to offer fetal scan screening in the 12th pregnancy week, despite a report from the Norwegian Knowledge Centre for the Health Services stating that this screening had little effect on fetal morbidity and mortality. The majority of the Council's members supported the equity argument; today, couples who are able to pay for this examination themselves already receive the service but the poorer do not. This is met by arguments that using public money to finance a service with little effect on mothers' and fetuses' health shifts health resources away from sicker patients to healthy women.

Rationing potentially life-prolonging treatment is especially difficult in an affluent country. Seriously ill patients, who are denied such treatment because of uncertain or very limited effect, will always cause anger in the public. Rationing of very expensive life-prolonging treatment is perceived as cruel and meaningless in one of the world's richest countries, even if the value of these treatments is uncertain. Politicians may have a hard time resisting such public anger.

In the summer of 2010, the director of the Norwegian Directorate of Health and chair of the National Council for Quality Improvement and Priority

Setting in Health Care tried to raise a public debate on whether there are upper limits to costs of treatment financed through taxation, such as home-ventilator support for neurological conditions and for patients with chronic respiratory failure. This debate was quickly silenced by politicians who assured the public that in a rich country like ours, everyone in need will receive treatment. Thus, a lesson learned so far is that successful and consistent resource allocation work is partly dependent on politicians who are able and willing to consider how their decisions may involve the use of health care resources and who are willing to say openly that there are limits to what a society can afford in order to protect a well-functioning health care system. In the spring of 2012, the Norwegian Health Directorate launched another publication on health care resource allocation aimed to raise public awareness on the necessity of rationing health care resources (Norwegian Health Directorate, 2012). The public response following this has so far been limited.

Clinicians are the ones who must struggle with expectations that are impossible to meet when politicians keep promising the public shorter waiting lists and more health care services without securing enough resources. In 2013 many clinicians felt that too much focus is on economics in Norwegian health care. A national health care workers movement ("Protect the welfare state") was established, claiming that the strong focus on efficiency and costs is a threat to quality and ethics in health care and that Norwegian health care actually is under financed.

A remarkable indication of the prominence of resource allocation as an issue in the public arena in Norway is the appointment in June 2013 of a new governmental resource allocation commission.

REFERENCES

Berge, Øyvind M., & Hyggen, C. (2012). *Framveksten av private helseforsikringer i Norden.* [The growth of private health insurances in the Nordic countries]. FAFO-notat 2010-11. Available at: http://www.fafo.no/pub/rapp/10107/10107.pdf.

Carlsen, B., & Frithjov Norheim, O. (2005). "Saying no is no easy matter" a qualitiative study of competing concerns in rationing decisions in general practice. *BMC Health Services Research,* Nov 9;5:70.

FOR 2000-12-01 nr 1208: *Forskrift om prioritering av helsetjenester, rett til helsehjelp fra spesialisthelsetjenesten, rett til behandling i utlandet og om klagenemnd (prioriterings-forskriften).* [Regulations concerning the prioritization of health services, the right to health care from specialist health services, the right to treatment abroad and the board of appeals]. Available at: http://www.lovdata.no/cgi-wift/ldles?doc=/sf/sf/sf-20001201-1208.html.

Førde, O. H., Breidablik, H. J., & Øgar, P. (2011). *Truar skilnadene i tilvisingsratar målet om likeverdige helsetenester?* [Are differences in referral rates a threat to the goal of fair health care?] *Journal of the Association,* 131, 1878–1881.

Førde, R., & Aasland, O. G. (2008). Moral distress among Norwegian doctors. *Journal of Medical Ethics*,34, 521–525.

Førde, R., & Aasland, O. G. (2013). Moral distress and freedom of speech among doctors. http://tidsskriftet.no/article/3032909/en_GBJ

Førde, R., Pedersen, R., Nortvedt, P., & Aasland, O. G. (2006). *Får eldreomsorgen nok ressurser?* [Are resources for health care sufficient?] *Journal of the Norwegian Medical Association*, 126, 1913–1916.

Gjerberg, E., Førde, R., Pedersen, R., & Bollig, G. (2012). Ethical challenges in the provision of end of life care in Norwegian nursing homes. *Social Science & Medicine*, 71(4), 677–684.

Gulbrandsen, P., Førde, R., & Aasland, O. G. (2002). *Hvordan har legen det som portvakt?* [What does it feel like to be a gate keeper?] *Journal of the Norwegian Medical Association*, 122, 1874–1879.

Hagen, T. P., Amayu, K. N., Godager, G., Iversen, T., & Henning, Ø. (2011). *Utviklingen i kommunenes helse- og omsorgstjenester 1986–2010.* [Development of health and care services 1986–2010].

Report from the Health Economic Research Programme at the University of Oslo, 2011/05. Available at: http://www.med.uio.no/helsam/forskning/nettverk/hero/publikasjoner/skriftserie/2011/2011_5.pdf.

Husebø, B. S., & Husebø, S. (2005). *Sykehjemmene som arena for terminal omsorg –hvordan gjør vi det i praksis?* [Nursing homes as arenas of terminal care: practical aspects] *Journal of the Norwegian Medical Association*, 125(10),1352–1354.

The Patient- and User's Rights Act of 2.7.1999 nr. 63. (Lov om pasient- og brukerrettigheter) (Pasientrettighetsloven). Available at: http://www.lovdata.no/all/hl-19990702-063.html. The Act is also available in an unofficial English translation: http://www.ub.uio.no/ujur/ulovdata/lov-19990702-063-eng.pdf.

Specialist Health Services Act *(Lov om spesialisthelsetjenesten) m.m. av 2.7.1999 nr. 61.* []. Available at: http://www.lovdata.no/all/hl-19990702-061.html.

Mørland, B., Ringard, A., & Røttingen, J-A. (2010). Supporting tough decisions in Norway: a healthcare system approach. *International Journal of Technology Assessment in Health Care*, 26(4), 398–404.

National Council for Quality Improvement and Priority Setting in Health Care. (2012). About us. Available at: http://www.kvalitetogprioritering.no/R%C3%A5det/About+us?language=english.

Norwegian Directorate of Health. (2008). *Skapes helse, skapes velferd—helsesystemets rolle I det norske samfunnet.* [Health creates welfare—the role of the healthcare system in the Norwegian society]. Report IS-1545. Available at: http://www.helsedirektoratet.no/publikasjoner/utviklingstrekkrapport-2008-skapes-helse-skapes-velferd-helsesystemets-rolle-i-det-norske-samfunnet/Publikasjoner/utviklingstrekkrapport-2008-skapes-helse-skapes-velferd-helsesystemets-rolle-i-det-norske-samfunnet.pdf.

Norwegian Directorate of Health. (2010). *Hva kan offentlig statistikk si oss om prioriteringer i pleie- og omsorgstjenesten?* Report IS-1863. [What can public statistics tell us about prioritizations in the health and care services?]. Available at: http://www.helsedirektoratet.no/publikasjoner/hva-kan-offentlig-statistikk-si-oss-om-prioriteringer-i-pleie-og-omsorgstjenesten/Publikasjoner/hva-kan-offentlig-statistikk-si-oss-om-prioriteringer-i-pleie-og-omsorgstjenesten.pdf.

Norwegian Directorate of Health. (2012). *Prioriteringer i helsesektoren. Verdigrunnlag, status og utfordringer.* Report IS-1967. [Prioritizations in the health sector. Value foundation, status, and challenges]. Available at: http://www.helsedirektoratet. no/publikasjoner/prioriteringer-i-helsesektoren/Publikasjoner/prioriteringer-i-helsesektoren.pdf.

Norwegian Electronic Health Library. (2011). *Prioriteringsveiledere for medisinske spesialiteter.* [Prioritization guides for medical specialities]. Available: http://www.helsebib lioteket.no/Retningslinjer/Prioriteringsveiledere.

Norwegian Knowledge Centre for the Health Services. (2014). Home page. Available at: http://www.kunnskapssenteret.no/Home.

Norwegian Medical Association. (2007a). *Lang lang rekke, hvem må vente, hvem skal få.* [Long, long line: who must wait and who will get]. Oslo: The Norwegian Medical Association.

Norwegian Medical Association. (2007b). *Legeforeningens policy nr. 3/2007–prioritering I helsetjenesten. Rett prioritering I alle ledd.* ["White paper" of the Norwegian Medical Association nr. 3/2007–prioritization in the health services. Right policy at all levels]. Available at: http://legeforeningen.no/PageFiles/28885/policynotat%20nr.%20 32007.pdf.

Norwegian Medical Association. (2012). *Godkjente spesialister per 14.5.2012.* [Licensed specialists as of 14.5.2012]. Available at: http://www.legeforeningen.no/id/171362.

OECD [Organisation of Economic Co-operation and Development]. (2014). Stat Extracts. Available online at: http://stats.oecd.org/BrandedView.aspx?oecd_bv_ id=health-data-en&doi=data-00543-en

OECD [Organisation of Economic Co-operation and Development]. (2011). Health at a Glance 2011: OECD Indicators. Available online: http://www.oecd.org/health/ healthpoliciesanddata/49105858.pdf

OECD [Organisation of Economic Co-operation and Development]. (2012). Health Data 2012. Partly available online: http://www.oecd.org/health/healthpoliciesanddata/ oecdhealthdata2012.htm.

Official Norwegian Reports. (NOU 1987:23). *Retningslinjer for prioriteringer innen norsk helsetjeneste.* [Guidelines for priority setting in Norwegian health care]. Available at: http://www.nb.no/utlevering/nb/d3afab5efd9c8269986bd2a7771bb2d8#&struc t=DIV12.

Official Norwegian Reports. (NOU 1997: 17) *Finansiering og brukerbetaling for pleie- og omsorgstjenster.* [Financing and user payment for nurse and care services]. Available at: http://www.regjeringen.no/nb/dep/hod/dok/nouer/1997/nou-1997-17.html?id= 140948.

Official Norwegian Reports. (NOU 1997: 18). *Prioritering på ny: Gjennomgang av retningslinjer for prioriteringer innen norsk helsetjeneste.* [Prioritizing again: Evaluating the guidelines for prioritizations in the Norwegian health services]. Available at: http:// www.regjeringen.no/nb/dep/hod/dok/nouer/1997/nou-1997-18.html?id=140956.

Statistics Norway. (2010). *Tabell 19. Dødsfall av underliggende dødsårsak, etter dødsted. Prosent. 2008.* [Deaths according to underlying cause, by place of death. Percentage. 2008]. Available at: http://www.ssb.no/dodsarsak/arkiv/tab-2010-02-19-19.

Statistics Norway. (2014). Online homepage: http://www.ssb.no/

Tønnesen, S., Nortvedt, P., & Reidun, F. (2011). Rationing home based nursing care: professional ethical implications. *Nursing Ethics*, 18, 386–396.

Wennberg, J. E. (2010). *Tracking Medicine*. NY: Oxford University Press.

6 The Italian Context

■ RENZO PEGORARO
AND ALESSANDRA BERNARDI

■ AN INTRODUCTION TO ITALY'S HEALTH CARE SYSTEM

The Italian National Health Service (INHS) was substantially reformed in 1978 by the law on the establishment of the INHS (Law n. 833/1978), based on three fundamental principles: universality of assistance, equality of access, and solidarity in funding. In particular, as described by Lo Scalzo et al. (2009), the National Health Plan for 1998–2000 prescribes that the whole INHS should be organized according to the following principles:

- Human dignity: every individual must be treated with equal dignity and have equal rights irrespective of his or her personal or social characteristics.
- Health needs: everyone in need has a right to health care, and resources should be allocated with priority given to satisfying the basic needs of the population.
- Equity: the INHS resources should be used to eliminate geographical and/or economic barriers that constitute an obstacle to citizens' demand for appropriate services. Behavioral and information gaps among the population should be reduced to provide the same opportunity for access to health care services.
- Protection: the INHS should give highest priority to protecting and promoting citizens' health status.
- Solidarity with the most vulnerable people: resources should be allocated primarily to the individuals, groups, or groups of diseases with the most relevant social, clinical, and epidemiological impact.
- Effectiveness and appropriateness of health interventions: resources must be channeled into services with scientifically demonstrated effectiveness and to individuals who can benefit the most from them.
- Cost-effectiveness: services should be provided by the relevant organizations pursuing financial balance through efficient and effective management.

The National Health Plan for 2006–2008 and for 2009–2011 confirms the importance of these general principles for the INHS.

A Regionally Based Health Care Service

The INHS is based on a decentralized organizational structure with national, regional, and local administration. The national government is responsible for determining the level of public resources to devote to health care and for planning the 3-year National Health Plan. In 2001 the Italian government established "essential levels of care" (*Livelli Essenziali di Assistenza* [LEAs]), which are a uniform basic package of health services that should be guaranteed to all citizens. Substantial progress in the definitions of LEAs was necessary to make sense of the overall strategy of redistribution of powers between the central government and the regions. This progress was made with the agreement between the regions and the central government, which was followed by a Governmental Decree (the so-called "LEA Decree"). At present this Decree is the pivotal element of the Italian health benefit catalogue. It defines the main areas of health care services to be guaranteed by the INHS (positive list), those completely excluded by public coverage (negative list), and those partially covered (only available for specific clinical conditions).

Previously, the Ministry of Health managed a National Health Fund (that is, the central government fund used to distribute health care financing to the regions) consisting of statutory withholding tax for health and general taxation. In 2000 the National Health Fund was abolished and replaced by various regional taxes (Legislative Decree n. 56/2000). Regional authorities are responsible, in a situation of absolute autonomy, for local planning according to health objectives specified at the national level, for organizing and managing health care services, and for allocating resources to the third tier of the system, a network of 200 population-based health units called *ASLs*, which are operational agencies responsible for providing services through their own facilities or through contracts with private providers and the related local hospitals.

In short, with regard to the organizational structure of the Italian NHS, the most important norms are Law 833/1978 (establishment of the NHS), Legislative Decrees 502/1992 and 517/1993 (first reform of the NHS), Legislative Decree 229/1999 (new regional reform that deepened the devolution process), and Decree of the President of the Council of Ministers of November 29, 2001 (the so-called "LEAs decree").

Primary and Ambulatory Care

All Italian citizens are registered with a general practitioner (GP) or, for under-16s, with a pediatrician of their choice, 'pediatra di libera scelta' (PLS), who is in charge of providing most primary care and prescribing diagnostic interventions and drugs. They may act as gatekeepers for access to secondary services. People can choose any physician they prefer at any time, provided that the physician's list has not reached the maximum number of patients allowed (1,500 for GPs and 800 for pediatricians). GPs and PLSs initially assess the patient and are expected to provide most primary care. Primary care is provided free of charge. In Italy the public system has the feature of paying general doctors a fee per capita per year, a salary system that does not reward repeat visits, testing, and referrals.

Although primary care physicians are given financial incentives to share clinic premises with their colleagues, they usually work in single practices. However, this attitude has been changing more recently. Primary care physicians are authorized to work in the INHS after successfully completing a 2-year specialization course in general medicine and acquiring clinical experience as temporary staff in INHS facilities. The major reform in 1999 introduced significant changes in primary health care services by reinforcing group practice, introducing economic incentives for GPs, and PLSs, and promoting integration between primary care physicians and district services such as social care, home care, health education, and environmental health. In particular, the law allows general doctors to work in a team in several ways: working in their own offices or sharing the same office, using the patient electronic health record system, adopting common guidelines or organizing workshops to assess quality, and prescribing appropriateness.

Specialist ambulatory services, including visits and diagnostic and treatment activities, are provided either by Area Health Authorities (ASLs) or by accredited public and private facilities with which ASLs have agreements and contracts. Services are listed in specific formularies that vary between regions. People are allowed to access specialist care in two ways:

- Indirect access (referral) after approval by their GP, who is responsible for the referral. Once the GP has authorized the visit or the procedure, people are free to choose their provider among those accredited by the INHS. Visits to a specialist and medical devices can be free (completely covered by INHS) or can require a copayment.
- Direct access: patients can obtain an appointment themselves through what is known as the Central Booking Point (*Centro Unico di Prenotazione* [CUP]) for the following health services: gynecology, dental care, pediatrics (for those who have decided not to register their children with a designated pediatrician), optometric services, and psychiatric services for children. In emergency cases, direct access is allowed for all health services. Urgency is established by a triage mechanism. Visits to a specialist and medical devices incur user charges.

Since waiting lists are very long and the quality of public services is not always satisfactory, especially in central and southern regions, many people seek ambulatory care in private clinics. Moreover, many people seek care outside their own regions, mainly going from the south to the north of Italy.

Inpatient Care

Hospital services are provided either by public and private hospital with which the INHS has agreements and contracts. The family doctor can refer the patient to a specific hospital department. The INHS allows a patient to have free access to any public hospital. Patients who do not want to wait can choose to go to a private hospital, where usually waiting lists are much shorter. In that case there is the option of being referred either to a private clinic (where the patient would pay the total cost of admission without any reimbursement by the INHS) or, alternatively, to a private accredited hospital where interventions are completely covered by the INHS in the same way as in public hospitals. Alternatively, patients can go directly to the nearest emergency department to obtain the necessary treatment. In case of an emergency, where patients require an ambulance to be taken to the closest hospital, this service is free of charge. In public and accredited private hospitals the urgency is established by a triage mechanism. Many regions apply copayments in cases of inappropriate use of hospital services (both treatments and transportation).

The "LEA Decree" defines seven chapters as broad categories of services to be delivered in the hospital: emergency services, ordinary admissions (including rehabilitative and long-term inpatient care), day hospital, day surgery, domiciliary care, control of blood components and transfusion services, and organ and tissue transplantation services. Torbica and Fattore (2005) reported that traditionally the services to be provided in hospital settings were never explicitly defined by the INHS. It has been, rather, implicitly recognized that all types of services deemed to be "appropriately" delivered at hospital level must be available to citizens. As a consequence it is explicitly recognized that some benefits are available in hospitals without charge, although not included in the positive list of outpatient services provided under public coverage (e.g., pharmaceuticals or diagnostic tests that can vary from hospital to hospital). While the detailed spectrum of services to be provided by hospitals is not explicitly defined, national and regional fee schedules regulate their funding.

Funding for Secondary Care Services

Since 1995 Italian hospitals have been financed mainly according to nationally predetermined rates. For inpatient care (ordinary and day-hospital treatments), patients are classified according to the diagnosis-related groups (DRGs) scheme, whereas for outpatient care, diagnostic services, and specialist treatments, reimbursement is based on fees for services. The only two forms of treatment for which a bed-day rate still applies are for rehabilitation and long-term care. These two types of hospital care have a progressive rate reduction scheme to prevent the unnecessary lengthening of hospital stay. A length of stay longer than a set limit (usually 60 days) triggers a 40% reduction in the bed-day rate.

Following discharge, each patient is assigned to a specific DRG by software based on information derived from the discharge letter, including the principal diagnosis, any procedures, and secondary diagnoses as well as information on gender, age, and status at discharge. There is no assessment of how effective or necessary a treatment/service is before assigning a tariff to it. However, for each DRG there exists a threshold value, expressed in days, giving the value beyond which a case is considered out of range (or "outlier"). It sets the threshold for a hospital length of stay whose duration of hospitalization deviates significantly from that of all the other patients with similar clinical features.

The rates of each DRG are set at regional level using the standard cost of production. The fees for each DRG relate to the average cost of care for all patients assigned to the same DRG. The pricing at the regional level will reflect the different composition of the benefits paid, which differs in each local and regional authority. This also allows use of tariffs as an instrument of regional health planning in terms of contribution to the address and control of the hospital in accordance with specific objectives and priorities. Regions are allowed to set up specific financing schemes aimed at providing additional funds for integrating hospital activities that cannot be completely financed by the DRG scheme. In particular, these include emergency wards, spinal cord units, burn units, organ transplant centers (transport, donor and receiver support and transplant activity coordination), AIDS centers, home-based care, training activities, and teaching and research activities, all of which receive additional funding from the regional government.

To a certain extent, DRG lists may be taken as the catalogue of hospital services and benefits covered by the INHS. This interpretation, however, should be made with some caution. DRGs are divided in two major groups, surgical and medical. The interventions to which surgical DRGs refer are expected to be offered and funded. Therefore, surgical DRGs define a sort of list of services available to patients. For medical DRGs the situation is different as the classification includes all possible diagnoses, comprising those for which hospital admissions may not have been appropriate. Therefore, medical DRGs do not define a list of services to be guaranteed but rather act as economic constraints according to which providers make decisions. Thus, albeit implicitly, the tariff values assigned to DRGs influence the specific content of the services provided in each diagnosis category such that some services may be excluded because their tariff is too low.

In response to the introduction of the DRG system in the early 1990s, the admission rate initially dropped, then peaked in 1995 and, finally, slowly fell to its lowest level in 2003. Changes in bed utilization are, together with the reduction in length of stay and in the number of admissions, a more recent result of the initiatives to control health expenditure, foster hospital efficiency, and reduce waste.

■ RESOURCE ALLOCATION POLICY PRIOR TO 2002

The general policy of resource allocation in the Italian health care system is based on the founding principles of the 1978 Act and is broadly the same today as in 2002. As we already said, the Italian health care system is required to guarantee the uniform provision of comprehensive care throughout the country. Nevertheless, responsibility for health care planning, organization, and financing is shared between the national government and the regions. The INHS's principles state that allocation of financial resources should be inspired by an equitable approach, so that every citizen should have equal opportunity of access to health care services. Basically, the INHS uses a mixed rationing approach mainly based on specification of budgets and financial incentives (implicit approach) linked to the specification of priorities for assistance.

The presence of fiscal federalism and the persistence of significant regional differences produce potential inequalities in resource allocation for health care among the regions. To avoid inequalities among regions and to provide equal access to the LEAs for the whole population, regions receive a quota (budget) from an equalization fund (the National Solidarity Fund), which aims to reduce inequalities between the northern regions (which are traditionally the richest and therefore have greater own-source tax revenues to guarantee the core benefits package, even if their population is older than the Italian average) and the southern regions (supported mainly by strong family networks).

By statute, each region defines its own internal allocation formula using criteria that may reflect potential resource utilization by the different population groups within the various ASLs. In fact, ASLs are financed by regions on the basis of a weighted capitation formula, following criteria congruent with those in the primary legislation. Nevertheless, each region is free to set its own specific formula taking into consideration other criteria (demographic, geographical, factors of social deprivation, health status indicators, and supply characteristics).

Models of Funding

The majority of health care expenditure (roughly 70%) is public, funded through general taxation, with most of the remainder financed by out-of-pocket expenditure. As a result of the near universal coverage, voluntary health insurance does not play a significant role in funding health care in Italy.

General Taxation

Before 1978, employers and employees were responsible for financing health care through a mutual health system. The system was fragmented into numerous health insurance funds and lacked unified regulation: there were many different financing methods and contribution rates, and often drastically different benefit packages. The 1978 reform not only granted a homogeneous benefit package to all citizens (actually identifiable with the LEAs mentioned earlier) but also rationalized the mutual health system by making contributions more uniform and pooling all resources into a single fund, the National Health Fund. The function of this fund was to guarantee the public resources required to meet the costs of providing health care to all citizens. The global amount of the National Health Fund was fixed yearly by the central government and came mainly from statutory withholding tax for health and general taxation. Additional resources were drawn from other sources such as regional and local taxes, revenue from services delivered privately by ASLs and hospitals, and user copayments. These various sources of funding were gradually transformed and simplified. Thus, in 1997, before fiscal reforms took place, the main funding sources were: payroll taxes (social insurance contributions) charged to employers in the public and private sectors and self-employed people with a regressive structure; copayment of ASLs' income for pharmaceuticals, diagnostic procedures, and specialist visits; and contributions from regions governed by special statute.

The Legislative Decree 446/1997 replaced the payroll tax and a few local other taxes with two new types of regional tax:

1) IRAP (*Imposta Regionale sulle Attività Produttive*): a regional corporation tax imposed on the production activities of companies (corporations, partnerships, and self-employed workers) and on the salaries paid to public sector employees.
2) IRPEF (*Imposta sui Redditi delle Persone Fisiche*): a regional tax imposed on top of the national personal income tax.

In fact, as already extensively described, several legislative measures approved during the period 1997–2000 have promoted the devolution of political power to the regions. During this same period, a process of transition toward federal reform of the state ran parallel to the progressive introduction of fiscal federalism, transferring the funding of the INHS from the central to the regional level, thus strengthening the fiscal autonomy of regional health departments.

Although Legislative Decree No. 56/2000 formally abolished the National Health Fund, to all intents and purposes, a fund of some sort (often it is still called the National Health Fund in official documents) operates as a kind of accounting container for money to be allocated to the regions. The Decree also stated that a fixed proportion of national value-added tax (VAT or consumption tax) revenue would be used to build a National Solidarity Fund to be used to redistribute funds to the regions unable to raise sufficient resources to provide the basic package.

Out-of-Pocket Payments

Italy currently has two main types of out-of-pocket payment. The first is demand-side cost sharing: a copayment for diagnostic procedures, pharmaceuticals, and specialist visits. The second is direct payment by users to purchase private health care services and over-the-counter (OTC) drugs. In 1993, a drastic reform classified pharmaceuticals into three categories according to a combination of their relevance (in terms of effectiveness) and cost (see the following section, Pharmaceutical Policy in Italy). The Budget Law for 2001 abolished all copayments for more cost-effective drugs, but there was a sharp impact on health expenditure levels. This led to a change in legislation in October 2001, which allowed regions to choose whether or not to introduce copayments on drugs, but only for the purpose of containing rising pharmaceutical expenditure. In 11 of the 20 regions, copayments were applied at a flat rate or a percentage of the price. It is estimated that in 2002, the first year of its application, this measure reduced drug expenditure by 5% compared with the regions that did not adopt copayments. For diagnostic and therapeutic procedures and specialist visits, users pay a proportion of the total cost per visit up to a ceiling fixed by law (the ceiling has changed several times and currently is €36.15 per single prescription). The prescription can be signed either by general or specialist doctors and can contain a maximum number of procedures.

Pharmaceutical Policy in Italy

In Italy the pharmaceutical market has usually been a favorite target for cost-containment interventions in the health care sector.

While in the 1980s Italy was one of the most generous countries in funding pharmaceuticals, Fattore and Jommi (1998) explained that, although the overall pharmaceutical market shrank in 1994 and 1995, a substantial part of NHS drug-bill savings resulted from cost-shifting from the public sector to patients, mainly because physicians have not aligned their prescribing behavior to the new positive list. The new Italian approach to containing pharmaceutical costs has been certainly effective, at least in the short run. However, new relevant issues were emerging regarding the fall of NHS pharmaceutical coverage, the centralized nature of the Italian pharmaceutical policy, and the gap between scientifically based policies and actual prescribing behaviors.

Bernardi and Pegoraro (2003) argue that the authorities find it easier to intervene in pharmaceutical expenditure since most of the health care budget consists of fixed costs (e.g., hospital services). As a consequence, regulatory authorities have aimed at short-term savings by imposing price cuts on reimbursable drugs. The 1993 reform made it possible for local health authorities (ASLs) to introduce expenditure targets and saving incentives to GPs. In 1997, a parliamentary commission created to check the macroeconomic viability of social expenditure relaunched the need to impose some kind of "mild" budget restrictions on GPs. Even so, most efforts are still in the direction of more information sharing between ASLs and GPs rather than explicit targets. With the aim of containing the growth of health expenditure, the juridical system provides the regions with a series of instruments and measures with which to manage their expenditure. Some of these are obligatory, while others may be used at the discretion of each region.

The main measures are the following.

- Copayment: Regions can levy a direct charge on "essential" medicines proposed by AIFA.
- Direct distribution: ASLs distribute medicines to patients who are receiving medical care at home, and public hospitals distribute prescribed drugs to patients for the first round after hospitalization and to outpatients who have consulted a specialist.
- Ceiling on pharmaceutical expenditure by the regions (for 2010 it was set at 13.3% of the total health expenditure). Upon successful completion of the ceiling on pharmaceutical expenditure, pharmaceutical companies, with wholesalers and pharmacists, compensate for cost overruns. The regions, in turn, are still required to take measures to avoid further overspend.
- Price reduction of 5% for drugs in the "group A" category.
- Introduction of unbranded drugs: those medicines whose patent has expired are reimbursed at the price of the corresponding cheaper generic drug (Legislative Decree 138/2002).

◼ CONTEXTUAL IMPACT ON PHYSICIANS' VIEWS OF RATIONING AT THE BEDSIDE: POSSIBLE EXPLANATIONS FOR FINDINGS OF THE VALUES AT THE BEDSIDE STUDY

The INHS has not yet established an expenditure budget for each GP, although some ASLs have created incentives and opportunities for making

GPs accountable for their prescribing activities, such as introducing methods to achieve defined targets (e.g., guidelines or protocols, lists of cheaper equivalent products, limited lists in critical areas such as antibiotics) and distributing a percentage of the savings to doctors as a "bonus." However, there is no standard system of control of GPs' prescribing, which, as for specialist prescribing, is managed at local and regional levels. Most commonly, Italian GPs make implicit rather than explicit rationing decisions. This is reflected in the Values at the Bedside study, which showed that Italian doctors are willing to participate in cost-containment decisions rather than be guided by administrative rules. As we have previously noted, attempts at sharing guidelines and improving efficiency are still at an early stage in Italian health care.

The majority of the Italian respondents perceived some resources as sometimes unavailable, especially with regard to intermediate and long-term care services, including interventions that are adopted in the post-acute and chronic phase of disease (e.g., rehabilitation, access to nursing home, mental services, etc.). These interventions require a high level of coordination in a multidisciplinary setting, and in several regions there is a scarcity of provision of this type of care. For instance, because of the limited number of beds, in order to gain admission to a nursing home a patient needs to make a request to his/her ASL, presenting a GP's prescription for the service. The GP makes a formal application, and the Nursing Home Assessment Unit evaluates whether or not the patient should be admitted. When admission is approved, costs are shared between the INHS and the patient based on the latter's income. Patient copayments vary from region to region.

With regard to the likelihood of patients being denied treatment based on group identity, Italian physicians identify a higher risk of rationing for patients who require chronic care or mental health care, and this finding is consistent with our previous comments on intermediate and long-term care. Less discrimination was reported for immigrants, which may reflect that legal immigrants have the same rights as Italian citizens and therefore should not be discriminated against. In contrast, illegal immigrants only have access to a limited range of free health care services—in particular, urgent specialist and hospital care following an illness or accident, health care schemes for babies and pregnant women, treatment for children, vaccination programs, and treatment for infectious diseases.

The Values at the Bedside study identified general overall agreement with the need for cost-containment policies. In particular, Italian physicians considered evidence-based practice, the criterion of urgency, and waiting lists for elective surgical operations to be more acceptable. These are all well-established interventions, which may be why physicians felt more comfortable with them. More recent work by Carelli (2010) has corroborated the finding that Italian GPs experience significant pressure to ration, reporting that Italian GPs are often "extremely frustrated" and feel "pulled and pushed by politicians and technologists with big and unrealistic decisions in the form of diktat".

■ NATIONAL DEVELOPMENTS SINCE 2002

An analysis of the dynamics of health care policy in Italy performed by France and Taroni (2005) suggests that in recent years the pace of change in the health care system has accelerated. Although the basic features of universalism, comprehensiveness, and funding from general taxation have remained remarkably constant, the capacity to innovate policy tools and their settings and to take account of domestic and international experience seems to have increased. The political will and capacity to combat entrenched interests may also have increased, although implementation is still weak. The imperative to contain public expenditure has heavily conditioned health policy and will continue to do so. This has occurred mainly at the national level, but as the principal locus of health policymaking progressively shifts to the regions, so too will the constraining effect of this imperative move downward. If the decentralization process continues, problems could arise due to interregional differences in capacities to formulate and implement appropriate policies and to tackle special interest groups.

Ghislandi et al. (2005) suggest that in the last decade, the Italian INHS has again been extensively reformed, mostly inspired by two major trends:

1. Increasing regional autonomy: this process culminated in the 2001 constitutional reform (Legislative Decree 300/2000), which modified the second part of the Italian Constitution, providing regions with more powers. Regions are now allowed to collect local taxation and finance extra health care services in addition to the basic package of health services that is guaranteed to all citizens by the National Health Plan.
2. Provision of managerial skills at a local level: local health authorities and hospitals were formerly administered by representatives of local institutions and thus dependent on political influence and party-political control. The 1992 reform injected managerial principles into the INHS. In fact, Legislative Decrees 502/1992 and 517/1993 were the first steps of a progressive pro-competition reform aimed at retaining universal coverage while introducing a financing system (budgetary approach) that would secure the macro-level objectives of containing costs and promoting equity, incorporating micro-level incentives for promoting efficiency, and enhancing responsiveness to consumers through competition among providers. At a local level the reform introduced general managers with renewable rolling contracts appointed by regions to run ASLs and major hospitals, both semi-independent public enterprises.

Pharmaceutical Policy Developments

Fattore and Jommi (2008) explain that pharmaceutical policy in Italy has been reshaped as a result of the 1993–1994 crisis in which it was revealed that pharmaceutical companies, policymakers, and top Department of Health (DOH) officers had constructed an illegal system to set prices. Following this crisis the rise of technical competency and leadership in the Italian Department of Health and, since 2004, in the drug regulatory agency (AIFA, *Agenzia Italiana del Farmaco*) has achieved major improvements in many aspects of pharmaceutical policy. These improvements have included increased transparency of decision making, the use of evidence-based medicine principles for reimbursement and pricing, and the use of generic drugs to lower prices.

Actually, the AIFA is the main national institution responsible for coordinating all the activities that concern pharmaceuticals: public research, private company investment in research and development, production, distribution, scientific information, monitoring of consumption, monitoring of adverse effects, pricing, and reimbursement policies. AIFA is also responsible for the drug reimbursement process.

After several revisions, at present drugs requiring a physician's prescription are classified into three groups:

- group A: drugs for severe and chronic illnesses that are totally reimbursed by the INHS
- group C: drugs that are not reimbursed by the INHS
- group H: drugs that are provided only by hospitals.

The criteria used for the classification of drugs are: effectiveness, safety and cost, (taken into account only when two drugs have presented the same benefit/risk ratio but different prices are available), and acceptability of therapy to patients. Many drugs with high cost or unfavorable benefit/cost ratio were excluded from class A. This criterion was seen as ethical and acceptable for people, as a suitable therapy is always available in class A. However, physicians did not always share the AIFA's opinion, and they continued to prescribe drugs in class C which were for paid by patients. In 2007, the government allowed OTC drugs to be sold outside pharmacies (such as in supermarkets), even though it expressly banned the sale of medicine requiring a physician's prescription.

Unlike many other European Union states, since 2010 Italy's reductions in health care spending have focused on price cuts for generic drugs and restrictions on reimbursements for more expensive medicines. Reimbursement of generic drugs has been limited to the cheapest version of a medicine, within four therapeutic categories, with the lowest price established by a tender system. Generic drugs have accounted for just 40% of patent-expired drug sales by volume in 2009 but were the only sector of the state-funded pharmaceutical market to see any growth last year, with rises of 18.4% by volume and 10.3% in terms of value according to IMS health data. On the basis of the austerity package, any purchase by the INHS that is greater than reference prices has to be substantiated. The cuts are intended to save the country around 600 million euros. Ferruccio Fazio, the Italian health minister, told the *Financial Times*: "The pharmaceutical industry is not happy but we feel [their prices] are well controlled. The problem is not discounts [of patented drugs] but volumes. We will consider giving incentives to GPs." Alongside price cuts to generic drugs, Mr. Fazio also announced plans for centralized procurement and administrative changes. The greatest weight, however, was placed on "rational prescribing," which will involve persuading doctors to cut prescriptions for unnecessary medications—most notably, antibiotics for nonbacterial infections—and increased use of cheaper generic drugs.

Espin et al. (Espin, 2011) suggest that Italy is one of the European countries where risk-sharing schemes (RSS) have been most widely implemented. RSS represent an innovative and important approach to the problems of rationing and achieving cost-effectiveness in high-cost or controversial health interventions. The key feature of RSS is to recognize that for any intervention, price (and therefore cost to the provider) may be variable, whereas effectiveness is fixed. The different schemes of risk sharing are described in detail in the following paragraphs. No specific legislation covers these innovative contracting instruments; rather, they are part of a negotiation procedure for pricing and reimbursement between the committee for pricing and reimbursement of the Italian Medicines Agency (AIFA) and the pharmaceutical industry. AIFA proposes different RSS on a case-by-case basis when the launch of a new high-cost pharmaceutical presents uncertainties concerning value, clinical results and/ or budget impact, and potentially inappropriate use. Italy has its own classification system for new innovative contracts that takes into account three schemes: "payment by results" (initial cycle of treatment fully reimbursed by marketing authorization holder (pharmaceutical company) for nonresponder patients), "cost-sharing" (discount on price of initial therapy cycle for all eligible patients), and "risk-sharing" (discount on price of initial therapy cycle for nonresponder patients). The "payment by results" scheme is the most frequent type of agreement in the oncology field, but the other schemes are also relevant.

Other Reforms

A recent national law (2011) has introduced a fixed payment for a GP's prescription to be added to the €3,615 ceiling for copayment, but only for patients with an annual family income over €29,000. The regions have the freedom to decide whether or not to apply this national legislation, on the condition that should they decide not to apply it they are able to provide full coverage of health care expenditure for other interventions. The issue of cost-sharing exemptions has also been debated within the Italian health policy arena. Currently, exemptions are established for specific categories of people: elderly people (>65 years old) with gross household income (family income) less than €36,152 per annum, people with chronic or rare diseases (as listed in the decree of the Ministry of Health approved in 1999), disabled people such as disabled ex-servicemen and people with work-related injuries, people with HIV, donors (for health services related to spinal cord donors or organ donors), prisoners, and pregnant women (health services are free of charge depending on the gestation week and specific diagnostic protocol).

■ CONCLUSIONS AND FUTURE TRENDS

Since the Values at the Bedside study, few changes to health care organization and public policy on resource allocation have taken place in Italy. The federal reform is still developing, and the main recent enhancements pertain to pharmaceuticals or concern the strengthening of a prospective payment system in-hospital. The regionalization of the health care system, together with the wide interregional differences in socioeconomic indicators typical of Italy, has produced a system that demonstrates large inequalities between regions. This discrepancy is constantly balanced by central interventions through the above-mentioned National Solidarity Fund.

Notwithstanding several differences among regions, some challenges remain common to them all and may have possible implications for physician bedside rationing. First, with regard to primary care GPs could, in principle, serve a gatekeeper function. But their ability to negotiate with downstream providers is actually limited, particularly given the recent movement to shift services from secondary to primary care. With more treatment occurring in primary care, there is likely to be more pressure on GPs to make rationing decisions. Recent proposals to provide incentives to GPs for providing 24-hour services to reduce inappropriate attendance in emergency departments could be seen as an example of this pressure. Second, the lack of efficient systems for monitoring and comparing quality and efficiency in LEAs leads to both inequity of services and cost inefficiency. Third, the lack of integration of health and social care services leads to inefficiencies and patient dissatisfaction. Improving integration could increase the value of local services for the elderly and patients with chronic diseases (rapidly growing in Italy), avoiding an excessive and sometimes inappropriate utilization of medical treatments and obtaining a subsequent reduction in health care expenditure.

The 1978 health care reform has been the focus of intense public debate in Italy for many years. The current period of scarce resources will require an even higher awareness of the dilemmas physicians face with microallocative choices but will also provide impetus for the development of new shared priority-setting guidance from central and regional authorities.

REFERENCES

Bernardi, A., & Pegoraro, R. (2003). Italian drug policy: ethical aims of essential assistance levels. *Health Care Analysis, 11*(4), 279–286.

Carelli, F. (2010). New competencies ignored: general practice is in danger in Italy. *British Journal of General Practice, 60*(578), 692–693.

Espín, J. Rovira, J., & García, L. (2011). Experiences and impact of European risk-sharing schemes focusing on oncology medicines. *Andalusian School of Public Health,* January.

Fattore, G., & Jommi, C. (2008). The last decade of Italian pharmaceutical policy: instability or consolidation? *Pharmacoeconomics, 26*(1), 5–15.

Fattore, G., & Jommi, C. (1998). The new pharmaceutical policy in Italy. *Health Policy, 46*(1), 21–41.

France, G., & Taroni, F. (2005). The evolution of health-policy making in Italy. *Journal of Health Politics, Policy and Law, 30*(1–2), 169–188.

Ghislandi, S., Krulichova, I., & Garattini, L. (2005). Pharmaceutical policy in Italy: towards a structural change? *Health Policy, 72*(1), 53–63.

Lo Scalzo, A., Donatini, A., Orzella, L., Cicchetti, A., Profili, S., Maresso, A. (2009). Italy: Health system review. United Kingdom: WHO/Europe.

Torbica, A., & Fattore, G. (2005). The "essential levels of care" in Italy: when being explicit serves the devolution of powers. *European Journal of Health Economics, 6*(Suppl 1), 46–52.

PART THREE

Analysis of Bedside Rationing

7 How Do Economic Incentive Schemes Influence Rationing Decisions by Primary Care Physicians?

■ THOMAS ALLEN, MATT SUTTON, AND RICHARD COOKSON

Prioritization or "rationing" of scarce resources is a ubiquitous feature of all health care systems and is accomplished through a variety of price and non-price mechanisms. Primary care physicians or "general practitioners" (GPs) play an important role in nonprice rationing, especially in health insurance systems like the UK National Health Service (NHS) that require GPs to act as "gatekeepers" to hospital services and other specialized and costly health services. In the NHS, rationing decisions in primary care begin at the reception desk, affect whether the GP sees patients for 5 or 10 minutes, influence whether and what brands of medicine are prescribed, and inform whether and where the patient is referred to specialist services—which then ultimately affects what specialist tests and treatments are received (Klein, 1993). Of course many important rationing decisions lie outside the control of the GP, including important decisions about investment in hospital buildings, staff, equipment, and other specialist facilities and infrastructure that influence the volume and quality of specialized health care services available. Furthermore, GPs are increasingly encouraged to engage in shared decision making with patients. Nevertheless, GP consultation, diagnosis, prescription, and referral behavior has an important influence over the allocation of scarce health care resources to particular patients.

How GPs make these rationing decisions will depend, at least to some extent, on the economic incentives they face. In recent decades, policymakers have become increasingly interested in reforms explicitly designed to change the economic incentives faced by primary care physicians in order to reduce costs and improve quality. A recent review of the effectiveness of health care incentives identifies four broad types of GP payment system that are commonly used, often in combination (Flodgren et al., 2011):

- salaries for working for specific time periods;
- fee-for-service paid on the basis of each unit of service provided;

- capitation payments based on the size and demographic structure of the treated population; and
- payments linked to specified performance measures.

In this chapter we focus on two mechanisms of the latter kind that have been used to influence rationing by primary care physicians: budget-holding and pay-for-performance schemes. Budget-holding gives GPs an incentive to make savings in pharmaceutical and hospital budgets by curbing their prescribing and referral volumes, and pay-for-performance gives GPs an incentive to deliver specific types of care to specific types of patients. We focus on experience of the use of these mechanisms in the UK NHS, which provides much of the international evidence base. Two main policy changes will be looked at in detail: the GP fundholding scheme, which was in place between 1991 and 1999; and the Quality and Outcomes Framework, which was introduced as part of a new contract in 2004.

■ BUDGET-HOLDING AND THE ENGLISH NHS FUNDHOLDING AND PRACTICE-BASED COMMISSIONING SCHEMES

Background to the Policy

The fundholding scheme was introduced as part of the NHS internal market reforms that started in 1990 (Department of Health, 1989). GPs were offered the choice of becoming a fundholding practice and, if they chose to do so, held a budget to purchase pharmaceuticals and a range of specialist nonemergency health care services. Fundholding ran for 9 years (1991 to 1999) with different practices becoming fundholders in different years. Not all practices became fundholders, and those that did so became fundholders at different times. This became an important feature that allowed researchers to estimate the effect of becoming a fundholding practice, but it also caused evaluation problems of "selection bias" as practices could choose to become fundholders if and when it suited them. Approximately half of practices eventually became fundholders. Fundholding was abolished in 1999, but involvement of family physicians in budget holding had a resurgence in England in 2005 under a new scheme called "practice-based commissioning."

Successful fundholder applicants were given a budget in order to procure secondary care services. The type of budget they would receive, and its coverage, varied depending on the size of the registered practice population (Dixon & Glennerster, 1995). Not all services were expected to be purchased with the fundholding budget. Emergency care was not purchased with this budget, only a selected group of elective procedures. Typically, these were common procedures taking up approximately 70% of elective admissions

(Propper, Croxson, & Shearer, 2002). Costs of prescribing were also covered by this budget.

Fundholding, among other aspects, aimed to incentivize GPs to increase rationing as they were made financially responsible for a range of elective admissions. The scheme also aimed to provide hospitals with an incentive to compete for the attention of fundholders, not with lower prices—as these were set equal to the average cost—but with lower waiting times (Propper et al., 2002). This is because GP fundholders typically paid hospitals on a case payment basis (i.e., for each patient treated), whereas patients from other practices were funded under a general system of "block contracts" awarded by the local funding body. Hence, hospitals stood to gain or lose revenue at the margin depending on how many GP fundholder patients they treated but received the same amount of income irrespective of how many patients they treated from non-fundholding practices. The possibility of losing GP fundholding patients thus gave hospitals an incentive to compete with each other on waiting times to attract additional referrals from GP fundholding practices.

Goodwin (1998) summarized the potential benefits of the scheme: higher quality of secondary care, reduction in drug costs, lowering the number of unnecessary referrals, better services for patients offered directly by practices, and a greater choice of services in general. One of the main arguments in favor of fundholding and other budget-holding schemes is that GPs have a relatively close connection both with their patients and with their local specialist health care providers, meaning they are able to make relatively well-informed decisions about patient care (Gillam & Lewis, 2009). Coupled with the GP's role as a "gatekeeper," a system was created whereby patients were referred to secondary care by those who decided which secondary services were most appropriate for the local area. In theory, budget-holding may therefore encourage GPs to tailor the specialist services they commission to the needs of their patients and in a more direct and comprehensive way than the larger local health care commissioning organizations introduced in the 2000s, called "Primary Care Trusts," which merely involved a few local GPs in management and governance functions (Smith et al., 2005).

Effect of the Policy

Fundholding ceased in 1999, and its effects have been researched extensively. Some of the early research was, however, subject to a number of methodological flaws. These flaws will be discussed in more detail, but common themes are small and potentially unrepresentative data as well as biases introduced into statistical analysis via the self-selected nature of fundholding practices. We present the evidence on fundholding as a narrative, first showing early research with its faults and moving on through time to later research that corrected these faults.

Concerns about whether fundholding practices were granted an unfair advantage in terms of funding were raised early on. The concern stemmed from the way in which the fundholding budgets for hospital care were set; this proportion of the budget was taken out of the total budget for all hospital care in the area. Therefore if fundholders overspent, the funds were effectively taken away from non-fundholding practices. Measuring the extent of this problem was the aim of Dixon et al. (1994). They used data on the level and costs of hospital care for both fundholding and non-fundholding practices in a single region (North West Thames). Only data from one year of the scheme (1993/1994) was used in this study, so the analysis lacks both breadth and depth. Overall, they found that funding was indeed more generously supplied to fundholding practices.

Another early study that also lacked a sufficient sample of patients is Maxwell, Heaney, Howie, and Noble (1993). They compared the prescribing volumes and costs of fundholding practices with those of non-fundholding practices that later became fundholders. They found evidence that fundholding practices controlled the unit costs associated with prescribing more effectively than non-fundholding practices. However, they failed to include practice characteristics in their analysis.

Dixon and Glennerster (1995) provided a review of much of the early research into the impact of fundholding across several areas—efficiency, equity, organizational change, patient choice, and quality of care. While they refer to methodological problems with some of the research, such as contaminated control groups, they suggest that fundholding did have an effect. Specifically, prescribing costs were reduced; more services were offered in primary care that were previously provided in secondary care; a two-tier health care system may have emerged; and capital seems to have been directed more toward fundholding practices. However, the key message from their research is that, as of 1995, not enough research had been done.

The impact that fundholding had on prescribing costs was investigated by Whynes, Heron, and Avery (1997). They found increased use of generic drugs and lower unit costs of prescriptions in fundholding practices. This appeared to be a short-term effect with no evidence of persistent cost-reducing behavior. Practices did not show evidence of increasing the costs prior to joining the scheme in the hope of acquiring larger budgets later. The paper's effective sample size is 700 practices, approximately 10% of the practice population, but practice characteristics were not controlled for.

In reviewing research on better cost control of prescribing, Goodwin (1998) found little evidence. This was attributed to the small scale of the initial research. Later, larger studies found that prescribing costs fell in fundholding practices in the early years, but the reduction in costs was not long-lived. This may reflect the incentives that fundholders faced over the longer term. Budgets were based on historic levels of spending so, once savings were made, budgets were reduced. Hence, the incentive to control costs existed only for a short time.

By making GPs more financially aware of the cost of their referral behavior, it was hoped that savings would be made for the NHS as a whole. Previously, GPs had borne no financial accountability for hospital costs (Goodwin, 1998). This became one of the rationales for the fundholding scheme. However, it had the potential to introduce conflicts of interest. With GPs now charged with the responsibility for paying for some secondary care, their incentive to ration on referrals became much stronger. There was a concern that this could result in patients not receiving the level of care needed. Goodwin (1998) also pointed out that patients may have suffered in two other ways: first, if GPs switched to a better value hospital, this increased the distance the patient had to travel; second, if the GP decided to delay treatment, sometimes an emergency admission was required, with the local funding body picking up the bill. Clearly, the latter had far more serious consequences. However, as GPs may have secured better quality treatment or a reduced waiting time, the effect on patients is ambiguous. As with prescribing costs, early evidence was based on small-scale analyses and was inconclusive.

With their new budgets, fundholders were able, and indeed encouraged, to provide a wider range of services; this could be in the form of bringing hospital services into general practice or purchasing services from outside the NHS. This shift might have constituted rationing if the volume of treatment had decreased. Shifts in the location of services were made in both fundholding and non-fundholding practices (Goodwin, 1998); whether this change produced a more cost-effective system, or one preferred by patients, had yet to be revealed. This point would be addressed by later research.

In summarizing mostly anecdotal evidence, Goodwin (1998) suggested that hospitals prioritized fundholding patients to a greater degree at the end of the financial year in order to bring in additional revenue once their "block contract" budgets had been spent. In a system with both fundholders and non-fundholders, patients from non-fundholding practices thus tended to receive lower priority throughout the year but more so at the year's end.

A potential danger of fundholding identified early on was that of "cream-skimming." This could materialize if fundholding GPs sought to increase their budget surplus by registering young and healthy patients likely to be relatively inexpensive to treat, and by avoiding registering elderly and sick patients likely to impose substantial costs on their budget (Le Grand, 1999). However, little evidence exists to support this, probably due to the cost caps for individual patients that were built in to the fundholding scheme to protect GPs from the costs of very expensive patients. Goodwin (1998) also points out the incentive fundholders faced to implement "cream-skimming" and cited anecdotal evidence that suggested some patients had been prevented from registering with practices due to potentially high medical costs. Despite this anecdotal evidence, however, no robust study shows the existence of cream-skimming. Goodwin (1998) attributes this to the same safeguards as does Le Grand (1999), and to the large fundholding budgets and the fact GPs would not suffer personal financial penalties for treating high-cost patients.

Although fundholding was abandoned in 1999, it was not until after this time that many questions were more definitely answered. Croxson, Propper, and Perkins (2001) used data on the number of referrals to hospitals over a 4-year period made by a large sample of GPs. Some of these GPs became fundholders, and those that did, did so at different times. As the size of the budget provided to GPs depended on the level of activity (i.e., referrals) in the year prior to gaining fundholding status, they hypothesize that there existed a financial incentive for would-be fundholders to increase the number of referrals in this year only to reduce them again afterwards. They found evidence that supported this hypothesis. Fundholding initially decreased rationing, in the form of increased elective referrals, only to increase it once fundholding status had been attained. The initial increase in referrals was in the order of 7%–10% depending on model specification. The decrease that followed was of similar magnitude.

Hospitals may have responded to their incentive to compete for fundholding patients with shorter waiting times. This was investigated by Propper et al. (2002). They found that when the referral related to treatment covered by fundholding, the waiting time was reduced. They did not find evidence of positive spillovers, which they defined as increased referrals for patients from fundholding practices but not having treatment covered by the scheme. Nor did they find substantial evidence to suggest that GPs moved patients to different hospitals once they became fundholders. The disparity in waiting times occurred both within fundholders and between fundholders and non-fundholders. It would appear that the scheme led to a two-tier system. The subset of patients who were both registered with a fundholding GP *and* had a treatment covered by the scheme benefitted most from shorter waiting times.

A common confounding factor when analyzing a policy such as fundholding is that participants can self-select into the policy. This may mean that comparing those affected by the policy with those not affected may not represent the desired like-for-like comparison: those participants are in some way different from the nonparticipants. Dusheiko, Gravelle, and Jacobs (2004) analyzed the waiting times experienced by patients of fundholding practices. They used a large dataset and controlled for self-selection bias, as fundholding practices are found to be different prior to joining the scheme when compared to non-fundholding practices. The main result was that waiting times were reduced for all types of admissions and not only those that were covered under the fundholding budget.

With the abolition of fundholding in 1999, budget-holding fell out of favor in the NHS until some commissioning responsibilities were delegated from Primary Care Trusts to GPs in 2005 (Department of Health, 2005). Following this there was a resurgence of research on the topic as well as a number of commentators reviewing the existing evidence. One such review, though not systematic, was that of Mannion (2005). The review suggests that, on the whole, the evidence is mixed: strong and weak evidence exists to both support and oppose fundholding. Evidence is strongest for lower elective referrals and inequality of access, due to the two-tier system. Evidence is weakest for an effect on emergency stays, improved dialogue and communication between practices, and higher management/transaction costs. It would appear that prior to the small resurrection of budget-holding in England in 2005, there were still questions needing answers regarding the appropriateness of such schemes. A subsequent review by Mannion of the evidence, again not systematic, published before the most recent GP budget-holding scheme (GP-led Clinical Commissioning Groups) found a similar mix of evidence (Mannion, 2011).

Dusheiko, Gravelle, Jacobs, and Smith (2006) approached the self-selection problem by using data on 7,000 practices in England from 2 years before and 2 years after the end of fundholding in 1999. The before and after element, coupled with fixed effects estimation,[1] allowed the authors to better control for the differences between fundholding and non-fundholding practices as well as differences over time. After fundholding ended, practices that previously were financially incentivized to ration elective admissions were seen to increase these admissions once this financial incentive was removed; this increase was between 3.5% and 5.1%.

Dusheiko, Gravelle, Yu, and Campbell (2007) investigated how the fundholding scheme affected patient satisfaction. They used a sample of patients taken from a cross-section of 60 English practices in 1998, the last year of fundholding. Findings suggest that fundholding did not adversely affect the quality of care provided, measured by self-reported health. However, patient satisfaction was lower in fundholding practices due to concerns regarding opening hours, GPs' knowledge of medical history, GPs' focus on cost controls, and lack of referrals and tests. It would appear that fundholding increased the incentive for GPs to ration on the basis of referral and tests, and that this change in behavior was detected by patients.

In reviewing the English NHS "internal market" reforms of the 1990s, Le Grand (1999) suggested that in general the reforms involved weak incentives and small effects but that the "fundholding" element of the scheme was an exception. Fundholders faced relatively strong incentives due to their ability to retain surpluses, and hence showed a relatively large response.

Clearly some aspects of budget-holding can work: the fundholding scheme promoted rationing in the form of reduced referrals and allowed fundholding practices to secure reduced waiting times. However, voluntary schemes like fundholding have the potential to lead to equity problems and a "two-tier system." An alternative approach would be to mandate the holding of budgets. However, this runs the risk of forcing budget-holding responsibilities on the inept and the unwilling.

■ PAY-FOR-PERFORMANCE INCENTIVES AND THE UK QUALITY AND OUTCOMES FRAMEWORK (QOF)

Background to the Policy

Prior to 2004, the way in which practitioners are contracted with the NHS had remained largely unchanged since the formation of the NHS in 1948 other than minor reforms in 1966 and 1990. However, the professional, academic, and political context aligned in 2004 to create a major new pay-for-performance scheme, the Quality and Outcomes Framework (QOF) (Roland, 2004). Prior to the QOF, practitioners did have experience with incentive schemes in other forms; for example, fees and bonuses for delivering certain forms of vaccination, screening, and prescribing. Indeed, the QOF was not even the first time GPs were incentivized based on their performance on chronic condition indicators: there was a small-scale policy implemented in East Kent between 1998–2000 (Smith & York, 2004). However, the QOF did represent a major shift in GP income away from capitation and salary payment and toward pay for performance.

The QOF is a pay-for-performance scheme introduced in 2004 as part of the General Medical Services contract. The contract was developed to address a number of aims identified in the NHS Plan 2000 (Department of Health, 2000). These aims included widening the range of services provided in primary care, improved access and choice in primary care, contracts that allow greater flexibility, and a great emphasis on paying for performance (NAO, 2008). It is clear that the new contract shared some of the same objectives as the GP fundholding scheme of the previous decade.

Under the new contract, practices themselves were contracted with the NHS. This represents a break from tradition as GPs' individual contracts meant they enjoyed significant autonomy and freedom (Smith & York, 2004). Practices are now paid based on four criteria: size of patient population, performance on the QOF, provision of enhanced services, and provision of out-of-hours care.

The QOF awarded points based on practice performance across four domains: clinical care, organizational characteristics, patient experience, and provision of additional services. Payments were then linked to the number of points achieved. Higher-scoring practices would earn higher incomes. The precise payment per point varied with the size of the treated population.

Effect of the Policy

Since its introduction in 2004, the QOF has been the subject of considerable research. New data were required to accurately measure performance, and then to pay on this basis. These data were made freely available on the QOF website[2] and have provided researchers with a valuable tool. However, these data were not collected before the introduction of the QOF. This meant that researchers could not use these data to analyze the effect of the introduction of the QOF. If researchers wished to analyze the impact of the QOF, they required comparable data from before and after payments were linked to performance.

Predictions about the possible effect of the QOF emerged soon after its introduction. Roland (2004) is a detailed early description of the policy from someone involved with the initial negotiations. Roland predicted a greater use of computer systems, a greater role played by nurses, improvements in health outcomes, reduced continuity of care, and increased administration costs. A similar early discussion of the policy is that of Smith and York (2004). Smith and York highlighted some potential benefits of the design of the QOF: it encourages teamwork throughout the practice, makes large increases in personal incomes possible, and provides a means to update the scheme regularly. However, these same benefits could also cause problems: individuals may *free ride*[3] due to payments being shared with colleagues, the large income increases may create too strong of an incentive to focus only on QOF areas, and frequent changing of indicators will impede analysis of changes in performance over time.

Due to the time delay in getting research published, it was not until 2006 that empirical research started to surface. The first published paper using QOF data was Sutton and McLean (2006). The study used data from 60 Scottish practices to analyze the factors that are associated with higher QOF scores. They found a number of significant associations. Interestingly, practices that were ex-fundholders scored higher in the first year of the QOF but, in the absence of data from before the QOF, it is not known whether this reflected an already higher level of performance or a greater response to the financial incentives.

Another example of this early research is Doran et al. (2006). The first full year of QOF data (2004/2005) were used and linked with practice characteristics and population characteristics from the census. The aim was to uncover what practice and population characteristics were associated with higher performance but also to ascertain if certain characteristics were associated with higher exception reporting. Practices are able to define some patients as ineligible for treatment, and therefore label them "exceptions," on various grounds: this could possibly create an incentive to exclude more patients from the eligible category in order to improve *reported* performance. Overall QOF performance was very high (95.5% of available points). Performance on the clinical indicators was even higher (96.7% of available points). Exception reporting was low (6%) but varied by a large degree across practices. This high performance meant that the first QOF payments were higher than expected. The models that used practice and patient characteristics to explain the variation in performance failed to explain more than 20% of this variation. Though some characteristics were significant, such as size of practice and whether the practitioner was educated outside of the United Kingdom (negative and positive correlation with performance, respectively), the effects were generally small. The largest single determinant of performance was the level of exception reporting. Practices that increased their exception reporting by 1% could expect an increase of 0.13% in performance.

Additional work based on the same first full year of QOF data was that of McLean, Sutton, and Guthrie (2006) and focused on the issues of inequality in delivery of care and whether the QOF contains adequate incentives to increase treatment in deprived areas. The study hypothesized that the use of exception reporting will mask inequalities because reasons to exclude patients are more common in deprived areas. Therefore, the QOF may not incentivize practices to ration care by providing it to the neediest areas—the areas with higher deprivation. Instead, the QOF may provide incentives to *restrict* care in deprived areas, a clearly negative effect of rationing. The study calculated performance for over 1,000 Scottish practices in 2004/2005 in two ways: first, based on the reported performance in the QOF, and second, based on a new measure that does not allow practices to exclude patients. They label this latter method *delivered quality* and find that practices serving more deprived areas had lower levels of this measure of performance when compared to the practices in less deprived areas. Their research suggested that the QOF failed to provide the incentives needed to adequately serve deprived areas; treating these areas will be more difficult, and providers clearly need additional incentives to do so.

As with fundholding and budget-holding more generally, the QOF has been the subject of much work that can be classified as the opinion of knowledgeable experts. These articles tend to review the literature somewhat selectively, and provide explanations and opinions for their findings. They do, however, act as a useful source of information and provide potential answers to questions that more rigorous research fails to address, perhaps due to a lack of data. Roland (2007) is one such article. Roland defends the £1billion annual investment in the QOF in England as a scheme that can measure and reward quality for many years to come. The results of McLean et al. (2006) are highlighted as clear problems with the scheme, but overall Roland felt that a 6% level of exception reporting was low.

Several of the QOF clinical indicators are designed to incentivize the prescription of certain types of drugs for certain types of patients, such as beta-blockers for patients with coronary heart disease. Research that compares the prescribing of drugs covered by QOF indicators with drugs not covered shows a faster increase in the prescribing of QOF drugs before and after the scheme's introduction (MacBride-Stewart, Elton, & Walley 2008). The non-QOF drugs also showed increases after the QOF but not to the same degree. This result is a similar to that of studies looking at other clinical indicators; improvements in performance predated the QOF. The study uses prescribing data for 2 years before and 2 years after the introduction of the QOF drawn from 92 practices in Scotland.

Steel and Willems (2010) reviewed the existing evidence on the QOF. They note that most studies have focused on the clinical domain: this is where over two-thirds of the total points are available and where the most interest lies. Despite a substantial body of research, studies lacked an experimental design, meaning it was difficult to determine what effect the QOF had. Gaps in the literature are identified as including a lack of panel data and more specific measures of socioeconomic status.

As the QOF developed over time, so too did the methods and data used to analyze it. Initial studies answered questions on performance, payments, and equality. However, these early studies used QOF data to measure performance that was only collected with the introduction of the scheme. Campbell et al. (2007) used data collected for several thousand patients from 42 representative practices in 1998, 2003, and 2005. The data measured performance on a range on indicators for asthma, coronary heart disease, and diabetes. Objective data were used, not publicly available data from the QOF, and the indicators included some incentivized by the QOF and others that were not. Their results showed statistically significant increases in performance post-QOF for asthma and diabetes indicators but not for coronary heart disease. However, coronary heart disease had higher levels of baseline performance, which might explain the insignificant improvements. Results also showed there were no differences between the performance of incentivized and nonincentivized indicators, perhaps due to positive spillovers from the latter to the former.

Generalizing about the successes and failures of the QOF is difficult due to the scale and scope of the indicators. Steel and Willems (2010) suggest that while some have shown above-trend improvements since the introduction of the QOF, others have shown below-trend improvements. As QOF indicators were selected due to a high quality of research in that area, they were already well targeted by practitioners. Nonincentivized indicators do not appear to have been overlooked as a result of the QOF.

In order to increase performance and quality, practices were expected to increase the number of patients treated for each clinical indicator. By doing so, they would achieve more points and therefore receive higher incomes. However, in the design of the QOF, practices could also increase points and income by decreasing the number of eligible patients. This is achieved by increasing the number of patients who are reported as exceptions. Specifically, a practice could increase its achievement on a given indicator without having to actually treat more patients by reducing the number of eligible patients. This was not the intended purpose of exception reporting. As explained earlier, exceptions were allowed so patients were not given inappropriate care. A common example is that of terminally ill patients: controlling cholesterol may not be a priority in this case. As with previous studies, Gravelle, Sutton, and Ma (2010) use data on approximately 1,000 Scottish practices for the first 2 years of the QOF. They investigate whether practices are systematic in their reporting of exceptions and prevalence rates. They hypothesize that genuine exception reporting should only be a function of patient characteristics and should not vary systematically with practice characteristics. However, they found a link between certain characteristics of practices such as number of patients, level of competition from other practices, and exception reporting. More troubling, they found that practices increased their exception reporting in 2005/2006 if they were below the maximum number of points in 2004/2005.

Where possible, the use of data from before and after the implementation of the QOF has been preferred by researchers as it provides a means of comparison. Difficulties arise as this form of data is often drawn from a small sample of patients from a small sample of practices. Using data from 315 Scottish practices representing almost 400,000 individual patients observed across five risk factors for up to 6 years, Sutton, Elder, Guthrie, and Watt (2010) address both issues of small sample and pre-intervention data.[4] The study aimed to measure the effect of the QOF on incentivized tasks, and if there were measurable spillovers onto these same tasks but for diseases not targeted by the QOF, and for totally nonincentivized tasks. In this study, performance was measured by the recording of risk factors that were covered by the QOF. Such high-powered incentives can often lead to unintended negative effects. For example, teachers in Chicago responded to financial incentives placed on exam performance by cheating on exams on behalf of students (Jacob & Levitt, 2003). This type of behavior may surface as a result of the QOF in the form of diverted effort from nonincentivized tasks to those with strong incentives. Sutton et al. (2010) found no evidence of effort diversion, as performance was seen to increase in all areas regardless of incentives. The greatest increase was found in the incentivized tasks for targeted patients, which was where the incentives were strongest. The QOF has managed to influence GP behavior, focusing on incentivized tasks, without neglecting the other areas of care that are measured in this study. However, it is possible that there were other negative consequences that were not measurable in the data used.

A possible avenue whereby the QOF may promote rationing and lead to cost savings is by lowering emergency hospital admissions, or the costs associated with these admissions, through better disease management in primary care (Dusheiko, Gravelle, Martin, Rice, & Smith, 2011). The study takes advantage of a number of large datasets and links them together to create a very large and unique dataset. Many individual, practice, and area level covariates are included. Once linked, a 10% sample of approximately 5 million individual patients is taken and the authors perform a range of cross-sectional and panel data models. In this way Dusheiko, Gravelle, et al. (2011) addressed one of the gaps in the literature identified by Steel and Willems (2010). Results showed that with respect to only one disease area incentivized by the QOF (stroke), better primary care reduced the number of emergency admissions to hospital for that disease. This may not represent a total saving to the NHS, as there are clearly additional costs associated with meeting the QOF targets as well as costs associated with patients living longer. However, the paper does present the most robust evidence available for a link between primary care quality and hospital costs.

The implications of improvement in the quality of primary care diabetes treatments (as measured in the QOF) on hospital costs relating to emergency admissions for diabetes-related problems was studied by Dusheiko, Doran, Gravelle, Fullwood, and Roland (2011). The study differs from previous research as it concentrated on the QOF indicators associated with one aspect of one disease area: the proportion of patients with diabetes receiving poor versus moderate versus good glycemic control. The paper lacked comparable data from before and after the introduction of the QOF, so could not make assertions about whether the QOF has resulted in better diabetes care. This is a point made clear by the authors. What they concluded from the analysis was that practices with a higher level of diabetes management were associated with fewer emergency admissions for short-term diabetic complications. Practices that reported more patients with moderate versus poor glycemic control had a significantly lower emergency admission rate. The same could not be said about practices that report more patients with good versus moderate glycemic control. Further evidence has been provided that suggests the QOF helped to reduce hospital admissions but, again, the evidence is limited to a specific disease area and may not be applicable to the entire QOF.

One of the aims of the new GMS contract was to reduce health inequalities by redistributing income from high-performing practices in affluent areas to low-performing practices in less affluent areas. However, in the early stages of negotiation of the contract it was decided that no practice would have its income reduced[5] (NAO, 2008). This decision meant that it was not possible to redistribute income as planned, which had the potential to increase health inequalities. Doran, Fullwood, Kontopantelis, and Reeves (2008) analyzed data from the first 3 years of the QOF (2004/5, 2005/6, and 2006/7) to uncover if health inequalities had been effected by the introduction of the framework. Their main variable of interest was the percentage of overall achievement of a practice. They calculated this as the percentage of points earned across 34 clinical indicators that all remained largely unchanged over the 3-year period.[6] A clear socioeconomic gradient was found in the first year of data. Practices in the most deprived areas report lower scores on the QOF, with scores increasing as deprivation decreases. By the third year of data, this socioeconomic gradient had all but disappeared. As with other papers analyzing the QOF, there is a lack of data from before the framework's introduction. It is not possible to detect if health inequalities increased between 2003/2004 and 2004/2005, only that they decreased in the second and third years of the QOF. It would appear that, to some extent, the QOF has helped to reduce health inequalities by incentivizing practices to treat patients with chronic diseases. Doran et al. (2008) point out that it is these chronic conditions that are the cause of 60% of the gap in life expectancy between the most and least deprived areas.

In a review of the evidence on the effect the QOF has had on health inequalities, Dixon, Khachatryan, and Boyce (2011) also conclude that the performance gap between the most and least deprived practices is narrowing. This is identified as a positive effect of the QOF, but that further work is required to untangle the impact of health inequalities when measured objectively and not simply measured using QOF performance.

One of the few before and after studies investigating the effects of the QOF on primary care quality was Campbell, Reeves, Kontopantelis, Sibbald, and Roland (2009). Detailed data on clinical quality was collected for three disease areas: coronary heart disease, asthma, and diabetes. Data were objective: unlike other research, quality was not measured by QOF performance. Instead, performance was measured using a range of indicators, some of which were incentivized under the QOF, some of which were not. Additional data on communication, access to care, and continuity of care was obtained using a customized questionnaire. The number of practices sampled was small (approximately 1%), but the authors claim the sample was representative. Findings suggest that performance was increasing in the three disease areas prior to the introduction of the QOF. Performance then increased for asthma and diabetes above the past trend; coronary heart disease increased but in line with past trends. Following these increases, the performance seemed to plateau. The authors suggested a number of causes for this plateau effect. Essentially, the incentives are reduced once a high level of achievement is reached. Within asthma and coronary heart disease, performance was higher in the indicators that are incentivized by the QOF. The scheme influenced the behavior of providers by incentivizing them to focus on certain areas of care.

Further research into how the QOF influenced incentivized and nonincentivized indicators has been conducted using a sample of 148 practices for which data were available from 2000 to 2007; a sample of 653,500 patients was then drawn from these practices (Doran et al., 2011). As with Campbell et al. (2009), the sample of practices is claimed to be representative, and evidence is included showing this to be the case in all relevant areas except patient population size. The sampled practices have larger populations owing to larger practices being overrepresented in the data available. Expert knowledge was used to select a range of indicators that could be used to objectively measure performance in the pre- and post-intervention period. Forty-two indicators were chosen, 23 incentivized by the QOF and 19 not incentivized by the QOF. This study, which used more frequent time points and a larger sample of practices and patients, finds similar results and draws similar conclusions to the study of Campbell et al. (2009). Performance on the chosen indicators had been increasing before the intervention. Following the intervention, incentivized indicators had significant increases in performance above trend before reaching a plateau in the third year of the QOF. However, nonincentivized indicators improved at a rate below the predicted trend and appeared to have been negatively affected by not having financial incentives attached to them.

■ CONCLUSION

The first economic incentive scheme we have considered is budget-holding, namely the granting of budgetary control to family doctors over pharmaceutical expenditure and routine hospital and other specialist health care services used by their patients. We focused on the evidence from the fundholding scheme implemented by the UK NHS between 1991 and 1999, which has been intensively studied. The scheme made practitioners more aware of the financial consequences of their decisions. As a result there was improved control over prescribing costs, including greater use of generic, off-patent drugs. Practitioners also responded by reducing the number of patients they referred to specialist hospital care and negotiating with hospitals to secure shorter waiting times for their patients. Without the budgetary responsibilities granted with fundholding, practitioners would have had little or no incentive to change these aspects of their rationing behavior.

However, the influences of fundholding extend beyond these intended behavioral changes. Patient satisfaction was adversely effected by the increased pressure practitioners faced to control budgets. Patients felt their doctor now lacked knowledge of their medical history and that their doctors were more reluctant to refer them for further treatment. Another concerning consequence of fundholding arose because of the voluntary nature of its implementation—practices had to choose to hold budgets. This created a "two-tier" health system with patients experiencing different degrees of rationing depending on whether the practice with which they were registered had chosen to be a fundholder or not.

Several lessons can be learned from the fundholding experiment that could help policy makers influence rationing behavior. In principle, the policy works. Rationing was increased when practitioners were given control of budgets and allowed to retain surpluses. The problem was that not all practices opted into the policy. It therefore might be tempting to recommend that future policies, along the lines of fundholding, mandate the holding of budgets. However, considering that 50% of practices chose not to participate in the scheme, a mandated policy may carry risks of alienating large numbers of GPs by forcing them to accept budget management responsibilities they do not want and are unable to discharge effectively. A potential solution might be to implement a compulsory policy on a gradual area-based time scale, starting with areas of the country where most GPs are willing to take part and then scaling up the scheme as providers become more comfortable with their newfound commissioning roles. It would also be important to build safeguards into such a scheme to prevent the negative effect on patient satisfaction seen in fundholding.

Paying GPs based on measured performance is a quite different approach to fundholding. In a sense, the QOF *protects* patients from rationing by providing practitioners with an incentive to treat more patients of particular kinds—although, on the other hand, the potential risk is that patients and treatments not incentivized in the scheme might become marginalized. So far, however, evidence of this has not materialized. However, it must be remembered that the QOF scheme was implemented in the mid 2000s at a time of accelerated NHS expenditure growth, when there was sufficient funding to do more activity and meet QOF targets without having to cut back on other aspects of GP activity. It remains to be seen whether QOF activity will result in marginalization of other activity in the current environment of public sector austerity and funding growth slowdown.

The QOF scheme explicitly encourages the provision of more and better quality care. The benefit of such a payment scheme is in benchmarking performance and then rewarding as necessary. Research on the QOF is ongoing, but so far this scheme has shown the potential to reduce health inequalities by lowering the performance gap between the more and least deprived areas. Nonetheless, studies have suggested that the additional gains in quality due to the QOF were small due to the increases in performance that were already occurring prior to the QOF. The QOF was introduced at a time of substantial increases in health spending, which may explain why the scheme had a smaller than expected negative effect on the nonincentivized areas.

One might expect significant diversion of effort given the level of income involved. However, the QOF has shown to induce some positive spillovers onto tasks and diseases that were not incentivized. On top of these effects, the QOF has also reduced the number of hospital admissions related to some of the diseases covered by clinical indictors. The scope of this effect is somewhat limited.

These modest benefits of the scheme have come at a cost. The QOF is an expensive policy. This expense was not unanticipated however; the scheme was designed to involve a large financial reward. Aspects that cause concern are the degree and speed in which practices engaged in unintended gaming of the system; specifically, the way in which they manipulated the exception-reporting feature.

In terms of lessons from QOF for policymakers, one lesson is that family doctors can respond strongly to highly powered performance incentives. Another lesson should be caution when targets are based on *levels* of performance rather than *changes*. The NHS paid significant amounts for preexisting activity. The QOF has shown that, when coupled with an environment with relatively high spending on health care, targeted performance payments may not result in practitioners diverting effort away from other aspects of care.

Although fundholding has ended, further research on the scheme can provide insight into the possible consequences of future policies that allocate budgets to practitioners. This research should focus on the effects on patients as well as providers. As the QOF is ongoing, there are many areas that still require evaluation. As more QOF indicators are added, it will be necessary to analyze their impact. In addition to this, more emphasis should be placed on how the effect on population and patient health can be measured.

The NHS experience with two forms of economic incentive schemes suggest that they do influence rationing by family doctors. Such schemes need to be carefully designed and evaluated, as both of the schemes we have reviewed had unintended consequences that reflected the design properties of the schemes. Economic incentives should therefore be used with care. They should be rigorously evaluated and be flexible in their implementation to allow their design to be adjusted to reflect both the intended and unintended behavioral responses of those they are seeking to influence.

Notes

1. Fixed effects estimation helps to control for factors influencing the analysis but for which we have no data. If these factors are fixed over time then they can be assumed constant. We can therefore control for them by looking at *time demeaned values*. What this involves is taking the year of interest and comparing it to the time trend for the same practice.

2. www.qof.ic.nhs.uk

3. When payments are shared among team members, there is an incentive for individuals to reduce effort and allow the rest of the team to take up the slack. This is known as the "free rider" problem.

4. Risk factors are: blood pressure, smoking status, cholesterol, BMI, and alcohol consumption. Years of data are from 2000/2001 – 2005/2006. Total observations are over 9 million.

5. This was known as the *Minimum Practice Income Guarantee.*

6. QOF indicators are often added, changed, and removed. The framework is designed to evolve, including indicators that were a priority at that time.

REFERENCES

Campbell, S., Reeves, D., Kontopantelis, E., Middleton, E., Sibbald, B., & Roland, M. (2007). Quality of primary care in England with the Introduction of pay for performance. *New England Journal of Medicine, 357*(2), 181–190.

Campbell, S., Reeves, D., Kontopantelis, E., Sibbald, B., & Roland, M. (2009). Effects of pay for performance on the quality of primary care in England. *New England Journal of Medicine, 361*(4), 368–378.

Croxson, B., Propper, C., & Perkins, A. (2001). Do doctors respond to financial incentives? UK family doctors and the GP fundholder scheme. *Journal of Public Economics, 79*(2), 375–398.

Department of Health. (1989). Working for patients. London: HMSO.

Department of Health. (2000). The NHS Plan: a plan for investment, a plan for reform. London: HMSO

Department of Health. (2005). Commissioning a patient-led NHS. London: HMSO.

Dixon, A., Khachatryan, A., & Boyce, T. (2011). The public health impact. In: Gillam, S., Siriwardena, A. N,, editors. *The Quality and Outcomes Framework. QOF—transforming general practice.* Oxford: Radcliffe Publishing.

Dixon, J., Dinwoodie, M., Hodson, D., Dodd, S., Poltorak, T., Garrett, C., Rice, P., et al. (1994). Distribution of NHS funds between fundholding and non-fundholding practices. *British Medical Journal, 309*(6946), 30–34.

Dixon, J., & Glennerster, H. (1995). What do we know about fundholding in general practice? *British Medical Journal, 311*, 727–730.

Doran, T., Fullwood, C., Gravelle, H., Reeves, D., Kontopantelis, E., Hiroeh, U., & Roland, M. (2006). Pay-for-performance programs in family practices in the United Kingdom. *New England Journal of Medicine, 355*(4), 375–384.

Doran, T., Fullwood, C., Kontopantelis, E., & Reeves, D. (2008). Effect of financial incentives on inequalities in the delivery of primary clinical care in England: analysis of clinical activity indicators for the quality and outcomes framework. *The Lancet, 372*(9640), 728–736.

Doran, T., Kontopantelis, E., Valderas, J. M., Campbell, S., Roland, M., Salisbury, C., & Reeves, D. (2011). Effect of financial incentives on incentivised and non-incentivised clinical activities: longitudinal analysis of data from the UK Quality and Outcomes Framework. *British Medical Journal, 342*, d3590

Dusheiko, M., Doran, T., Gravelle, H., Fullwood, C., & Roland, M. (2011). Does higher quality of diabetes management in family practice reduce unplanned hospital admissions? *Health Services Research, 46*(1p1), 27–46.

Dusheiko, M., Gravelle, H., & Jacobs, R. (2004). The effect of practice budgets on patient waiting times: allowing for selection bias. *Health Economics, 13*(10), 941–958.

Dusheiko, M., Gravelle, H., Jacobs, R., & Smith, P. (2006). The effect of financial incentives on gatekeeping doctors: Evidence from a natural experiment. *Journal of Health Economics, 25*(3), 449–478.

Dusheiko, M., Gravelle, H., Martin, S., Rice, N., & Smith, P. (2011). Does better disease management in primary care reduce hospital costs? Evidence from English primary care. *Journal of Health Economics, 30*(5), 919–932.

Dusheiko, M., Gravelle, H., Yu, N., & Campbell, S. (2007). The impact of budgets for gatekeeping physicians on patient satisfaction: Evidence from fundholding. *Journal of Health Economics, 26*(4), 742–762.

Flodgren, G., Eccles, M. P., Shepperd, S., Scott, A., Parmelli, E., & Beyer, F. R. (2011). An overview of reviews evaluating the effectiveness of financial incentives in changing healthcare professional behaviours and patient outcomes. Retrieved June 3, 2012, from http://onlinelibrary.wiley.com/doi/10.1002/14651858.CD009255/abstract.

Gillam, S., & Lewis, R. Q. (2009). Practice based commissioning in the UK. *British Medical Journal, 338*, b832–b832.

Goodwin, N. (1998). GP fundholding. *Learning from the NHS Internal Market. A review of the evidence.* London: King's Fund Publishing.

Le Grand, J. (1999). Competition, cooperation, or control? Tales from the British National Health Service. *Health Affairs, 18*(3), 27–39.

Gravelle, H., Sutton, M., & Ma, A. (2010). Doctor behaviour under a pay for performance contract: treating, cheating and case finding? *The Economic Journal, 120*(542), 129–156.

Jacob, B. A., & Levitt, S. D. (2003). Rotten apples: an investigation of the prevalence and predictors of teacher cheating. *Quarterly Journal of Economics, 118*(3), 843–877.

Klein, R. (1993). Dimensions of rationing: who should do what? *British Medical Journal, 307*, 309–311.

MacBride-Stewart, S. P., Elton, R., & Walley, T. (2008). Do quality incentives change prescribing patterns in primary care? An observational study in Scotland. *Family Practice, 25*(1), 2–32.

Mannion, R. (2005). Practice based commissioning: a summary of the evidence. *Health Policy Matters,* (11). Retrieved from http://www.york.ac.uk/media/healthsciences/documents/research/HPM11final.pdf.

Mannion, R. (2011). General practitioner-led commissioning in the NHS: progress, prospects and pitfalls. *British Medical Bulletin, 97*(1), 7–15.

Maxwell, M., Heaney, D., Howie, J. G., & Noble, S. (1993). General practice fundholding: observations on prescribing patterns and costs using the defined daily dose method. *British Medical Journal, 307*(6913), 1190–1194.

McLean, G., Sutton, M., & Guthrie, B. (2006). Deprivation and quality of primary care services: evidence for persistence of the inverse care law from the UK Quality and Outcomes Framework. *Journal of Epidemiology and Community Health, 60*(11), 917–922.

NAO. (2008). *NHS Pay Modernisation: New contracts for general practice services in England.* National Audit Office. Retrieved January 24, 2012, from http://www.nao.org.uk/publications/0708/new_contracts_for_general_prac.aspx.

Propper, C., Croxson, B., & Shearer, A. (2002). Waiting times for hospital admissions: the impact of GP fundholding. *Journal of Health Economics, 21*(2), 227–252.

Roland, M. (2004). Linking physicians' pay to the quality of care—a major experiment in the United Kingdom. *New England Journal of Medicine, 351*(14), 1448–1454.

Roland, M. (2007). The Quality and Outcomes Framework: too early for a final verdict. *The British Journal of General Practice, 57*(540), 525–527.

Smith, J., Dixon, J., Mays, N., McLeod, H., Goodwin, N., McClelland, S., Lewis, R., et al. (2005). Practice based commissioning: applying the research evidence. *British Medical Journal, 331*(7529), 1397–1399.

Smith, P., & York, N. (2004). Quality incentives: the case of U.K. general practitioners. *Health Affairs, 23*(3), 112–118.

Steel, N., & Willems, S. (2010). Research learning from the UK Quality and Outcomes Framework: a review of existing research. *Quality in Primary Care, 18*(2), 117–125.

Sutton, M., Elder, R., Guthrie, B., & Watt, G. (2010). Record rewards: the effects of targeted quality incentives on the recording of risk factors by primary care providers. *Health Economics, 19*(1), 1–13.

Sutton, M., & McLean, G. (2006). Determinants of primary medical care quality measured under the new UK contract: cross sectional study. *British Medical Journal (Clinical Research Ed.), 332*(7538), 389–390.

Whynes, D. K., Heron, T., & Avery, A. J. (1997). Prescribing cost savings by GP fundholders: long term or short term? *Health Economics, 6*(2), 209–211.

8 The Legal Context of Bedside Rationing

■ KEITH SYRETT

In the context of the provision of medical care, the role for law has traditionally been to regulate the relationship between doctor and patient. This is reflected in the importance which is attached, by both the legal literature and the case law, to questions of autonomy and consent to treatment, duties of care owed by medical professionals to those whom they treat, matters relating to birth or death, donation of organs and transplantation, and reproductive choice. Issues of a broader, systemic nature, such as the appropriate role for legal and regulatory tools in ensuring the conditions for the health of the population—the field of study known as public health law—have occupied a much more subsidiary place in both teaching and research of law. This is in part because such measures are regarded as being "political" rather than "legal" in character. That is, they represent (possibly transient) choices made by the elected branches of government in response to specific societal problems, or strategies for the realization of a particular (possibly ideologically driven) vision of what constitutes a good society. As such they can be distinguished from the purportedly neutral and enduring rules that function to establish a framework within which relations between individual and physician are mediated.

One deficiency of this bifurcation between individual-oriented medical law and population-focused public health policy is that it is unclear where resource allocation fits. On the one hand, distribution of finite resources between competing claims is pre-eminently a function of the political branches of government: indeed, one influential academic account of politics describes it simply as being concerned with allocative questions of "who gets what, when and how" (Lasswell, 1936). If that view is accepted, it is arguable that law has no part whatsoever to play in regulating the manner in which decisions are made as to how, and to whom, funds for the provision of healthcare services and treatments are apportioned. Such matters should simply be resolved by elected politicians or appointed officials for whose actions and decisions elected politicians are responsible, in however indirect a manner. From another perspective, however, allocation of resources may be viewed as fundamental to the physician–patient relationship and thus very properly the subject of legal intervention. Given that the demand for health care services is highly elastic—or, possibly, infinite—whereas the supply of resources, both financial and physical, is relatively inelastic, the scope and nature of treatment which the doctor is able to provide to the patient, and the quality of care which is offered, will inevitably be shaped by limitations on the resources that are available. Since law provides a framework within which the social relations between doctor and patient are managed and disputes that arise from that relationship are adjudicated, it follows that law must, at the very least, take account of the resource constraints which impact upon it. More controversially, it could be argued to be within law's remit to establish a set of principles that provide guidance to the physician when making decisions on how s/he should allocate the limited resources that are available when determining what is best for the patient within their care.

The objective of this chapter is to explore the function performed by law with respect to the allocative dimension of those social relations which form the subject matter of this book: that is, the nexus between doctor and patient. One obvious difficulty which presents itself is that legal processes, principles, and institutions differ from jurisdiction to jurisdiction, albeit that certain common features may present themselves, particularly where legal systems share historical origins. It is accordingly not possible to definitively state *what the legal position is* in each instance, at least in the absence of highly detailed knowledge of each of the countries that are discussed here. However, this need not prove especially troubling: after all, this is not a practitioner text whose aim is to explicate the law as guidance for action in a practical context. Instead, the analysis will be pitched at a more theoretical or conceptual level, with the goal being the identification of the nature of the "law job"—that is, the societal function performed by law—in this instance (Llewellyn, 1940). While the precise manner in which that function is performed will vary according to geographical location, it is intended that a reader of this chapter will nonetheless gain an insight into the potential contribution which law may make, and that this may serve in part to stimulate some rethinking as to the appropriateness of legal intervention, which has frequently been regarded as an annoyance rather than an asset.

A further caveat that must be mentioned prior to commencement of analysis is that the relevant form of legal regulation of allocative decisions will vary according to the manner in which health services are funded. In a system funded by general taxation, such as the National Health Service (NHS) in the United Kingdom (UK), the applicable processes are those of public law—specifically, administrative law—whose function might be broadly described as the regulation of the relationship between the individual and the state. Under the "Bismarckian" model of insurance coverage (under which health insurance is mandated, normally being jointly funded by employers and employees through payroll deduction), special social courts applying principles of social security law are likely to have a key role, as is the case in Germany. And in a privately funded system, rationing decisions will be litigated as questions of private law, applying—at least in broad terms—principles of contract law, as happens in the United States. This alerts us to the importance of the sociopolitical context in which law operates, an issue that will be developed in the next section of this chapter.

This contextual variety renders it difficult to identify a universally applicable "law job" with respect to the rationing of scarce health care resources. Nonetheless, certain commonalities may be identified. For example, Jost (1998) notes that the approach taken by the courts in the United States toward private health insurers has increasingly tended to resemble judicial review of the reasonableness of decisions of regulatory agencies that are imposed upon individuals, rather than interpretation of contractual agreements entered into by parties with putatively equal bargaining power. This brings the United States closer to the German and (especially) UK models of legal intervention, despite a different mode of funding health care. Accordingly, the primary—albeit not exclusive—focus of this chapter will be upon the processes and principles of public law from which, it is argued, the most valuable generalizable lessons as to the role of law in bedside rationing can be learned.

■ CONCEPTUALIZING THE FUNCTION OF LAW

Modern legal scholars tend to reject the idea—perhaps most closely associated with the ancient and widely venerated principle of the rule of law—that law stands above and beyond politics as an objective and wholly neutral system of rules. Rather, the dominant contemporary view is that law operates within a social, political, and economic environment through which it is shaped but which it also functions to steer in a particular direction. This is most self-evidently true with respect to legislation, since statutes are made by legislative assemblies that are dominated by political parties that themselves reflect particular coalitions of interest groups and that seek to pursue certain policy goals through the enactment of laws.

It is less straightforward to apply this analysis to the law made by the judiciary when called upon to adjudicate disputes in court, this activity being of especial significance in those "common law" systems (such as England and Wales, the United States, and Australia) which do not possess codified statements of legal principles in given fields. Widespread commitment to the constitutional doctrine of the separation of powers would suggest that the judiciary must function in a manner that is clearly independent of government, although the extent to which such independence is, in fact, realized may depend upon particular constitutional arrangements (for example, the identity of the person or institution by whom the judiciary is appointed). In principle, the system of precedent limits the capacity for judges to exercise choices based upon their individual policy preferences, and may indeed retard the progression of legal principle in response to changing sociopolitical developments, albeit that the incremental nature of the evolution of judge-made law may render it more malleable than statutory law in many situations.

However, a strong strand of "legal realism," especially within the United States, has argued that judicial decisions are shaped by political beliefs and opinions (Segal & Spaeth, 1993), which in turn are heavily influenced by social factors such as education, class, gender, and ethnicity (Griffith, 2010). Furthermore, a functionalist approach to law has (at least since the interwar period) been highly influential in shaping the "context-located" view of law that was described above as enjoying hegemony among contemporary scholars. In this approach law does not operate as a neutral, autonomous control mechanism that restricts and restrains certain actions, policies, and decisions of the executive branch (and/or, where constitutional provisions or principles permit, those of the legislature). Rather, it can only be understood as a product of the social, political, and economic environment within which it sits and, from a more dynamic standpoint, operates in an instrumental fashion as a tool for shaping that environment.

One possibility is that law may be used in a *facilitative* manner, assisting officials in the discharge of their duties and thus contributing to the realization of the public good (Loughlin, 2005). Those who would endorse such a role for law might well be uncomfortable with entrusting it to the judiciary rather than to the political branches of government, given that the former is not popularly elected and that it may be unsympathetic toward the pursuit of collective social goals such as those which are at stake in the provision of publicly funded healthcare (Laski, 1926). Nonetheless, judicial involvement is in practice unavoidable: first, it is implausible to assume that legislative intervention can cover every conceivable form of activity in a field as diverse as health; second, it is inevitable that disputes as to the services and treatments that are provided (or, more likely, denied) will arise and will necessitate adjudication.

If viewed from this realist, functionalist perspective, it would seem to follow that changes in the manner in which scarce health care resources are allocated—that is, in the context in which law operates—will be reflected in changes in the way in which law responds to this social, political, and economic activity. More proactively, law may act in a facilitative manner as a tool that can assist those charged with making allocative decisions to fulfill their duties in this changed environment in a way that is most conducive to the achievement of the collective goals of the community at large.

In order to assess the validity of this "context-located" model of law, and to identify the precise role as facilitator which law might play in this field, this chapter will consider the impact of the progression from implicit to explicit rationing strategies that has occurred in various health systems over the course of the past two decades or so. As a brief preliminary side note, however, it may be thought helpful to distinguish regulation through legal means and processes (which are the subject of attention here) from standards of conduct laid down by professional bodies or other applicable ethical codes. The latter may, of course, perform a function comparable to law in so far as they operate to guide the behavior of physicians. At the extreme, in cases of noncompliance, such standards of conduct can be used to impose sanctions that may lead to suspension of a practitioner's license. However, they are not laid down by institutions, such as the judiciary or legislature, which possess authority to make binding rules for society as a whole. Nevertheless, such standards may be highly pertinent to bedside rationing, particularly as they are frequently directed expressly at the doctor–patient nexus. For example, the Hippocratic Oath contains an injunction to the physician to "follow that system of regimen which, according to my ability and judgment, I consider for the benefit of my patients, and abstain from whatever is deleterious and mischievous." On the face of it, this might suggest that any denial of access to beneficial treatment to a patient on cost grounds is ethically unacceptable (Newdick, 2005, pp. 17–18; Bloche, 2011),[1] but as Newdick observes, doctors are, in practice, aware that they bear responsibility for groups of patients rather than single individuals, with the consequence that "the idea of *absolute* clinical freedom may long ago have been an unaffordable myth" (Newdick, 2005, p. 18).

■ IMPLICIT BEDSIDE RATIONING AND THE LAW

A classic account of the nature of implicit bedside rationing is that presented in Aaron and Schwartz's *The Painful Prescription* which, although seeking to compare allocation of resources for health care in two countries, the United Kingdom and the United States, provides a description that is much more broadly applicable. The authors argue that physicians tend to "internalize" resource limits, "gradually redefin[ing] standards of care so that they can escape the constant recognition that financial limits compel them to do less than their best" and presenting the decision as the optimal or routine in the clinical circumstances of the patient's case (Aaron & Schwartz, 1984, p. 101). Rationing in such circumstances was implicit in that it amounted to an "unacknowledged limitation of care" (Coast, 1997, p. 1118) in which "the reasoning involved [was] not clearly stated to anyone except . . . the person making the decisions, or active decision-making [was] avoided altogether" (Locock, 2000, p. 93). This represented the predominant mode of resource allocation in most health systems at least until the early 1990s.

In an environment in which allocation of resources was undertaken in this unacknowledged manner, the role for law was essentially a passive one. This is well illustrated by a decision of the Court of Appeal of England and Wales in 1988. In this case (*R v Central Birmingham Health Authority*, ex parte *Collier* [January 6, 1988], see Newdick, 2005, pp. 99–100; Syrett, 2007, pp. 164–67), a 4-year-old child with a heart defect required open heart surgery, the treating physician indicating that such intervention was "desperately needed" and placing the child at the top of the hospital's waiting list as a consequence. However, owing to a shortage of intensive care beds, the operation was cancelled on four separate occasions. The child's father sought a legal order requiring the responsible health authority to provide the surgery or some other form of treatment. This application was rejected by the court, which stated that it was "in no position to judge the allocation of resources by this particular health authority." The three judges expressed considerable sympathy for the family's plight but indicated that it was not the function of the court to require "that somehow more resources should be made available to enable the hospital authorities to ensure that the treatment is immediately given." They indicated that no criticism had been, or should be, directed at the surgeon or any other doctor at the hospital, and that the health authority could not be accused of "dragging its feet"; rather, there may have been "good reasons why the resources in this case do not allow all the beds in the hospital to be used at this particular time." The court was not prepared to investigate these reasons more closely, since it was considered important that it should not "substitute its own judgment for the judgment of those who are responsible for the allocation of resources."

It is notable that, in this case, the court made no serious attempt to disentangle the allocative function (provision of intensive care facilities) from the clinical function (recommendation of the appropriate form of treatment for the patient), merely commenting that no criticism could be leveled at any party involved. In principle, it might have been possible to do so, since there were, in effect, two allocative decisions at play: the initial decision on prioritization by the child's surgeon (that is, to place the patient at the top of a waiting list for treatment) and the subsequent failure to allocate beds such that the patient could be given surgery. The first might be seen as an archetypal instance of bedside rationing, implicit in so far as allocation of positions on the waiting list (which, to use the typology advanced by Klein [1993], amounts to a form of rationing by delay) were rationalized as exercises of clinical judgment rather than considerations of cost. The second choice (which, arguably, took the form of a *failure* to allocate in the patient's favor rather than a conscious decision to deny access) appears more managerial in character and may not have directly involved the treating physician at all. However, the court rested content with observing that there were "good reasons" for the allocation of beds which it declined to analyze further: it is therefore unclear whether the justification was clinical, resource-driven, or a combination of the two.

The Court of Appeal's unwillingness to attempt any degree of meaningful penetration into the decision-making process in order to establish the factors that may have driven it is entirely consistent with the environment in which the law was operating at the time. Implicit rationing—especially in its bedside variant—was ambiguous in character, being composed of an amalgam of clinical and financial factors, the precise relationship between which was opaque to the patient and, to some degree, the physician. Arguably, this lack of transparency served a legitimate sociopolitical purpose in that disguising the nature of the choices made served to minimize the "deprivation disutility" (the anguish suffered by patients who know that something could have been done, but was not because of concerns about cost; see Coast, 1997, p. 1119). At the health systems level, this may be seen as "more conducive to stable social relations and a lower level of conflict" than explicit rationing, which "inevitably gives preference to some who care less about treatment than others who are excluded...[and which] results in many disaffected people...challenging either the rules of allocation or decisions to withhold greater investment in the area" (Mechanic, 1995, p. 1658). A refusal on the part of the judiciary to dissect the nature of the choice thus served to preserve the "merciful lie" (Schmidt, 2004, p. 976) that denial or restriction of access to treatment was premised upon clinical judgment rather than scarcity of resources, and thereby reinforced the relationship of trust between patient and physician. It was this bond, which rested upon the exercise of expertise by the doctor, coupled with the Hippocratic obligation to act as advocate for the patient (Mechanic, 1998, p. 661), that rendered implicit rationing feasible as a strategy, and it inevitably placed the doctor–patient nexus analyzed in this book at center stage.

▪ THE TOOLS OF JUDICIAL PASSIVITY

A noninterventionist stance of the type discussed in the preceding section may therefore be said both to be reflective of, and to reinforce, an allocative environment in which the nature of rationing was unclear and in which clinical judgments exercised by physicians ostensibly shaped the distribution of resources. Judicial unwillingness to reopen allocative decisions for wider public scrutiny had the consequence of containing the suspicion, distrust, and resistance that might ensue if patients became aware that treatments and services which might be medically beneficial to them were being denied on grounds of cost. In this manner, an approach characterized by judicial passivity toward implicit rationing choices might serve to preclude emergence of the "legitimacy problem" which Norman Daniels and James Sabin (1997; 2008) have identified as impacting upon systems of privately managed health care, such as that which exists in the United States.

Of course, courts, once they have commenced adjudication upon a case, must provide reasons for the conclusions they reach, even when they consider that no legal wrong has occurred. A noninterventionist stance in cases in which the basis of challenge is the allocation of scarce health care resources may be explained on the basis that the issues being litigated are not justiciable; that is, that they are not "amenable to the judicial process" (*Council of Civil Service Unions v Minister for the Civil Service* [1985] 1 AC 374, p. 418 [Lord Roskill]; see further King [2007]). Nonjusticiability may be a factor of the lack of constitutional or institutional competence of the court to resolve the issue in question (Jowell, 1999). The former relates, in essence, to the separation of powers and to the democratic (il)legitimacy of an unelected judiciary. As outlined previously in this chapter, decisions on the allocation of resources may be regarded as archetypally political in character and therefore best assigned to the other branches of government. The latter relates to the procedural suitability of the judicial process to address the distributive choices involved in these cases, given that "problems in the allocation of economic resources present too strong a polycentric aspect to be suitable for adjudication" (Fuller, 1979, p. 400). In the case of health care, polycentricism manifests itself in the fact that provision of resources to treat one patient carries opportunity costs insofar as insufficient resources may remain to treat others. Courts may therefore indicate their unwillingness to intervene on this basis, in terms such as this:

> I would also stress the absolute undesirability of the court making an order which may have the effect of compelling a doctor or health authority to make available scarce resources (both human and material) to a particular child, without knowing whether or not there are other patients to whom those resources might more advantageously be devoted (*Re J* [2002] 4 All England Law Reports 614, p. 625 [Balcombe LJ]).

Nonjusticiability affords a justification for nonintervention that is grounded in legal and constitutional principles. By contrast, the notion of deference to medical professional judgment is best understood as a *social* construct, which can be applied with greater or lesser vigor depending upon the inclinations of the judge and upon other contextual factors. A former Lord Chief Justice of England and Wales has explained the propensity of courts to adopt an attitude of "doctor knows best" as reflective of the particular environment in which the emergence of medical law occurred. This constituted a period when medical decisions gave rise to relatively little public controversy, and advocates possessed insufficient expertise in medical matters to successfully challenge health authorities or medical practitioners (which in turn were vigorously defended by bodies providing professional insurance). Medical experts were unwilling to give evidence against colleagues, and courts wished to avoid encouraging defensive medicine (Woolf, 2001, pp. 1–2). While this stance gradually changed with respect to cases of medical negligence, it was somewhat slower to do so in the sphere of resource allocation, in part because the predominance of implicit forms of rationing defused the controversy that such decisions might otherwise have engendered. Thus, as late as 1995, in the leading English case of *R v Cambridge Health Authority*, ex parte *B*, the court felt itself unable to resolve between conflicting medical opinions as to the likely effectiveness of a particular course of treatment and the consequent allocation of funds that would ensue if the treatment were adopted. It stated that "the courts are not, contrary to what is sometimes believed, arbiters as to the merits of cases of this kind. Were we to express opinions as to the likelihood of the effectiveness of medical treatment, or as to the merits of medical judgment, then we should be straying far from the sphere which under our constitution is accorded to us" ([1995] 2 *All England Law Reports 129*, p. 135 [Sir Thomas Bingham MR]).

However, this case also provides a valuable illustration of the complexity of the judicial task in adjudicating upon disputes arising from bedside rationing decisions. The "merciful lie" inherent in implicit rationing is that decisions upon access to treatment are taken solely upon clinical grounds. The *Cambridge Health Authority* case exposes the reality: while there were powerful clinical arguments militating against provision of the treatment, including doubts as to its effectiveness, the suffering which it might cause to the patient, and the experimental nature of the treatment, these were intertwined with an allocative argument—namely, that treating the patient might cost £75,000, which money could be used to provide treatment for others. Choices made by physicians at the bedside are, in practice, very frequently *mixed* allocative and clinical judgments. This was further illustrated by a somewhat surprising decision of the US Supreme Court in *Pegram v Herdrich* (530 U.S. 211 [2000]), in which an aggrieved patient challenged the decision of a physician to delay treatment which, it was claimed, had been motivated by financial incentives offered by the patient's health maintenance organization to limit access to care. The Court conceptualized the role of a physician offered such incentives as one which concerned *both* treatment and eligibility for treatment, the former being clinical and the latter—relating as it did to the control of costs—managerial. While the courts had previously construed decisions involving the coverage offered by a health maintenance organization as precluded from legal liability by the Employee Retirement Income Security Act, the Supreme Court indicated that the comingled clinical and allocative decisions taken by physicians in circumstances such as these would not be so barred (see Bloche & Jacobson, 2000).

Once the courts had accepted that bedside decisions are mixed in this manner, the argument for judicial nonintervention which springs from deference to professional medical judgment becomes less potent, simply because physicians are acting in more than just a clinical capacity: they are gatekeepers of resources as well as patient advocates. It remains the case that there is justification for a passive judicial stance from the perspective of nonjusticiability. While courts have traditionally not tended to regard decisions on allocation of resources in other fields of activity as requiring professional expertise which they do not possess, they may nonetheless still regard such choices as being inherently political or problematically multifaceted. However, the recognition of an allocative component to the physician's work opens the possibility of a more nuanced and active judicial response to rationing choices than was evident in the English *Central Birmingham Health Authority* or *Cambridge Health Authority* decisions. That such a development was appropriate in light of the social, political, and economic context in which the law now operates becomes apparent once we have considered the evolving nature of rationing over recent years, as the next section of this chapter seeks to do.

■ TOWARD EXPLICIT RATIONING?

The prevailing trend in health systems over the past two decades or so has been in the direction of greater visibility in the process of allocation of scarce health care resources. As Ham and Coulter (2001, p. 163) observe, there is a "menu of possibilities" available to policymakers who wish to develop a more systematic approach to allocation of resources, a development which is regarded as necessary in order to exercise some degree of control over spiraling expenditure on health care. These range from the attempt made in Oregon to draw up a list of core treatments and services (Oregon Health Services Commission,1991), through the development of national frameworks to guide priority setting (as in the Netherlands [Ministry of Welfare, Health and Cultural Affairs, 1992] and New Zealand [National Advisory Committee on Core Health and Disability Services, 1994]) to attempts to establish an ethical platform upon which rationing choices could be made (as in Norway [Government Commission on Choices in Health Care, 1987] and Sweden [Swedish Parliamentary Priorities Commission, 1995]).

These strategies were necessarily pursued at a "macro" national or state level, but other modes of explicit rationing have emerged elsewhere in the health system. At the "meso" level, where decisions are made as to which health services or treatments are to receive priority, a move toward separating the function of provision of health care from that of the purchase (or commissioning) of treatments and services in order to enhance supply-side efficiency might lead certain bodies exercising the latter function to choose to exclude access to particular services or treatments. This would render them unavailable to patients in the locality, at least in the absence of proof of exceptional circumstances. Such a strategy was adopted by a number of health authorities in the NHS in the United Kingdom in the early 1990s (mainly in relation to treatments at the margins of heath provision, such as tattoo removal or breast augmentation) (Klein, Day, & Redmayne, 1993, pp. 68–70), and it has recently reemerged as a response to significant financial pressures that are being placed upon the Service, this time in relation to more frontline treatments. Additionally, or alternatively, explicit rationing might take the form of "rationing by guideline" (Ham, 1995, p. 1483), entailing the development of statements to assist practitioners and patients in reaching decisions as to appropriate health care in particular circumstances. Such guidelines may function as rationing tools in situations where they operate to deny access to treatments or services on the ground that they are ineffective (or less effective than alternatives) despite the fact that they may offer *some* clinical benefit to *certain* patients.

Since guidelines have a nonbinding character they can be considered as amounting to a form of rationing at the bedside, as it is the physician who makes the final decision as to which service or treatment will be made available to the patient, exercising discretion to depart from the guideline if the circumstances require it. The guideline strategy is thus politically useful for policymakers, as it enables blame for unpopular allocative choices to be diffused and diverted to physicians, with a view to retaining the benefit of systemic stability that implicit rationing strategies offer (Ham and Coulter, 2001, p. 165). However, the picture has altered from that which characterized the era of implicit rationing in various respects. First, the existence of the guideline renders the fact of rationing more visible: a statement exists as to which treatments or services should be used in a particular clinical context (and, by extension, those which should not be used) with the consequence that it is more widely apparent—particularly to medical professionals but also to patients and the public—that restrictions on access exist. Second, rationing by guideline frequently exists alongside rationing by exclusion at "macro" or "meso" level. In particular, agencies may be established to undertake appraisal of new and existing health technologies and to provide guidance on their clinical and cost effectiveness to policymakers, purchasers, and providers of health care (Morgan, McMahon, Mitton, Roughead, Kirk, et al., 2006). In some instances (for example, as is the case with the National Institute for Health and Clinical Excellence [NICE] operating in England and Wales), the recommendations made by such agencies directly impact upon the scope of coverage of a health system. These decisions are thus high profile and controversial, attracting considerable media interest, especially in view of the fact that they frequently concern innovative but expensive treatments that promise some clinical benefit to those patients close to the end of life. They might be regarded as the epitome of explicit rationing.

It is therefore most accurate to view the recent evolution of rationing strategies as marked by a transition from a predominantly implicit model, in which physician choice played a central role, to one which synthesizes explicit and implicit approaches (Ham & Coulter, 2001, p. 167). Such an analysis recognizes the continuing significance of rationing at the bedside and the application of clinical judgment. However, it acknowledges that these now operate within an environment in which decisions beyond the physician's direct control—such as those made by local or regionally based bodies with responsibility for commissioning health care for particular populations, by the developers of clinical guidelines, or by agencies undertaking health technology appraisal—may in practice serve to constrain what the physician can, or feels able to, provide to the patient.

■ LAW'S ROLE IN THE NEW RATIONING ENVIRONMENT

In analyzing the part played by law with respect to allocative decisions reached by physicians in this "hybrid" environment of explicit and implicit rationing, it may be useful as a preliminary observation to recall the distinction previously drawn between ethical and legal frameworks. It was noted that, while the ethical frameworks might exhibit some of the characteristics associated with law—notably, an impact upon behavior and the attachment (in certain instances) of sanctions in the event of noncompliance—they could not be said to amount to law because they did not emanate from a source (such as the legislature or judiciary) with constitutional authority to make and enforce general rules for the conduct of society.

The existence of clinical guidelines serves further to obfuscate the already opaque boundary between different forms of "rule." It is quite clear that guidelines which articulate best practice in the management of patient care are intended to establish normative standards of conduct for the physician in the same manner as a legal obligation might do: as Eddy (1990, p. 2243) notes, their purpose "is to modify the behavior of practitioners to steer their decisions toward actions that the policy-makers consider desirable." In principle, the two forms diverge insofar as guidelines possess a non-obligatory character, physicians retaining discretion to depart from the guideline without sanction in circumstances in which, in their clinical judgment, such departure serves the interests of the patient. In practice doctors may consider themselves to be bound by the terms of the guideline, which may therefore best be described as constituting a form of "soft law" (Campbell & Glass, 2001).

Furthermore, the guideline may achieve indirect legal enforcement if the courts determine that it represents the appropriate standard of care for determination of liability in negligence (Campbell & Glass 2001, pp. 482–486). If this is the case, the physician's autonomy in determining the appropriate form of care for a patient—and the attendant decision as to how resources will be allocated—will be severely constrained. The precise status of clinical guidelines in establishing a legally enforceable standard of care is, however, somewhat uncertain (Semanta, Mello, Foster, Tingle, & Semanta 2006, p. 322). This can be illustrated by reference to the clinical guidelines issued by NICE to the NHS in England and Wales. The Institute has stated as follows:

> Guidance that does not recommend a treatment or procedure, or that recommends its use only in defined circumstances, is not the same as a ban on that treatment or procedure being provided by the NHS. If, having considered the guidance, a health professional considers that the treatment or procedure would be the appropriate option in a given case, there is no legal bar on the professional recommending the treatment or on the NHS funding it…As NICE guidance is based on a robust assessment of the clinical evidence and/or reflects a consensus of current medical opinion, one would expect that a health professional who acts in accordance with NICE guidance would be able to count on that fact to help with his or her defense. While a health professional who *follows* NICE guidance might be able to count on that fact to help their defense, it does not necessarily follow however, that health professionals who *deviate* from NICE guidance are negligent. Whilst there is always likely to be a "responsible body" of health professionals supporting the recommendations made in NICE guidance, there may be other health professionals who subscribe to a different view (NICE 2004, pp. 3–4. Emphases in original).

The tentative conclusion that might be drawn from this analysis is that guidelines are not *determinative* of the legal standard of care, a view that is borne out by empirical research which "suggests a degree of judicial skepticism about the weight of guidelines in determining the legal standard. Judges may feel that guidelines are for guidance rather than prescription in this determination."[2] This stance would seem a plausible one for the judiciary to adopt given the widespread concerns that exist within the medical profession as to slavish adherence to "cookbook medicine" (see, e.g., Holoweiko, 1989), coupled with the existence of a legal principle that a decision maker should not "fetter its discretion" by over-rigid application of policies or guidance (*British Oxygen Co. Ltd v Board of Trade* [1970] UKHL 4). If correct, it underlines that clinical guidelines do differ—albeit to a relatively limited degree—from "hard" legal rules. The consequence is that, while a physician may feel bound by a guideline, as a normative standard of good practice, to deny or permit access to a given treatment or service to a particular patient, such denial or permission cannot straightforwardly be regarded as mandatory in a legal sense.

Indeed, not only does the law not mandate compliance by the physician with clinical guidelines, it actually operates to preserve a degree of clinical autonomy in the making of allocative choices. This is apparent from a number of cases in which the judiciary has declared "blanket" exclusions of particular forms of treatment to be unlawful. While the courts have conceded the utility of establishing a list of priorities for funding in situations where resources are scarce (*R v North West Lancashire Health Authority*, ex parte *A, D and G* [1999] EWCA Civ 2022), they also seek to ensure that patients who present with exceptional circumstances which might warrant a departure from the rationing policy may receive treatment (*R (Rogers) v Swindon Primary Care Trust* [2006] EWCA Civ 392). Consequently a physician remains, in principle, free to exercise judgment as to the most appropriate treatment for a patient notwithstanding that it has been allocated low priority for funding, provided that atypical clinical considerations can be demonstrated. This autonomy is preserved even in cases in which a decision not to fund a particular treatment or service is taken at "macro" level—for example, by a minister of health (*R v Secretary of State for Health*, ex parte *Pfizer Ltd.* [1999] EWHC Admin 504), or an agency undertaking health technology appraisal. However, in such instances the likelihood of the physician successfully demonstrating clinical exceptionality such that the "macro" level decision is overriden appears statistically to be considerably lower.[3]

However, while compliance with guidelines may not be legally obligatory, a court will ensure that any departure is justified by the physician by reference to the particular circumstances of the patient. For example, NICE (2004, p. 4 quoting the Medical Defence Union; see also Syrett, 2010, pp. 416–417) has advised that "ignorance of NICE guidance is a poor defense, but a reasoned and reasonable decision to reject the guidance in an individual case, together with a good record, made at the time, may be acceptable." It notes that, in such an instance, full discussion with the patient and/or their guardian or caregiver is recommended. An explanatory duty imposed by a court serves a number of purposes. First, with respect to the patient, it ensures that the physician is obliged to explore choices as to appropriate treatment and allocation of resources in a careful and considered manner, with proper reference to evidence of effectiveness. This will additionally assist the discharge of the obligation to provide sufficient information to enable the patient to exercise consent to the treatment rather than the alternative set out in the guideline. Second, with respect to the court itself, it facilitates the task of ascertaining whether the required standard of care has been met insofar as the physician is required to proffer explanation for deviating from the guidance in order to demonstrate that the actions taken were reasonable. Third, with respect to other stakeholders (such as patient groups or other professionals) and the wider public, an account presented in court of why the guideline has not been followed enhances understanding of the clinical and allocative decision-making process undertaken by the physician and, in particular, of the criteria that have impacted upon the choice which has been reached and the relative weight that has been attached to these.

We are now in a position to identify the key function undertaken by the law in the contemporary health care rationing environment. Its primary role is to *ensure transparency in allocative choices*. This goal is pursued at all levels at which decisions that have the effect of restricting or denying an individual access to a service or treatment is taken. Thus, in addition to the "micro" level of bedside rationing considered above, there is legal precedent for judicial intervention at the "meso" level, with courts requiring bodies responsible for the local commissioning of health care to explain the reasons for noncompliance with national guidance. For instance, the law required that a policy which restricted beta-interferon treatment for patients with multiple sclerosis to those willing to participate in randomized controlled trials be fully explained, since it departed from national guidance which specified that patients be referred to secondary care services for assessment and, where appropriate, treatment (*R v North Derbyshire Health Authority*, ex parte *Fisher* [1997] EWHC Admin 675). Similarly, in *R v North West Lancashire Health Authority*, ex parte *A, D and G* [1999] EWCA Civ 2022, the court decided that a decision by the Health Authority to allocate low priority to reassignment surgery as a form of treatment for gender identity dysphoria was unlawful in part because no explanation had been provided for departure from a strong body of medical evidence that such treatment was effective. There is also authority for judicial imposition of explanatory obligations upon decision makers making rationing choices at a "macro" level, including a ministerial decision to exclude Viagra from the scope of coverage of a publicly funded health system (*R v Secretary of State for Health*, ex parte *Pfizer Ltd.* [1999] EWHC Admin 504) and recommendations by national-level agencies undertaking health technology appraisal which have the impact of restricting access to specified interventions (*R (Eisai Limited) v NICE* (2007) EWHC 1941 (Admin)/(2008) EWCA Civ 438, *R (Servier Laboratories Limited) v NICE* (2009) EWHC 281 (Admin)/ (2010) EWCA Civ 346, *Pfizer Pty Limited v Birkett* (2000) FCA 303/(2001) FCA 828: Syrett, 2011).

Furthermore, although (as previously noted) the applicable legal principles and processes will differ in systems where allocative decisions rest primarily with private health insurers, litigation appears to provide a similar spur to openness in such situations, offering a form of public accountability that might otherwise prove elusive in an atomized marketplace. Thus, Bloche and Studdert (2004, p. 39) argue that the Supreme Court decision in *Pegram v Herdrich* functioned to oblige insurers to be more "upfront" about cost considerations underpinning the denial of coverage for treatments and services, rather than sheltering behind the opaque contractual language of "medically necessary" care.

The insistence upon transparency represents a significant shift from the previous, largely passive, position adopted by the judiciary. Yet, as in those earlier cases, the stance taken by the courts is entirely consistent with the social, political, and economic context in which the law is functioning. The shift toward greater explicitness in resource allocation that began in the early 1990s means that cost considerations have become more clearly visible to physicians, patients, and public alike. In such an environment, opacity in decision making is more troublesome than was previously the case; while some implicitness may remain, widespread attempts to disguise the nature of decisions in an arena in which transparency is relatively commonplace risk generating suspicion and distrust. Accordingly, the judicial function can once again be seen as assisting allocative decision makers in the quest for legitimacy. Although the legal process will usually be initiated by those who are dissatisfied with a rationing decision (and, if the claim that explicit rationing is more socially unstable than the implicit form is accurate, one might anticipate an increase in the incidence of litigation), judicial enforcement of an explanatory requirement may serve to temper that dissatisfaction by enhancing understanding of the criteria that have impacted upon the decision, reassuring those affected by it (and, by extension, the wider public) that it has been reached on the basis of careful consideration of all relevant factors.

Furthermore, since court decisions possess precedential value, imposition of standards of good decision making in one case should encourage others who are engaged in rationing to embrace transparency and reasoned articulation of choices in their work, thus enhancing consistency and accountability in decision making in the health system as a whole. In these ways, law in general, and judicial adjudication in particular, may be said to operate as a means of enforcing the "publicity" condition (public accessibility of rationing decisions and their rationales) of the "accountability for reasonableness" model of procedural justice that Daniels and Sabin (1997; 2008) have prescribed as a means of responding to the "legitimacy problem" which arises as a consequence of the socially unstable nature of explicit rationing.[4]

It is important to note that the role of the courts is restricted to review of the *procedural* dimensions of the rationing decision. The courts are not empowered to substitute their view on the question of whether resources should be allocated to a particular patient or group of patients in place of that of the original decision maker. To do so would be to exceed the competence they possess within the constitutional arrangements of a particular society,[5] and would raise questions of institutional capacity to adjudicate upon polycentric questions. However, since judicial articulation of certain procedural qualities of decision making does not entail prescription of a particular substantive outcome, the argument against intervention that springs from nonjusticiability is not particularly potent. Indeed, it has been cogently argued that such an obstacle need not have precluded a proceduralist approach on the part of the judiciary to the earlier cases (Newdick, 2005, pp. 99–100; James & Longley, 1995). The failure of the courts to move in such a direction at that time is, therefore, best understood not in terms of the existence of an abstract legal principle that precluded judicial intervention in all such cases, but rather as a sociopolitically constructed response to the opaque milieu in which the law was operating and which, for reasons of systemic legitimacy, it was considered important to preserve. Once that environment had changed as a consequence of developments beyond the reach of legal principle, the rationale for continuing judicial passivity on procedural matters no longer held.

This having been said, courts remain acutely conscious of their limited democratic legitimacy in a field that inevitably generates significant political controversy. In some instances, therefore, they have viewed their role more in terms of catalyzing wider democratic debate upon rationing questions in general than imposing specific procedural requirements in individualized cases. Litigation from South American countries is especially instructive in this regard. In Colombia, the Constitutional Court has called for a participatory, transparent process of determination of the health treatments and services that are covered by the national insurance scheme (Yamin, Parra-Vera, & Gianella, 2011, p. 177); while in Brazil, the Supreme Court made use of a public audience to promote discussion of the appropriate solution to a case concerning the state's obligation to provide medicines (Gargarella, 2011, p. 243).

■ CONCLUSION

Physicians who seek to provide appropriate, effective, and affordable treatment for patients in an environment in which rationing has a more explicit character will inevitably find their autonomy more constrained than might have been the case in the past. Clinical guidelines, while not mandatory, lay down best practice for treatment and are influential—albeit not determinative—in establishing the legal standard of care. Funding may, in practice, be unavailable for certain treatments or services absent proof of exceptionality. Decisions that impact upon access to treatment (particularly where treatment is being denied) will need to be recorded, communicated, and justified, especially when these conflict with guidelines.

Such physicians might be forgiven for considering the law to be an unwelcome irritant to their work. Yet law's capacity to establish a framework of principles for fair decision making should not be overlooked. Its commitment to transparency both responds to and reinforces an environment in which rationing decisions, and the reasons for them, have gradually become more visible to all. Within this potentially socially unstable context, the law's enforcement of an obligation to provide reasoned justifications for allocative choices both ensures that proper respect is shown for the autonomy of the affected patient and contributes to building broader societal understanding of the need for hard choices in health care, and of the criteria that underpin these choices. Hence, and paradoxically, a mechanism that is often invoked by those who would seek to challenge decisions on resources may constitute a means whereby the fairness and legitimacy of those decisions can be secured.

Notes

1. It is notable that professional bodies are frequently more ambivalent about the relationship between the Oath and the need to manage scarce healthcare resources. For example, Opinion 2.03 of the *Code of Medical Ethics* of the American Medical Association states that "a physician has a duty to do all that he or she can for the benefit of the individual patient…Decisions regarding the allocation of limited medical resources among patients should consider only ethically appropriate criteria relating to medical need": see http://www.ama-assn.org/ama/pub/physician-resources/medical-ethics/code-medical-ethics/opinion203.page (accessed 14 November 2011).

2. Samanta, Mello, Foster et al (2006, p. 340) also give brief consideration to litigation involving the use of clinical guidelines in the United States, concluding that "the role of guidelines as a standard for legal liability is not straightforward. However, one principle that emerges with relative clarity from the US experience is that guidelines function as a facet of evidence that is informative, rather than determinative, of the legal standard of care."

3. For example, a survey conducted by the Department of Health in England (2008, p. 63) showed that only 13% of Primary Care Trusts (which were responsible for commissioning healthcare for their local populations) had funded treatments which had not been recommended by NICE on the basis of the existence of exceptional clinical circumstances. See Department of Health. 2008. *Improving Access to Medicines for Patients.* London: Department of Health.

4. Daniels (2008, p. 330) has recently characterised "accountability for reasonableness" as requiring "transparency for all aspects of the process, including the rationales for the priorities adopted": Daniels, Norman. 2008. *Just Health.* Cambridge: Cambridge University Press.

5. Courts do not lack such competence in jurisdictions in which a right to health or a right to access healthcare is afforded constitutional protection, as is the case in more than two-thirds of the countries of the world: see Kinney, Eleanor and Brian Clark. 2004. Provisions for Health and Healthcare in the Constitutions of the Countries of the World. *Cornell International Law Journal* 37: 285-355. However, even in such jurisdictions courts may remain reluctant to intervene in allocative choices, according the decision-maker a discretionary area of judgment in such cases. For discussion of some of these issues, see Yamin and Gloppen (2011).

REFERENCES

Aaron, H., & Schwartz, W. (1984). *The Painful Prescription.* Washington, DC: Brookings Institution.

Bloche, M. G. (2011). *The Hippocratic Myth.* New York: Palgrave Macmillan.

Bloche, M. G., & Jacobson, P. (2000). The Supreme Court and bedside rationing. *Journal of the American Medical Association, 284*(21), 2776–2779.

Bloche, M. G., & Studdert, D. (2004). A quiet revolution: law as an agent of health system change. *Health Affairs, 23*(2), 29–42.

Campbell, A., & Glass, K. (2001). The legal status of clinical and ethics policies, codes, and guidelines in medical practice and research. *McGill Law Journal, 46*, 473–489.

Coast, J. (1997). The rationing debate: Rationing within the NHS should be explicit: the case against. *British Medical Journal, 314*, 1107–1111.

Daniels, N., & Sabin, J. (1997). Limits to health care: fair procedures, democratic deliberation, and the legitimacy problem for insurers. *Philosophy and Public Affairs, 26(4)*, 303–350.

Daniels, N., & Sabin, J. (2008). *Setting Limits Fairly.* New York: Oxford University Press.

Eddy, D. (1990). Clinical decision-making: from theory to practice. Guidelines for policy statements: the explicit approach. *Journal of the American Medical Association, 263(3)*, 2239–2240.

Fuller, L. Winston KI (1978). The form and limits of adjudication. *Harvard Law Review, 92(2)*, 353–409.

Gargarella, R. (2011). Dialogic justice in the enforcement of social rights: some initial arguments. In Yamin, A., & Gloppen, S., eds. *Litigating Health Rights: can courts bring more justice to health?* pp. 232–245. Cambridge: Harvard University Press.

Government Commission on Choices in Health Care (Norway) Guidelines for prioritization in Norwegian Health care. (1987). Oslo: Universitetsforlaget NOU.

Griffith, J. (2010). *The Politics of the Judiciary.* London: Fontana Press.

Ham, C. (1995). Health care rationing. *British Medical Journal, 310*, 1483–1484.

Ham, C., & Coulter, A. (2001). Explicit and implicit rationing: taking responsibility and avoiding blame for health care choices. *Journal of Health Services Research and Policy, 6(3)*, 163–169.

Holoweiko, M. (1989). What cookbook medicine will mean for you. *Health Economics, 66*, 118–120.

James, R., & Longley, D. (1995). Judicial review and tragic choices; *ex parte B. Public Law Aut, 367*–373.

Jost, T. (1998). Health care rationing in the courts: a comparative study. *Hastings International and Comparative Law Review, 21(3)*, 639–714.

Jowell, J. (1999). Of *vires* and vacuums: the constitutional context of judicial review. *Public Law Aut*, 448–460.

King, J. (2007). The justiciability of resource allocation. *Modern Law Review, 70(2)*, 197–224.

Klein, R. (1993). Dimensions of rationing: who should do what? *British Medical Journal, 307*, 309–311.

Klein, R., Day, P., & Redmayne, R. 1993. *Managing Scarcity.* Buckingham: Open University Press.

Laski, H. (1926). Judicial review of social policy in England. *Harvard Law Review, 39(7)*, 832–848.

Lasswell, H. (1936). *Politics: who gets what, when, how.* New York: Whittlesey House.

Llewellyn, K. (1940). The normative, the legal, and the law-jobs: the problem of juristic method. *Yale Law Journal, 49(8)*, 1355–1400.

Locock, L. (2000). The changing nature of rationing in the National Health Service. *Public Administration, 78(1)*, 91–109.

Loughlin, M. (2005). The functionalist style in public law. *University of Toronto Law Journal, 55(3)*, 361–403.

Mechanic, D. (1995). Dilemmas in rationing healthcare services: the case for implicit rationing. *British Medical Journal, 310*, 1655–1659.

Mechanic, D, (1998). The functions and limitations of trust in the provision of medical care. *Journal of Health Politics, Policy and Law, 23(4)*, 661–686.

Ministry of Welfare, Health and Cultural Affairs (Netherlands). (1992). *Choices in Health Care: a Report by the Government Committee on Choices in Health Care, the Netherlands.* Rijswijk: Ministry of Welfare, Health and Cultural Affairs

Morgan, S., McMahon, M., Mitton, C., Roughead, E., Kirk, R., et al. (2006). Centralized drug review processes in Australia, Canada, New Zealand and the United Kingdom. *Health Affairs, 25(2)*, 337–347.

National Advisory Committee on Core Health and Disability Services (New Zealand). (1994). *Third Report: Core Services for 1995/96.* Wellington: Core Services Committee.

Newdick, C. (2005). *Who Should We Treat?* Oxford: Oxford University Press.

NICE [National Institute for Health and Clinical Excellence]. (2004). *Legal Context of NICE Guidance.* London: NICE.

Oregon Health Services Commission. (1991). *The 1991 Prioritization of Health Services.* Salem: Oregon Health Services Commission, 1991, no. 8746.

Schmidt, V. (2004). Models of health care rationing. *Current Sociology, 52*, 969–988.

Segal, J., & Spaeth, H. (1993). *The Supreme Court and the Attitudinal Model.* Cambridge: Cambridge University Press.

Semanta, A., Mello, M., Foster C., Tingle, J., & Semanta, J. (2006). The role of clinical guidelines in medical negligence litigation: a shift from the *Bolam* standard? *Medical Law Review, 14(3)*, 321–366.

Swedish Parliamentary Priorities Commission. (1995). *Priorities in Health Care: Ethics, Economy, Implementation.* Stockholm: Ministry of Health and Social Affairs.

Syrett, K. (2007). *Law, Legitimacy and the Rationing of Health Care.* Cambridge: Cambridge University Press.

Syrett, K. (2010). Institutional Liability. In Grubb, A., Laing, J., & McHale, J., eds. *Principles of Medical Law*, pp. 395–438. Oxford: Oxford University Press.

Syrett, K. (2011). Health technology appraisal and the courts: accountability for reasonableness and the judicial model of procedural justice. *Health Economics, Policy and Law, 6(4)*, 469–488.

Woolf, H. (2001). Are the courts excessively deferential to the medical profession? *Medical Law Review, 9(1)*, 1–16.

Yamin, A, Parra-Vera, O., & Gianella, C. (2011). Colombia: Judicial Protection of the Right to Health. In Yamin, A., & Gloppen, S., eds. *Litigating Health Rights: can courts bring more justice to health?*, pp. 103–131. Cambridge: Harvard University Press.

9 Bedside Rationing or Rational Planning

In Search of Perspective on Medical Benefit and Safety

■ YECHIEL MICHAEL BARILAN

I will make the case that "rationing" in healthcare may have three distinct, but sometimes overlapping meanings.

1. Withholding medical care because society does not have enough resources. It will be argued that we have good reasons to suppose that affluent societies (e.g. OECD nations) have enough material resources to universally provide (even if by means of private markets) for the level of health care required by respect for human dignity and human rights, and that perceptions of insufficiency are derived from inappropriate regulation and from publicity pressures coming from self-interested stakeholders.

2. Withholding medical care because other patients need it (i.e., rationing within a closed health care economy). It will be argued that triage is the appropriate method for such rationing, and that its morality depends less on the criteria of triage but on its external conditions—the structuring of health care in society and freedom from conflicts of interest. The external conditions pertain to proper separation between market and nonmarket modes of governance, granting each sphere its due roles in societies that respect human dignity and rights.

3. Withholding medical care that the patient feels entitled to at the time of rationing. When done by the patients' clinicians, this is usually referred to as "bedside rationing." Due to the values of beneficence, respect for autonomy, and fiduciary obligations, it is the most vexing form of rationing psychologically, morally, and politically. The media, tort law, and forces of the market exacerbate this perception to the point where many believe that clinicians must never carry it out. However, it will be argued that when the health care system is properly structured it is possible, even desirable, to construe the third meaning of rationing as moral, even respectful of patients' autonomy. Motivations to do so might be either protection of patients' salient interests as well as commitment to patients in greater or more urgent need. Indeed, when the health care system is properly structured, the two kinds of motivations significantly overlap.

This chapter does not build on new moral teachings and political ideals. Rather, I wish to show that a broad-view reflection on already accepted values, ideas, and policies, as well as careful reading of clinical research, compel a synthetic and coherent approach in which reform of some valuable aspects of society (e.g., the regulation of markets) is dictated by other, no less valuable aspects of society (e.g., respect for life and for personal autonomy). We have to acknowledge that the diverse values and structures of liberal societies tend to limit each other, and that proper regulation sets limits on each. In this light, when properly constructed and governed, "bedside rationing" is moral, respectful, empowering, and sometimes beneficial, even to the rationed patient.

■ SCARCE RESOURCES OR PROFLIGATE HEALTHCARE?

The bioethical discourse on distribution of health care resources is beset by two conflicting narratives. According to one, health care costs keep rising; the aging of the population boosts demand, and somebody must set limits on public spending on care simply because even rich societies cannot afford all the wonderful benefits of biomedicine. Hence, rationing occurs at all levels of the health care system; even doctors at the bedside cannot help making tough decisions such as which patient to send to intensive care and which not; whom to prescribe a cutting edge anticancer drug or a sophisticated pacemaker and whom not to.

According to the second narrative, despite the growth of the biomedical sector, health indices such as infant mortality and life expectancy have stopped rising in a significant manner. More and more of the health care budget goes to administration and less and less to direct care (Riley, 2001, pp. 106–121; Watts, 2003, ch. 10; Woolhandler & Himmelstein, 1997). Even direct care has been drifting away from genuine benefit. Many find the most expensive aspects of care (i.e., keeping hopelessly ill patients in ICU, NICU) futile and even offensive to human dignity. The rate of hospitalization due to drug interactions and complications is staggering (Lau et al., 2005). The biomedical industry and the medical profession are accused of "disease mongering," of making the public believe that people suffer from conditions that fit the biomedical services in the market (McNally, 2011, ch. 2). According to this second narrative, doctors' real duty is to focus on clearly beneficial care and to shield their patients from the dreadnaught of biotechnology.

It is tempting to find in these dual meta-narratives a reflection of the image of contemporary affluent societies. On the one hand we admire the richness and variety of products and possibilities; on the other hand, much of this abundance is unhealthy and contributes little to personal fulfillment and happiness. Although promoted incessantly, consumption of many advertised products does not improve well-being (Offer, 2006, ch. 2). The more medical care is part of the free market, the more one expects its services to be similarly alluring yet superfluous and even counter to the aim of promoting health.

On top of these two apparently incompatible narratives of health care, policymakers have to confront two apparently incompatible perspectives on the notion of good care. While both private and public health care planning takes the perspective of the insurance buyer with regard to budgeting and marginal analysis (Gibson et al., 2006), under current legal doctrines of professional liability, caregivers are guilty of malpractice whenever they fail to prescribe care that, according to prevailing medical practice, offers some net medical benefit to the patient and that the sick patient wants to have (Aaron, 2008).

According to the prevailing legal frameworks in the West, health insurance policies are considered "adhesion contracts." This term applies to contracts whose terms and conditions are dictated by one side, usually the one that is significantly stronger and better informed, while the other party to the contract is in a position of "take it or leave it." This means that people buy insurance policies because they feel obliged to have health insurance, not that they consciously agree with every term and condition in the policy. Because of this imbalance, in cases of dispute about the meaning of adhesion contracts the courts tend to interpret them in favor of the weak party. As Clark Havighurst observes, this is the reason why courts find the "patient's reasonable expectations at the time of treatment prescription" to be the standard of interpretation of health insurances (Havighurst, 1992). The outcome is a cultural construction according to which patients' health care choices when sick constitute a gold standard of their needs; any kind of "rationing" is by default an exploitation of the weak, the unreasonable fear of small risks and the low chances of success notwithstanding. This means that we have grown culturally to hold every marginal utility a patient might desire when sick a kind of basic right, even if it is risky and even if he or she did not anticipate the desire for it while still healthy. Altogether, we need an alternative conceptualization of health insurance in order to come up with a fair, autonomy-oriented instrument of planning and allocating resources. The conception of insurance must also reflect the special roles of health and life in democratic societies as well as the psychological and economic biases that are typical of coping with life crises.

In this paper I approach the problem of bedside rationing from the broader perspective of the kinds of insurance schemes for which people may and may not be able to contract. I will show that even libertarian markets are not open to every kind of insurance scheme chosen by buyers and providers, and that proper understanding of reasonable health care contracts illuminates schemes of bedside rationing that are reasonable, even desirable, from the point of view of the autonomous patient.

I will first explore different kinds of rationing and different conceptualizations of "health needs." By pointing out some gaps in the current discourse on both issues, I will import insights from psychology and economics in order to proffer an approach to decisions regarding resource consumption in clinical care. Arguably, other challenges to allocation policies exist, but the problem in hand is special because it undermines the very instrument of allocation policies—public deliberation. The literature on allocation asks: "who should make the decision" and "whose interests may play a role in allocation decisions." Some authors believe that clinicians must never make such decisions (Levinsky, 1984); others point out that physicians cannot avoid rationing and that the public trusts physicians more than administrators and other potential decision makers (e.g., Hall, 1997b). I will argue that in a properly hedged insurance scheme, the physician's perspective may be regarded as the most representative of patients' genuine health care interests. This requires high standards of freedom from conflicts of interest, separation of the basic interests of life and health from other interests, especially financial ones, and understanding the psychology of personal autonomy.

■ THE TRIAGE MODEL

Perhaps the oldest system of health care rationing is triage. Napoleon's chief medical officer, Baron Dominique Jean Larrey, realized that a fair and rational approach had to be applied to the care of battlefield casualties (Winslow, 1982, ch.1). Today, triage is divided into the conventional and the nonconventional (Gross, 2006, p. 145). In conventional triage, all patients receive the care they need because those who are made to wait have no urgent needs and those who need immediate lifesaving care are treated with urgency. In nonconventional triage, due to lack of sufficient resources some patients will not receive all the care they need because others will be cared for. When a health care provider performs a nonconventional triage, he or she knowingly lets a patient suffer health damage because another patient will receive care.

The staple answer to problems of allocation is the one formulated by the oldest system of triage. First, conventional triage aims at the selection of those who cannot wait. Then, nonconventional triage is performed with the selection of those whose health care needs are more salient. Philosophers and policymakers debate the criteria of saliency, but an additional aspect of the problem is that regardless of expert opinion, few patients consider their needs as "less salient." When denied a service and when requested to wait, patients often feel profound resentment. Especially in the age of autonomy-oriented medicine, clinicians feel morally and psychologically uncomfortable when they seek to withhold a medical service from a patient who articulates his or her entitlement to it. When this is done for the benefit of another person, a sense of exploitation aggravates the situation. When done for the sake of saving money, nothing seems more vexing.

In order to seek a way out of this impasse, let's revisit the notion of "health care need." In the context of this chapter it is not necessary to explicate fully the notion of "health care need" in general, but to observe that a health care need *that stands a chance in competing for scarce resources* must be an objective need (Barilan, 2012, pp. 105–106). Objectivity means that the judgment of need can be established independently of anybody's attitudes, feelings, and valuations. The reason why objectivity is an essential property of any need that is going to compete for scarce resources is the incommensurability of subjective goods. Public reason can compare, even if roughly, objective properties, not subjective ones. When subjective claims are struggling for attention we are talking primarily about wishes, not needs. Moreover, as Bernard Williams explains, the moral and political value of liberty is not about granting equal consideration to every wish and desire, but rather about an "impartial standpoint" from which desires are evaluated and considered (Williams, 2005, p. 94). In reference to health care, the "impartial standpoint" is the objectivity of needs.

As defined by Norman Daniels, a basic good is objectively known as a human need and it is objectively attributable to persons. Food, shelter, and cure of many diseases are known to be goods for human beings, and a need for any may be identified even without asking the needy about their wishes (Daniels, 1981). It seems that typically, objective needs are also "basic needs," because they are those things every human needs and can identify in oneself and others.[1]

But Daniels' definition is insufficient for problems of allocation. Let us consider a set of services according to four parameters: expected benefit, the chances that the expected benefits are realized, risk of harm, and financial costs. Resuscitation of a drowning person typifies the "Rule of Rescue"—the benefit is enormous (saving a whole life and restoring full health), the chances of success are quite high, harm is negligible, and the costs to the performer are minor.

Relative to rescuing a drowning person, hospitalizing a patient with metastatic cancer and pneumonia in the ICU is expected to yield much less benefit, with lower levels of confidence. A stay in the ICU might produce complications such as nosocomial infection, and the costs are huge. It is tempting not to admit this patient on grounds of safety (worry about complications), while cost awareness is a factor as well.

Some cutting-edge immunotherapies for cancer offer minor benefits (e.g., increased survival in the range of a weeks) at very low risk (they do not have the toxic effects of traditional chemotherapy), but the chances of success are low (in some studies no more than 10% of patients benefit) and the costs are skyrocketing.

A routine CT scan following head trauma might bring substantial benefit (early detection of intracranial bleeding), but rarely (the vast majority do not bleed). But every CT scan also brings with it a minor but measurable risk of harm from radiation and minor costs that, when multiplied by all those who sustain head injury, amount to an immense burden on few patients (who will be harmed) and the health care system.

Consider immediate availability of PET scanning for the detection of possible metastases. There is evident psychological benefit in not letting patients anxiously await information about their disease status for weeks; the accuracy of the exam and the chances of risk are the same (i.e., they do not change if the patient waits for a few weeks), but immediate availability of PET scanning is quite expensive.

Some emerging immunotherapies are especially challenging. Suppose drug A is immensely effective, side effect–free, and very costly. As long as the number of patients needing it is very low, provision of this drug falls under the Rule of Rescue; it would be exactly like spending millions on rescuing a person from a burning skyscraper. But once the projected burden on society rises significantly, the Rule of Rescue does not apply anymore because the circumstances cannot be considered "extraordinary" (see Cookson, McCabe, & Tsuchiya, 2008). Policymakers must incorporate such costs in their ordinary planning (see Fleck, 2009, ch. 6).

It is not difficult to see that all of the services just listed meet Daniels's criteria of "basic need," and that the patients described would wish to be resuscitated, to be cared for in the ICU when they have cancer and pneumonia, to have a chance with a risk-free chemotherapy, to rule out bleeding after a head injury, to have their PET scan as soon as possible, and to receive the medicine that will certainly help them substantially without producing side effects.

However, if we consider people's real choices the picture becomes more complicated. When faced with a choice of a health insurance plan, many people are likely to opt for a cheaper premium at the price of not having access to the novel immune-modulating therapies for cancer or waiting list free–health care. In the same vein, by means of democratic deliberation the state might exclude such treatments from its socialized health care coverage. On the one hand, the doctor is expected to act upon the informed choice of the patient (either choice of insurance or democratic decision making); on the other hand, physicians are educated to conduct shared decision making during the clinical encounters with their patients. Does a doctor act ethically when she withholds from the uninsured patient a medically reasonable treatment that he now wishes to receive? Before we try to tackle this question, let's consider the following two thought experiments.

Imagine a person who wishes not to have medical insurance at all, and even waives his right to resuscitation in exchange for a tax break by the state. This proposal is a hypothetical thought experiment precisely because nobody has the liberty to contract away the right to life. Even if the person in question has no health insurance, and has evaded paying taxes all his life, he will be resuscitated; and in situations of triage, the urgency-of-need criteria will prevail, not the kind of insurance he and other patients in need of the same health service might have.[2] Patients have the power to refuse lifesaving medical care; some countries and states recognize a right to assisted suicide and euthanasia. But this is not the thought experiment I have in mind. I am talking about a person who has waived his right to resuscitation in exchange for some money, but upon collapsing in the street he does wish for care and does not want to die. He is just like millions of young men and women who smoke and drink and engage in reckless activities against the explicit warnings of their health care professionals, but once they become sick and injured they also consider themselves entitled to health care, no matter how costly. Societies that abide by the values of human dignity respect the wish for care, because life is a higher value than honoring a contract; health is irreducible to pecuniary losses.

Here is the second thought experiment. Suppose a wealthy and health-minded person is willing to pay as much as asked for the best health insurance policy conceivable, an insurance plan that will grant him all health services possible with no waiting or rationing at all. Whatever procedure doctors recommend will be available at high quality and immediately. Nevertheless, it seems unlikely that this person will be given an MRI scan indicated for the detection of residual disease before an uninsured patient is scanned for a medical emergency (e.g., aneurysm of a blood vessel in the brain). Once again, we confront a deeply entrenched social norm according to which money and personal preferences cannot trump the commitment of clinicians to the salient health needs of their patients. Prior to any business contract in health care comes the implied contract between the profession and the public and between doctor and patient (Haakonssen, 1997, 125; Barilan, 2009). This implied, unspoken contract does not allow doctors to grant a minor health benefit higher priority than a lifesaving intervention. It is also true that part of the implicit contract between the medical profession and the public is the liberty to offer in the private market any licensed service; however, this liberty does not encompass services whose very nature takes priority over other needy people, such as a promise to always receive medical care before the less insured.

Three Categories of Health Care Services

In the light of the above thought experiments, and in accordance with the formative role of the values of life and dignity in society, I suggest we divide all health care services into three categories:

1. Services that cannot be waived (cannot be contracted away or alienated—see Radin, 1987), only refused in real time and under strict regulations.

2. Services that cannot be bought even when the prospective buyer and an able and legal provider agree on the price.
3. Services that doctors provide only if the patient pays for them directly or has contracted for them through a specific commitment (private or public insurance for specific services).

The scope of the third category varies from societies that subscribe to state-funded universal and equal health care to societies that do not. But the pattern persists. For example, an individual residing in the United States will receive emergency care from any hospital emergency department as required by the federal government, regardless of whether he has insurance). Nobody can sell to the public his or her right to emergency care.

As for the services in the third category, the literature offers a few principles for ethical rationing based on fairness and participatory rational deliberation. If we recall Daniels' definition of "health care need," it depends on attribution. It must be "objectively attributable to persons." Any deliberative scheme includes the patient (either as a private customer or as indirectly represented through democratic governance) as a contributing party to the process of attribution. The problem is that people's ascriptions of needs vary considerably. When a person contemplates whether to purchase insurance that covers an implantable cardiac device, he might deem this unworthy of the money; when the very same person is given a diagnosis of a propensity to fatal arrhythmias, he suddenly considers the device an absolute necessity. But this is not all. In the waiting room sits another patient who had invested in a better health insurance plan, who needs the very same implantable device, but whose risk for contracting a fatal arrhythmia is five times lower than the person who does not have the appropriate coverage. The doctor is haunted by the fundamental question of whether the device should be classified under either the first or second health care service category that I have specified above, or both. The answer is not likely to be found by means of public deliberation, unless we have compelling reasons to give more weight either to the moment when the healthy person is buying insurance, as more representative of the autonomy of the person, or the moment when treatment is needed and prescribed.

We have reached a kind of *aporia*. We have learned that the prevailing methods of accountable public deliberation and liberty-based personal choices may result in conflicting outcomes, depending on two crucial factors—the circumstances of both public and personal deliberation, and choice relative to the occurrence of the need. Because circumstances influence people's choices, policymakers need to know which circumstances of deliberation are more authentic in terms of moral probity, democratic legitimacy, or respect for personal autonomy. Because of its recursive nature (it is a question about the very structuring of public deliberation), it does not make sense to subject this question to public deliberation. In the absence of a fuller understanding of human choice and democratic governance, we are at risk of wavering between one mode of reasoning and another, of suffering the throes of doubt about whether allocation is moral and prudent or unjust and harsh. I will now try to mobilize insights from moral psychology and philosophy in order to sketch a way out of this conundrum.

A recurrent theme in psychology and economics is that people tend to make myopic choices, which means that they prefer immediate gain, even if puny, at the expense of sacrificing much greater good in the long run. Only later on, when they have to face the consequences of their myopic choices, do they regret them (Ainslie, 2001; Offer, 2006, ch. 4). People are also poor predictors of their future state of well-being, which means that people's projections of their levels of happiness and misery onto a future scenario (e.g., when I am 64) tend not to match their actual reports (e.g., reported wellbeing at 64) (Gilbert, 2006). The bioethical discourse appreciates now the challenge of reconstruction of the authentic autonomy of patients (so-called "effective autonomy") as opposed to the wishes of the moment (Schwab, 2006; Barilan, 2011).

Admittedly, people have the right to change their minds "autonomously." But they do not have the right to exploit respect for autonomy to "game the system" for personal advantage at the expense of others who have paid premiums into the system for many years. But this is not my concern here; I do not address manipulation and free riding, but the more fundamental problem of determining the proper timing of allocation decisions that are made in good faith.

I may spend lots of money on fashion, not saving toward future needs, downplaying my projected needs in old age. When the future need is personally or socially critical, society might force me not to spend irresponsibly. By means of democratic deliberation we institute obligatory pension plans in the same way individual people pledge in advance a monthly allotment for saving. Such ploys are "commitment devices." One of the simplest such devices is an alarm clock. People who anticipate their own laziness often remove the snooze button or ask a friend to shake them out of bed. When the person keeps control over the device, or when the interference with autonomy is minor (forcing you to wake up), the commitment devices are weak. When the person has no option at the time of action (it is illegal not to set aside money in a pension plan or public health insurance), the device is stronger. It receives its legitimacy from a combination of four factors—first, during a significant period of his or her life, the person endorses the device; it is compatible with his/her authentic autonomy. Second, the device is the best way known to protect a fundamental and objective good of the person. The more fundamental and self-evident the value is, the less likely are we to believe that other personal or social considerations might be stronger. Hence, saving life by means of curative care is clearly more fundamental a goal than extending life by a few months only; 80 chances out of 100 of success are self-evidently more compelling than 10 chances out of 100. The third factor is legitimization by means of direct personal choice or indirect democratic legislation and governance. Public deliberation is also necessary for determining proportionate judgments, such as the classification according to the above three categories of treatment that bear 50% chance of extending life by 2 years. The fourth factor is the restriction of coercion to a milder kind of enforcement. Compulsory taxation is much less obnoxious, morally and psychologically, than imposition on the body and mind.

Turning our attention back to the allocation problem of the uninsured individual's need for the implantable cardiac device, we may observe that a man who squanders all of his salary on beer and computer games cannot blame anybody for not having saved enough money to buy a car. He should do without it. But if the implantable cardiac device belongs to the first category, the irresponsible person should receive it nevertheless. If the implantable device belongs to the second category as well, he is entitled to have it at the expense of responsible people who need the device much less. Put in other words, it is up to the doctor to calculate the risk-benefit ratio of different patients in order to determine whether one "needs" a medical service "much less" than the other. This is an inevitable task of every doctor who is committed to saving life before she is committed to specific business and labor contracts.

Things become even more complicated when we realize that conventional triage is hardly evidence based and, consequently, it depends on very wide safety margins and deep trust in doctors. Busy doctors may allow a febrile) but not septic) patient to lie 2 hours in the waiting area of their emergency department, but not 2 days. Health care systems in affluent countries do not corner doctors to decide whether 10 or 15 hours of waiting are safe as well. Since it is unethical to conduct controlled studies that aim to trace the curve of safety as it slopes down in proportion to patients' waiting time, our epistemological blindness dictates generous margins of safety. But unless checked somehow, margins of safety may become too costly, too risky of nosocomial harm, and impractically wide.

From "Rationing" to Sophisticated Decision Making

At this stage I wish to collect my observations into a more coherent approach toward the problem of "bedside rationing." A reasonable health care program should delineate with a broad brush health care needs that fall into the first and second categories—those treatments that must be put beyond the powers of the market and unchecked free choice. But, on the other hand, over-generosity that bites too deeply into the third zone is problematic. Beyond its humongous costs, it is likely to shower patients with risky and unnecessary medical interventions and to eliminate personal choice from the planning of care.

In one recent study in a geriatric hospital, researchers discontinued 311 medications from a cohort of 70 patients following predetermined criteria. The results were striking: 88% of patients reported globally improved well-being and there was no increase in mortality (Garfinkel & Mangin, 2010). Had these drugs been discontinued with the intention of saving money, an outcry condemning ageism would have broken out. In another study, researchers followed acutely ventilated patients who had been denied hospitalization in the ICU on grounds of limited resources. It was found that these patients fared quite well on the medical floor (Lieberman et al., 2010). This fascinating study has all sorts of ethical problems (Barilan, 2010). Among other things it showed a worrisome pattern of patient discrimination on the basis of age. Yet, without attempting to justify or condemn the practice it documented, I allow myself to conjecture that had these patients been approached 10 years earlier and offered to invest a certain amount of money so as to guarantee them an ICU bed in case they needed mechanical ventilation at old age, many of them would have declined. But had they been told on the day before falling ill that they were going to be sent to a regular floor while a younger patient is admitted to the ICU, they would have been exasperated. People are "myopic," and those who experience suffering and anxiety are even more so. They grant excessive priority to the wish of the moment, as if they have little insight into long-term values and needs.

On top of the myopia bias, two additional factors confound public deliberation and rational choice on health care allocation. The first is the publicity bias. A halo of media hype accompanies services that are paid for directly and are marketed by for-profit sellers, while little is done to advertise other health care goods. We are bombarded by messages on the value of prescription drugs for health and happiness, while nobody promotes the importance of the time a nurse and a doctor spend with a single patient or the value of foot care for diabetic patients. Economists have described the publicity bias in general (Frank, 1999, pp. 174–177; Offer, 2006, ch. 6). I think it is even more consequential in medicine. Precisely because a well-ordered society guarantees a minimum tier of healthcare to everyone (first category), goods associated with this level of care are never promoted publicly. They are always at risk of marginalization. A patient feels abused when he is not prescribed a drug about which he has learned from an ad or a TV program. No publicity underscores the value of foot care, of safety measures in the bathroom, and of many other items whose impact on health and life is exceedingly more important than other marketable medical services. Sale promotions are likely to accompany treatments and procedures that are less likely to be prescribed by doctors and accepted by patients. Such promotions tend to describe goods as essential needs and to divert attention from futile and risky use. One more example is the drug *varenicline* (Chantix), which is prescribed in order to help quit smoking. Quitting is a highly valued health behavior worthy of much investment, but the marketing campaign downplays the fact that unaided cessation is the most common and efficient method known so far (Chapman & MacKenzie, 2010). When the choice of drug is presented in this light, the side effects as well as the costs might look very different. It might be preposterous to consider "rationing" the withholding of effective treatment because of the availability of a free and safe alternative. It is quite possible that some patients cannot quit without pharmacological assistance, but it is also possible that an "effective drug" might fail as well. All in all, the "free market" environment of health care marginalizes the impact of noncommercialized but still immensely valued goods such as self-help and thorough doctor–patient counseling.

Thus, despite a tradition that values personal care for the sick, a growing number of patients are prescribed expensive medical services but cannot have somebody to listen to them properly and to help them wash and eat. The publicity bias shifts everybody's attention (i.e., public, patients, clinicians, providers, advocates) from the very essence of care as an interpersonal event to commodified care and even more powerfully toward commercialized services. We are driven to spend less on the basic and absolutely necessary and to feel more obliged to the marketable. Consequently, we shift our priorities toward the less needed and more preference-sensitive aspects of care.

An offshoot of the publicity bias is the public and professional enthusiasm for technology in general and information technology (IT) in particular. Technological advances reduce the price of services (e.g., each CT scan is cheaper) but tend to increase spending overall (many more CTs and many more ancillary expenses related to false-positive results and iatrogenic complications). This is known as the Jevon effect or "Jevon's paradox"—technological progress that increases the efficiency with which a resource is used tends to increase (rather than decrease) the rate of consumption of that resource (Alcott, 2005). Besides, in the consumerist culture, painstaking and laborious care of pressure sores in the hospital or home calls by primary care providers are much less inspiring than computerized telemedicine. Despite the fact that there is no definitive evidence that investment in hospital computing causes reduced costs and improved quality of care (Himmelstein, Wright, & Woolhandler, 2010; Restuccia et al., 2012)[3], academics as well as the public are more open to rationing care than to diversion of health care moneys to basic interpersonal health care and preventive medicine.

Related to the publicity bias is the personalization bias. When people are denied personal services such as medicines, exams, and appointments, they feel personally offended. We are much less sensitive when a nonpersonal— but no less needed—good is compromised. A policy favoring generic over patented drugs might be considered "rationing," but reduced standards of hospital hygiene are not. Patients do not say much when health care moneys are diverted to management and marketing, but they respond with moral rage when made to wait for an exam or make a copayment (see Frank, 1999, ch. 4).

A third complication is the unnatural pricing of health care. According to neoclassical economics, prices are set "naturally" following the balance of supply and demand. A fundamental tenet of economics is that prices are negotiable, never fixed like facts of nature. When set too high, demand wanes accordingly; when too low, overconsumption erodes availability. But in health care the most expensive goods and services are expensive because, due to patent laws and market failures, the supply side enjoys a monopoly while the demand side is psychologically incapable of not procuring the promises of health and life (the choice is unconscionable or close to it). Whenever society commits itself to the provision of a certain service (suppose it is considered obligatory by the rule of rescue to provide the implantable cardiac devices), two outcomes ensue. There is less pressure on sellers to control prices, and there is a hidden incentive for consumers to ask for more. When these consumers are exposed to publicity efforts on behalf of the sellers, a vicious circle ensues. It accelerates health care costs and confounds autonomous judgments. Additionally, as long as the supply side is not competitive, the more "needed" a health care service becomes the more likely it is that society practically pushes it to the limits of affordability. In the industrialized nations, much of the need to "ration" health care is a product of market failures and inflated perceptions of "health needs," and much less is due to genuine lack of resources in society.

There are two ways to cope with this self-defeating situation. One way is to make supply more flexible (for example by altering patent laws; see Pogge, 2005), directing public spending toward research and development, structuring care that is not based on fee-for-service). Indeed, it has been argued forcefully that an "imperfect", flexible patent regulation, best promotes technological and economic development (Dutton, 1984). The other endorses the morality of refusal of the public to pay, even at the price of some people's lives, but with the intention of lowering prices and thus saving many more people in the long run.[4] Neither method looks promising unless an independent and effective examination of the structure of clinical decision making is made by the public, patients, clinicians, and administrators.

An illustrative example of a structural failure is the pricing of patented medicines; some cost in the range of dozens of thousands of dollars a year (Goozner, 2012). The universal justification for these high prices is not marginal production costs of each pill, but the enormous burden of research as well as the high risk of failure that accompanies the development of every new potential drug. Much of this research is carried out in the form of clinical experiments on volunteers. It is unethical to represent participation in research as beneficial ("the therapeutic misconception"); paying patients "market" fees for participation is highly controversial and rarely done, mainly because ethics and research regulations require that consent to participation in clinical trials occur under circumstances that minimize the possibility of undue influence (Grady, 2005). Here is the paradoxical structural failure. Because significant sums of money might distort the judgment of patients, they are "protected" from being paid for their role in the development of a new drug. But when the drug is already on the market, the desperate situation of many "incurable" and suffering patients is not considered a potential distortion of their consent to buy very expensive and risky drugs. In this way, the public market share in the development of new drugs is eliminated, and the pricing power of the pharmaceuticals goes unbridled. (Nothing has been said yet about the clinicians' inability to ask "market" fees for their roles as clinical investigators and the government's investment in grants that contribute to basic research).

The last bias is the status quo bias (Kahneman, Knetch, & Thaler, 1999). When applied to allocation of health care, there is a prevailing impression that current or recent practice is the "gold standard" and any new policy aimed at efficiency amounts to "rationing" and downgrading of care. Interestingly, a considerable body of research shows that many patients do not receive recommended and nonrationed care (McGlynn et al., 2003). One notorious example is underprescription of cheap drugs, "beta blockers," to patients who need them in order to avoid heart attacks and early death (Egred, 2005; Soumerai, 1997). Patients and policymakers might better seek methods to optimize use of nonrationed and necessary care, rather than focus on optimizing inclusions of "new technologies".[5]

All in all, with the problems of myopia and biases in mind, we find ourselves facing two interrelated problems; namely, how doctors allocate resources at the bedside, and which hypothetical voice of the patient should count in the processes of allocation should we wish to avoid both reckless spending and undertreatment. The question is not merely "who decides." The framing of our question is this: With acceptance of the inevitable fact that resentment is unavoidable (moments of disagreement with allocation decisions are inevitable), which structure of decision making best represents patients' autonomy and the values of medicine?

A Reasonable Range of "Ulysses Contracts" of Allocation of Health Care Resources

The emerging answer is that a certain range of health care services or needs fall in between the absolutely necessary and the dispensable. Ideally, informed patients should discuss the available knowledge with their clinicians and develop an informed health care plan. The problem is that every patient and pressure group promotes aggressively the services they care about, usually ignoring other personal needs and the needs of other patients and stakeholders.

Nobody takes responsibility for developing aggressively and self-assuredly comprehensive health care planning that is endorsable both at the time of deliberating the coverage of insurance policies and at the bedside.

I wish to contend that, given a reasonable delineation of the first two categories, any fair (i.e., unbiased and democratically governed) rationing of services within the third category will be reasonable as well. It is not necessarily harmful and unjust. Put in other words, if a well-ordered society allows people to opt out of insurance coverage for certain procedures (say, treatment A for indication B in circumstances C), it is also reasonable for doctors to withhold such treatments from patients without specific coverage (i.e., if there is no specific mentioning of treatment A in indication B in the insurance policy) on grounds of limited resources. When put this way, clinicians at the bedside will have a sound argument that is also compatible with the ethics of clinical decision making. They will understand that saying no at the bedside is not necessarily opposed to autonomy and the overall good of the patient. The elimination of rationing in the first two categories will also diffuse much of the claim patients may raise in the name of contracts of adhesion. If it is possible to ration care whenever any healthy reasonable patient is likely to endorse it, then it is not unreasonable to argue that the rationing that is carried out at the bedside is indeed according to the patient's autonomous choice and respectful of his human dignity.

This key contention is neither a direct statement about the nature of "human needs" nor about circumscribing the range of claim rights in a given sociocultural context. It is about the implications of the social acceptance of certain needs as "basic" in the sense that their presence makes a strong moral claim on society. Such needs are placed beyond anybody's subjective choice—they are given to everybody, and nobody has the power to contract them away (only to refuse them in real time—Barilan, 2012, pp. 180–189). Once it is reasonable to neglect a foreseeable need, there cannot be an absolute moral claim by the unprepared needy to get it. Their claim to assistance is only *prima facie* and, consequently, subjected to constraining considerations as well, even at the bedside. It is natural for human needs to have a subjective valuation built into them, but because our commitment to meet claim rights is anchored in a sense of duty to meet basic needs, not personal desires, we have to realize that whereas an objective need may create a claim right, a qualified need makes a qualified claim right. Classifying health care services into any of the three categories requires public deliberation that is informed by scientific knowledge and commitment to the ethos of human dignity.

Any moral claim to health care is a claim for money. When claim rights are contaminated by wishes of the moment (either the moment of health care planning or the moment of the clinical encounter at "the bedside"), financial considerations regarding the benefit of no less salient needs of either self or others may bear on the decision at the bedside. If we wish to keep decisions of allocation free from nonmedical considerations, clinical judgments regarding urgency and saliency of services should prevail. This is not a novel task for caregivers. Since the invention of conventional triage, the wise and fair division of attention and other resources of care has always been at the heart of clinical practice.

The decision whether to start dialysis for an 80-year-old patient with heart failure, diabetes, and some other problems—or whether to provide mechanical ventilation when, on top of all of these problems, this old man contracts pneumonia—is far from straightforward. Hence, although we are dealing with the possibility of a basic need (saving life), it is not an objective need. The pairing of "dialysis" with "the condition of the patient" cannot produce a "health care need" without a considerable input of the patient's values, preferences, and psychosocial situation.

So far, the concept of "health care need" is detached from considerations of costs. It must only be established on scientific grounds that the matching of the intervention to the particular patient is likely to produce a substantial health benefit. But the disconnection of need from costs also entails the nontransitivity of duty from need. Having recognized renal failure and respiratory failure as possible health needs of the patient does not mean that the public must pay for dialysis and mechanical ventilation (see Hasman, Hope, & Østterdal, 2006). If it is reasonable for the patient to decline such treatments and if it is reasonable for the person not to procure health insurance that covers them in such circumstances, then it is not immoral for the public to refuse to underwrite them, at least as long as the money saved is channeled to health care needs that are more reasonable to tend to.[6] At this very point, it is crucial to distinguish between profit or incentive-oriented and other kinds of financial considerations. For the reasons listed above, market-oriented modes of reasoning are likely to produce biased and inefficient care. But efficient management of resources is crucial for the provision of more needed care to more needy patients; it may also help protect patients from the harms of overtreatment.

Regardless of the considerations of costs, precisely because at least in certain situations it is reasonable for such patients to forgo dialysis and mechanical ventilation, doctors have a clinical duty not to administer them automatically. Rather, they should attempt a process of shared decision making with the patient or his proxy. The worst misconception might result when doctors infer from the administrative availability of very expensive services that it is also obligatory to prescribe them, that if a dialysis machine or an ICU bed is available for everybody then it is necessarily immoral not to let the patient have them. One must also not infer from availability the default status of treatment. Society might decide to provide dialysis care to the very aged should patients choose it following proper counseling, and yet it may not be true that doctors should recommend such treatment and frame it as the default practice (see Barilan, 2010b).

A recent study showed that mortality did not increase among patients who declined to initiate dialysis at the time recommended by their nephrologists. They fared less well in terms of biological and quality of life indexes (Thilly et al., 2011). However, because of the very burdensome nature of dialysis, its impacts on quality of life, and its psychosocial aspects, it is very difficult to tell whether the patients who were labeled "noncompliant" actually chose badly for themselves. They certainly did not risk human lives. And the tendency to delay dialysis was not exclusively a choice among a subset of patients (16% in the study); in many cases doctors understood and supported such choices. It follows that, although dialysis is considered a basic health service, delay of dialysis could be a reasonable choice for many patients.[7] I infer that it can also be a reasonable act intended to reduce health care expenditure, provided that even less reasonable services have been eliminated first and that the money saved is channeled toward services that are more reasonable to provide. Otherwise we risk unfair treatment of the vulnerable (those whose care is easily cut) for the benefit of the strong (those who will not let you cut costs).

What would constitute reasonableness in such circumstances? When a significant number of ordinary persons choose a course of action, we have a necessary but not sufficient condition for reasonableness. But this is not enough, because many people smoke, drink, and overeat in ways that medicine (and they themselves) consider unhealthy. Hence, reasoning based on scientific knowledge and moral values is another condition. Third, reasonable choices must be coherent with other choices and values. Although "reasonableness" and public deliberation are "incompletely theorized" and incompletely theorizeable, they have their own standards of coherence, and the bodies of knowledge it appeals to have theirs (see Ruger, 2010, chap. 3 on Kenneth Arrow's impossibility theorem).

Ethical Bedside Rationing

At this stage, I wish to lay out more fully the conception I propound of ethical bedside rationing. If we have a health care system that provides for services that are deemed unreasonable to refrain from buying insurance to cover, then we have a domain of indications (an indication is a match between a service and a patient thickly described[8]) in which it is reasonable both to provide the service and to withhold it (even though the default recommendation might be either to prescribe or not to prescribe it). The choice might be motivated by cost considerations, public health (e.g., worry about the production of resistant strains of bacteria), or other values of medicine. As long as the health budget is a relatively hermetic and rational apparatus, and every penny saved would be directed toward meeting more salient or more urgent health needs, the scheme would be moral.

It is still possible that one day society will not be able to afford even the services in the first two categories. However, there is plenty of data indicating that most health care expenditure is produced by the third category. Besides, I have suggested that in order to reduce prices it is moral to alter the legal and regulative structure of our health care system—for example, to decline the purchase of expensive services even if they belong to the first two categories. So there is much to do in the way of cutting costs before the most needed services become candidates for rationing.

For this scheme to work well and ethically, five conditions should apply. First, citizens ought to be empowered politically and financially so as to be able to contract for themselves health insurance for the basic tier of services, namely those it is unreasonable not to have when needed. This process is labeled "effective citizenship" (Rhys et al. 2006). Second, as explained in the previous paragraph, the health budget should be a closed and rational apparatus. In this context "rational" means "reasonable" as defined in the previous section. Third, the health system contains enforceable and adequately broad categories one and two.

The fourth condition touches upon the background ethos of health care in a society. If health care is merely a marketable good like many other consumer products and services, without any background value to it other than freedom of creativity and choice, consumers (the market name for patients) might think that the highest degree of health possible is a meaningful personal goal; that they need to achieve this goal; that they should be able to spend as little as possible on healthcare (i.e., be economically efficient); and that when specific health needs show up, they should receive the maximum relevant health services their personal and tax moneys entitle them to. Providers (the market name for caregivers) have the duty to give nothing beyond the mere words on the insurance policy. When consumers and providers maximize their respective interests (more services for less money vs. more money for fewer services) health care reaches Pareto optimality—a state of allocation of resources in which it is impossible to make any one individual better off without making at least one individual worse off. Within such a paradigm, rationing does not exist at all: either the consumer receives what their providers owe them by contract or not. The market is either efficient or not. Medicine has little interest in this paradigm, because the fundamental values of medicine—health, welfare, and human dignity—do not correlate with Pareto optimality at all (Sen, 1993).

Indeed, in all known societies, health care has a very strong background value that prevails upon society to extend some basic care even for those who have not contracted any insurance, and to regulate insured care so as to protect some basic needs of people regardless of the written word or the financial interests of the provider, whose duty is to factor in these risks in its business model (Brown, 1991). This is borne out by the historical emergence of triage. The French Republic had a clear background, even if implicit, of commitment to its wounded soldiers. The earlier methods of battlefield care, which ranged between nothing to preferential care to the nobility, had to be done away with in favor of a need-oriented scheme. Today, every well-ordered society considers itself committed to some level of health care for its citizens, even for aliens who happen to pass by. This background ethos renders the problem of "bedside rationing" both meaningful and manageable. It entails a commitment to divide fairly a common pie of care. Any method of division that is free from bias and that is "reasonable" would be "fair."

Virtually every human society has a hard core of cheap and unquestionably beneficial medical services (cheap in the context of the material culture of that society). Compliance with some of these services is partial. In the industrialized countries, one notable example is amputation of a diabetic foot, especially when the patient is old and afflicted with other serious conditions. However, within the hard core of care, the service is so cheap and its expected impact so marked (a saved life), that compliance status does not affect the moral claim of the service relative to others.

At the edge of this core lie services whose overall desirability is less evident and consequently in need of exploration, deliberation, and pluralistic approaches. Since people tend to downplay health needs while healthy and overemphasize desire for anything even remotely labeled treatment while sick, allocation schemes cannot rely on people's articulated preferences exclusively. It is not merely a question of finding a hypothetical deliberative moment that is the most representative of citizens' autonomy; rather, it is to acknowledge that in both consumer and solidarity contexts every practical deliberative point of view is distorted, and reliance only on the output of preference-based deliberation is incompatible with the values of medicine.

Hence input from public health, evidence-based medicine, and similar disciplines should aid the healthy to appreciate future risks. Good clinical practice should protect desperate and suffering patients from overconsuming health resources in futile and even harmful patterns. This is the fifth condition, which is the institution of a scientifically informed commitment device involving health care planning that allows bedside rationing to be representative of patients' autonomy even if they do not think so at the point of sickness

We can now see the three conditions for successful bedside rationing. The first is a distributive system in which routine bedside rationing occurs only in the third category (above, p. 12)[9]; the second is reliance on reasonable criteria and an unbiased decision process. The choice might be private or by means of democratic deliberation. The third is that doctors, and hopefully also patients and the public, understand the process of rationing as a commitment device representing people's genuine values. Genuine values are the values a person endorses systematically, over relatively long periods of time, over a broad range of circumstances (see Schwab, 2006). The latter two conditions support each other. Precisely because the acceptance of a commitment device entails the suspension of direct self-control, trust in those who are entrusted with control must be quasi absolute. In the next and last section, I will elaborate on the notion of a commitment device.

Inserting a Wedge between "The Market" and "Rationing"

If we conceive of health care only in terms of the market, then patients wish to maximize the goods they receive in exchange for their money (fee-for-service, insurance and taxes paid) and consider the withholding of care as unjust denial of basic needs. Within the paradigm of the market, every denial of a health care service is the subjugation of the value of life to the value of money and the subordination of the health of the vulnerable to the financial interests of the strong.

But it is possible to construe the situation in a different way. We might regard health care plans and clinical guidelines as "commitment devices" (Offer, 2006, pp. 48–52). The oldest known such device is Odysseus' order to his sailors to tie him to the mast of his ship and not to release him no matter how strongly he might beg them to do so. This scheme made Odysseus the only mortal who enjoyed the magnificent singing of the sirens, whose lure was so strong as to make every sailor steer his ship in their direction and crash it on the rocks, without dying (*Odyssey*, book 12).[10] "Ulysses contracts" (Ulysses is the Latin name of Odysseus) are very strong commitment devices because they entail direct imposition on the person while he or she is mentally competent, adequately informed, and nevertheless actively resisting the imposition. Such devices could be moral only when they serve a desire on a significantly and clearly higher order than the one it frustrates (see Davidson, 1981[1969]). The desire to stay alive is at a higher order than the cravings to hear the music of sirens or rush in their direction. Hence, prudent sailors employ a simple and weak commitment device, which is avoidance of approaching the area where the tempting music is heard. The cunning Odysseus managed to achieve more. He enjoyed the music and stayed alive, but only at the price of a stronger commitment device—being tied to the mast, remaining at the mercy of his crew, and undergoing the distressing experience of having his own freedom denied precisely at the moment when craving for it is as strong as can be.

The desire to have a stable and dignified pension is at a higher order than the desire to spend weekly on soccer and beer. The desire to be healthy and alive certainly ranks very high in any hierarchy of human values. Hence, in terms of health care planning, when supported by the five conditions listed in the previous section the choice of a health plan may be considered as a kind of commitment device.[11] If we wish for sustainable health care, we cannot help but contemplate strong, unbiased, and complex commitment devices.

The first commitment device is the commitment to a certain kind of health insurance—a commitment to levy taxes and to enforce the first two categories of care. The second commitment is to accept at the bedside choices made at the time of deliberation. It would be either the insurance plan chosen privately or the solidarity-based public coverage, decided by indirect democratic participation. Doctors cannot avoid their role in advising impartially during the formulation of the first commitment and in assessing patients' situations at the bedside while fulfilling the second. When an informed citizen decides that certain kinds of services are not worth the potential side effects or that the money would be better spent on different services (an "economic informed consent"— Hall, 1997, ch. 9) then, when sick and needy, the predetermined health care plan protects the patient from risky and unjust services that he might now crave. Thus rationing becomes just, rational, and respectful of the autonomy of the rationed patient. Odysseus trusted the navigation of his sailors because they were competent, loyal, and because he had ordered them to plug their ears with wax so as to make them deaf to the enchanting songs of the sirens. Patients would trust doctors' judgments only if they were skillful and shielded from financial and other external influences that might cloud judgment. This is not an easy task. According to the Medical Professionalism Charter, the renewed attention to professional and ethical values in medicine comes as a response to increasing financial pressures (ABIM, ACP-ASIM, 2002).[12]

In sum, when properly hedged and when appropriately protected from financial and political biases, the need to allocate scarce medical resources is not bad in itself. Finitude is part of the human condition. Sharing the inevitable implications of this finitude is emblematic of the values of solidarity and care that are the bedrock of medical practice. Considerations of cost might remind us that medicine is not innocuous and that when the evidence is skimpy or questionable, doing less is caring more—despite psychological biases and ploys of marketing. Societies that do not allow money to decide who will live and who will die have the moral power and structural capacity to use monetary considerations as means toward rational decision making that is efficient, safe, balanced, and promotes solidarity and justice.

Notes

1. For a literature survey on the definition of "basic needs" see Braybrooke, 1987, pp. 307–309 and Griffin, 2008, pp. 88–90.

2. According to the Geneva Convention, it is forbidden to care for less urgent fellow soldiers at the expense of more urgent wounded of the enemy. See Article 12 in the 1949

Protocol, http://www.icrc.org/ihl.nsf/FULL/365?OpenDocument (for further discussion see Barilan & Zuckerman, 2013). Only when resources are clearly not sufficient, as in the case of organ transplantation, are there ethicists who believe that noncontributors should receive low priority.

3. This is a very difficult question to answer at least because "investment" in information technology and quality control may assume protean meanings and forms.

4. Elsewhere I provide fuller argument in favor of refusal to cooperate with manipulation (e.g., even at the price of life it is moral to withhold available funds and not pay whenever there is deliberate exploitation of de facto monopoly in order to inflate prices of necessary commodities) (Barilan, 2012, pp. 210–211).

5. For additional market failures in health care see Hall, 1997, ch. 2. For a precautionary approach to cognitive biases in decision making see Jussim 2012.

6. Roughly, it may be said that a reasonable choice meets two conditions: (1) a substantial number of people choose this way, and (2) the choice has support by some recognized form of rational reasoning (e.g., economic and moral theory). Fairness in this context would entail good faith and, as much as possible, lack of bias.

7. Although in my view and in light of my clinical experience a 16% rate is quite considerable, in this chapter I argue in favor of a theoretical principle, not trying to establish whether this or that figure in this or that circumstance should make us conclude that it is reasonable to decline physicians' advice; that is, it might be in the genuine benefit of the patient to choose otherwise.

8. It is evident that the pair "end stage renal failure" and "dialysis" is too thin an indication. A thick enough description may include comorbidities, overall prognosis, and other relevant factors to the construance of the patient's well-being, at least terms of a holistic conceptualization of health.

9. Health care planning is always a matter of probabilities. Hence while a need to ration respiratory care on a daily basis might be an unacceptable routine, it might be reasonable to plan a health care system in which such a tragic choice occurs once a year. This observation brings forth the conclusion that clinicians cannot avoid events of bedside rationing, and consequently that explicit deliberation and education the matter is integral to, not a deviation from, excellence in medical practice.

10. Another early version, in the Talmudic literature. The sages infer the right of the government to levy taxes (Exodus 25) to the administration of necessary but very unpleasant medical care: "It is like a physician who ties a patient to a tree in order to cauterize a foot [ulcer]." (*Tosefta, Shekalim* 1:6).

11. Mark Hall (1997b, ch. 4) has already proposed medical insurance as a kind of commitment device. However, he does not distinguish between insurance as a means to balance personal financial interests with personal health and insurance as a means to balance the ante-factum tendency to accept undertreatment and neglect preventive measures with the post-factum tendency to cling to overtreatment. In my scheme the professional role of physicians is intrinsic to the insurance scheme, while Hall endorses bedside rationing by physicians because the public trusts bureaucrats less. Additionally, inspired by Havighurst, Hall combines the insurance companies' power to set limits on the costs of the insured with the socially beneficial outcome of reducing the overall burden of health care. But people do not save on insurance policies in order to divert resources to others while they take ill; rather, they wish to spend the appropriate amount on the insurance they need so as to be protected from both undertreatment and overtreatment while in

need. Hence, central to my scheme is the proper division of health care services follow-ing the three categories of care, even if this requires aggressive reduction of the prices currently asked by health care providers (e.g., physicians, pharmaceuticals) and the extra attention given to the maximally possible removal of physicians' conflicts of inter-ests. Scholars and court rulings incline to respect "Ulysses contracts" when they clearly benefit the patient, such as detox treatment that requires waiver upon admission of the right to check out from the hospital before the prescribed hospitalization period is over (Ryan, 2003; Davis, 2008). Even then, some argue against the legality of commitments to self-deny such a basic good as freedom in the future (e.g., Dresser, 1981–1982). Although Hall mentions this debate (p. 168), he fails to appreciate the unlikely acceptance of antici-patory commitments whose goal is pecuniary (paying less for insurance) and whose out-come is not in the clear benefit of the person. Rather, it is likely to deprive the person of a basic human value that is protected by human dignity and rights. Even more crucially, while the psychiatrists act with the good of the patient in mind, rationing is carried out for the good of other patients only.

Lastly, Hall and other writers on Ulysses contracts in health care do not distinguish between strong Ulysses contracts—in which, due to the contract, lucid and fully informed pleas are denied by means of force (e.g., Ulysses pleading with his sailors to untie him from the mast or to direct the ship to the sirens; a drug addict who adamantly demands his release from hospitalization)—and milder contracts such as insurance schemes that deny coverage for certain procedures but do not prohibit out-of-pocket expenditure on the uninsured service.

12. See also Mechanic (1986), Hall (2003) and Rodwin (2011).

REFERENCES

Aaron, H. J. (2008). Healthcare rationing: inevitable but impossible? *Georgetown Law Journal, 96*, 539–558.

ABIM, ACP-ASIM, and European Federation of Internal Medicine. (2002). Medical pro-fessionalism in the new millennium: a physician charter. *Annals of Internal Medicine, 136*(3), 243–246.

Ainslie, G. (2001). *Breakdown of Will.* Cambridge: Cambridge University Press.

Alcott, B. (2005). Jevons' paradox. *Ecological Economics, 54*(1), 9–21.

Barilan, Y. M. (2009). Responsibility as a meta-virtue: truth-telling, deliberation and wisdom in medical professionalism. *Journal of Medical Ethics, 35*(3), 153–158.

Barilan, Y. M. (2010a). The dilemma of good clinical practice in the study of compromised standards of care. *Critical Care 14*, 176.

Barilan, Y. M. (2010b). Informed consent: between waiver and excellence in responsible deliberation. *Medicine Health Care and Philosophy, 13*(1), 89–95.

Barilan, Y. M. (2011). Respect for personal autonomy, human dignity and the problem of self-directedness and botched autonomy. *Journal of Medicine and Philosophy, 36*(5), 496–515.

Barilan, Y. M. (2012). *Human dignity, human rights and responsibility: the new language of global bioethics.* Cambridge (MA): MIT Press.

Barilan, Y. M., & Zuckerman, S. (2013). Revisiting medical neutrality as a moral value and as a doctrine in international law. In Carrick, D. & Gross, M., eds. *Military Medical Ethics.* Aldershot: Ashgate.

Braybrooke, D. (1987). *Meeting Needs*. Princeton: Princeton University Press.

Brown, D. E. (1991). *Human Universals*, Chapter 6. New York: McGraw Hill.

Chapman, R., & MacKenzie, R. (2010). The global research neglect of unassisted smoking cessation: causes and consequences. *PLoS Medicine 7*, e1000216.

Cookson, R., McCabe, C., & Tsuchiya, A. (2008). Public resources allocation and the rule of rescue. *Journal of Medical Ethics, 34*(7), 540–544.

Daniels, N. (1981). Health care needs and distributive justice. *Philosophy and Public Affairs, 10*(2), 146–179.

Davidson, D. (2001[1969]). How weakness of the will is possible. In *Essays on Actions and Events*. 2nd ed., pp. 21–42. Oxford: Clarendon.

Davis, J. K. (2008). How to justify enforcing a Ulysses contract when Ulysses is competent and refuses. *Kennedy Institute of Ethics Journal, 18*(1), 87–106.

Dresser, R. S. (1981–1982). Ulysses and the psychiatrists: a legal and policy analysis of the voluntary commitment contract. *Harvard Civil Rights-Civil Liberties Law Review, 16*, 777–854.

Dutton, H. I. (1984). *The Patent System and Inventive Activity during the Industrial Revolution*. Manchester: Manchester University Press.

Egred, M., Shaw, S. Mohammad, B. Waitt, P. & Rodrigues, E. (2005). Under-use of beta-blockers in patients with ischaemic heart disease and concomitant chronic obstructive pulmonary disease. *QJM*, 98(7), 493–497.

Fleck, L. (2009). *Just Caring: Healthcare Rationing and Democratic Deliberation*. Oxford: Oxford University Press.

Frank, R. H. (1999). *Luxury Fever: Weighing the Costs of Excess*. Princeton: Princeton University Press.

Garfinkel, D., & Mangin, D. (2010). Feasibility study of a systematic approach for discontinuation of multiple medications in older adults. *Archives of Internal Medicine, 170*(18), 1648–1654.

Gibson, J., Mitton, C., Martin, D., Donaldson, C., & Singer, P. (2006). Ethics and economics: does programme budgeting and marginal analysis contribute to fair priority setting? *Journal of Health Services Research & Policy, 11*(1), 32–37.

Gilbert, D. T. (2006). *Stumbling on Happiness*. New York: Penguin.

Goozner, M. (2012). New cancer drugs: affordable by the 1 percent? *The Fiscal Times*, January 23rd. Available at: http://www.thefiscaltimes.com/Articles/2012/01/23/New-Cancer-Drugs-Affordable-by-the-1-Percent.aspx.

Grady, C. (2005). Payment of clinical research subjects. *Journal of Clinical Investigation, 115*(7), 1681–1687.

Griffin, J. (2008). *On Human Rights*. Oxford: Oxford University Press.

Gross, M. (2006). *Bioethics and Armed Conflict: Moral Dilemmas of Medicine and War*. Cambridge (MA): MIT Press

Haakonssen, L. (1997). *Medicine and morals in the enlightenment: John Gregory, Thomas Percival and Benjamin Rush*. Amsterdam: Rodopi.

Hall, M. A. (1997b). A theory of economic informed consent. *Georgia Law Review, 31*, 510–586.

Hall, M. A. (1997a). *Making Medical Spending Decisions: The law, ethics and economics of rationing mechanisms*. Oxford: Oxford University Press.

Hall, T. S. (2003). Bargaining with Hippocrates: managed care and the doctor patient relationship. *Southern Carolina Law Review, 54*, 689–740.

Hasman, A., Hope, T., & Østerdal, L. P. (2006). Healthcare need: three interpretations. *Journal of Applied Philosophy, 23*(2), 145–156.

Havighurst, C. C. (1992). Prospective self-denial: can consumers contract today to accept health care rationing tomorrow? *University of Pennsylvania Law Review, 140,* 1755–1808.

Himmelstein, D. U., Wright, A., & Woolhandler, S. (2010). Hospital computing and the costs and quality of care: a national study. *American Journal of Medicine, 123*(1), 40–46.

Jussim, L. (2012). *Social Perception and Social Reality: Why Accuracy Dominates Bias and Self-Fulfilling Prophecy.* Oxford: Oxford University Press.

Kahneman, D., Knetsch, J. L., & Thaler, R. H. (1991). The endowment effect, loss aversion and the status quo bias. *Journal of Economic Perspective, 5*(1), 193–206.

Lau, D. T., Kasper, J. D., Potter, D. E. B., Lyles, A., & Bennett, R. G. (2005). Hospitalization and death associated with potentially inappropriate medication prescriptions among elderly nursing home residents. *Archives of Internal Medicine, 165*(1), 68–74.

Levinsky, N. G. (1984). The doctor's master. *New England Journal of Medicine, 311*(24), 1573–1575.

Lieberman, D., Nachshon, L., Miloslavsky, O., Dvorkin, V., Shimoni, A., Zelinger. J., et al. (2010). Elderly patients undergoing mechanical ventilation in and out of intensive care units: a comparative, prospective study of 641 ventilations. *Critical Care, 14,* R48.

McGlynn, E. A., Asch, S. M., Adams, J., Keesey, J. Hicks, J. DeCristofaro, A., & Kerr, E. (2003). The quality of care delivered to adults in the United States. *New England Journal of Medicine, 348*(26), 2635–2645.

McNally, J. M. (2011). *What is Mental Illness.* Cambridge (MA): Harvard University Press.

Mechanic, D. (1986). *From Advocacy to Allocation: The evolving American healthcare system.* New York: Free Press.

Offer, A. (2006). *The Challenge of Affluence: Self-Control and Well-Being in the United States and Britain Since 1950.* Oxford: Oxford University Press.

Rhys A, Cowell, R., Downe, J., Martin, S. and Turner, D. (2006). *Promoting Effective Citizenship and Community Empowerment.* London Office of the Deputy Prime Minister.

Pogge, T. (2005). Human rights and global health. *Metaphilosophy, 36,* 182–209.

Radin, M. J. (1987). Market inalienability. *Harvard Law Review, 100,* 1849–1937.

Riley, J. C. (2001). *Rising Life Expectancy: A global history.* Cambridge: Cambridge University Press.

Rodwin, M. A. (2011). *Conflict of Interest and the Future of Medicine: The United States, France and Japan.* Oxford: Oxford University Press.

Ruger, J. P. (2010). *Health and Social Justice.* Oxford: Oxford University Press.

Restuccia, J. D., Cohen, A. B., Horwitt, J. N. and Shwartz, M. (2012). Hospital implementation of health information technology and quality of care: are they related? *BMC Medical Informatics and Decision Making, 12,* 109 doi:10.1186/1472-6947-12-109

Ryan, S. (2003). Reviving Ulysses contracts. *Kennedy Institute of Ethics Journal, 13*(4), 373–392.

Schwab, A. P. (2006). Formal and effective autonomy in healthcare. *Journal of Medical Ethics, 32*(10), 575–579.

Sen, A. (1993). Markets and freedoms: achievements and limitations of the market mechanism in promoting individual freedoms. *Oxford Economic Papers, 45*(4), 519–541.

Soumerai, S. B., McLaughlin, T. J., Spiegelman, D., Hertzmark, E., Thibault, G., & Goldman, L. (1997). Adverse outcomes of underuse of β-blockers in elderly survivors of acute myocardial infarction. *Journal of the American Medical Association, 277*(2), 115–121.

Thilly, N., Boini, S., Soudant, M., Kessler, M., Briaçon, S. & Frimat, L. (2011). Outcomes of patients with delayed dialysis initiation: Results from the AVENIR study. *American Journal of Nephrology, 33*(1), 76–83.

Watts, S. (2003). *Disease and Medicine in World History*. New York: Routledge.

Williams, B. (2005). *In the Beginning Was the Deed: Realism and moralism in political argument*. Princeton: Princeton University Press.

Winslow, G. R. (1982). *Triage and Justice*. Berkeley: University of California Press.

Woolhandler, S., & Himmelstein, D. U. (1997). Costs of care and administration at for-profit and other hospitals in the United States. *New England Journal of Medicine, 336*(11), 769–774.

10 Just Caring

The Ethics Challenges of Bedside Rationing

■ LEONARD M. FLECK

Is it ever morally permissible for physicians to make bedside rationing decisions with regard to their own patients, thereby compromising what might be regarded as the "best interests" of their patients? This is the key moral question I will address in this chapter. One response that has been given by Levinsky (1984) and has become a *locus classicus*—a standard view—on this issue is the following: "I would argue the contrary, that physicians are required to do everything that they believe may benefit each patient without regard to costs or other social considerations. In caring for an individual patient, the doctor must act solely as that patient's advocate, against the apparent interests of society as a whole, if necessary."

David Eddy (1996) takes a very different point of view. He notes that physicians never care for individuals who are "merely" patients; they are always patient/payers. As individuals afflicted with a potentially serious illness, we see ourselves primarily as patients. But as healthy individuals attached to an insurance plan of good quality, costing perhaps $13,000 per year for a family and increasing in cost at 7% per year, we see ourselves primarily as payers who may not feel we are getting very much in the way of tangible benefits for all that money. As members of costly insurance plans, what we ought to demand are serious efforts to control health costs related to services which we cannot control and that offer little in the way of obvious benefit to ourselves. These are the social and economic and moral realities of belonging to a health plan. In effect, what we say to our physicians *as healthy individuals* is, "Please do not lavish all manner of health services in our health plan on these other patients who are entirely strangers to me."

How is a "good doctor," whom we expect in general to be a loyal patient advocate, supposed to respond to such a plea? The answer Eddy gives to this question, in essence, is that the best interests of patients are complex; they are both medical and monetary. Consequently, physicians must be sensitively responsive to these complexities, although their responses ought to be governed primarily by considerations of cost-effectiveness (which best represent a larger societal perspective, even though that is rarely the perspective of a patient with serious and immediate medical needs). Is this a morally satisfactory response? Is this a practically workable response? I will answer both these questions in the negative.

Levinsky is correct, to a point. Patients want physicians who will be strong, loyal advocates of their best interests. But it is reasonable to ask whether patients have a *moral right* to literally have their *best* health care interests met, especially in light of the fact that under any insurance scheme, whether in the United States (with its highly fragmented insurance mechanisms) or in Europe (with more centralized and uniform insurance mechanisms), it is *social* resources to which they are seeking to lay claim. Eddy is correct on this latter point. Think of politicians who reward their friends and family with public resources over which they have control and then "justify" their behavior by saying this was required by their sense of loyalty. Few nonpoliticians would regard this as anything but transparent ethical sophistry.

How should we (patients/payers) and our physicians think about this issue of bedside rationing? Are all instances of bedside rationing intrinsically morally objectionable because core moral commitments of the medical profession are violated? Or are only some instances of bedside rationing open to justified moral criticism? If so, what criteria may we invoke for purposes of distinguishing morally permissible from morally impermissible forms of bedside rationing? And what exactly should "count" as an instance of bedside rationing? Is every denial by a physician of some health care intervention demanded by a patient, who sees that intervention as something that he needs, an instance of bedside rationing? Is it possible for physicians to simply avoid doing any bedside rationing, thereby dissolving the problem?

■ THE UNBEARABLE NECESSITY OF BEDSIDE RATIONING

The answer to this last question is that it is impossible for physicians to avoid doing bedside rationing (Morreim, 1991; 1989; Aaron & Schwartz, 1984, ch. 1). Patients may request interventions to which they have no just claim, or which are very unlikely to succeed, or whose likely benefits are minimal in relation to extraordinarily high costs. If physicians refuse to acquiesce to such requests, they have made a rationing decision. In addition, any physician who is responsible for caring for some significant number of patients over the course of a day will have to ration her time and energy over the patients who need her care that day (Ubel, 2000, ch. 7; Orentlicher, 2010). Not all health needs require an equal amount of medical attention.

Physicians are ultimately responsible for judging which patients will have access to absolutely scarce medical resources, such as the last bed in the ICU or the last respirator (or any respirator, if we were talking about a pandemic). No hospital or health care system can afford to have all the ICU beds that might be needed during relatively infrequent super-peak demands for those beds. This will be as true in Europe as in the United States. So some physician will have to make some decisions about how those absolutely scarce resources will be allocated among all the patients who have serious medical needs for those resources. I am quite confident that few patients would endorse the idea of philosophers or administrators making these allocation decisions on the basis of either favored philosophic theories or pressing economic factors. The expectation of patients is that physicians will somehow make these allocation judgments fairly and in accord with values central to the practice of medicine. Again, this is bedside rationing and it is inescapable as a moral responsibility of physicians.

Some analysts have argued that rationing decisions should be made at the macro level by bureaucrats or administrators or other policymakers (Veatch, 1986; Abrams, 1986; Hiatt, 1975). Physicians then would be mere implementation cogs who would transmit rationing decisions to patients as opposed to being responsible for making those rationing decisions themselves. They would just be good soldiers carrying out orders in the war to control health care costs. However, this is a very specious moral perspective. Physicians are rightly expected to be enduring moral agents (as opposed to occasional moral agents), who do not surrender their moral responsibilities for patients to administrators who have other goals unrelated to the interests of particular patients.

In addition, what needs to be appreciated is that any rationing protocol generated at the macro level will necessarily be general in character. Every rationing protocol at the macro level will require judgments in its application at the micro level. Someone needs to make a judgment about whether that protocol aptly applies to the very distinctive clinical circumstances of an individual patient (Orentlicher, 2010, p. 454). This is as true for rationing protocols as it is for clinical guidelines.

Part of the moral puzzlement about bedside rationing pertains to the issue of what counts as being loyal to the "best interests" of the patient. Related to that is the issue of who gets to define the content of that notion. Should that be the physician? Or the patient? Or some professional or social body charged with setting standards? Atul Gawande has described in an essay (2009) two cities in Texas with radically different approaches to delivering health services. In McAllen, Texas, Medicare spent almost $15,000 per enrollee, the second highest amount for any health care market in the United States. In El Paso, Medicare spending was only slightly more than half that per enrollee. More of virtually everything medicine had to offer was lavished on Medicare patients in McAllen. Compared to El Paso Medicare patients, McAllen Medicare patients were 66% more likely to see 10 or more specialists in a 6-month period, get 20% more abdominal ultrasounds, 30% more bone density scans, 60% more stress tests, and 200%–300% more pacemakers, implantable cardiac defibrillators, cardiac bypass operations, carotid endarterectomies, and coronary stent procedures (Gawande, 2009). For all this medical care that was lavished upon

Medicare patients in McAllen, they did not seem better off in terms of survival, functional status, or patient satisfaction relative to Medicare patients in El Paso.

Were physicians in McAllen deserving of the highest moral praise for satisfying to the maximum degree the "best interests" of their patients? And were physicians in El Paso deserving of substantial moral criticism for compromising the "best interests" of their patients? Gawande himself is clearly on the side of the physicians in El Paso. He compliments them for working together as a team, thinking more strategically about how best to meet patient health needs, and putting community needs above their own self-interest. He does not accuse them of having engaged in morally objectionable bedside rationing. Instead, he sees them as offering key lessons for the reform of the US health care system: If there is an interest in covering everyone in the US with a comprehensive package of health services at a cost that is sustainable into the foreseeable future, which is what the Affordable Care Act aims to accomplish, then it will be necessary to follow the example of physicians in El Paso. That is, physicians will have to take the lead in reorganizing the US health care system fundamentally so that health services are delivered with much greater efficiency and appropriateness. This is a reasonable example of the parsimonious style of care advocated by the American College of Physicians (2012). A large number of proponents of health reform have echoed this same sentiment (Luft, 2009, 2008; Emanuel, 2008; Daschle, 2008).

What we need to recognize is that the need for health care rationing is inescapable. I and many other health policy analysts have argued for precisely that point (Fleck, 2009; 2006; Daniels & Sabin, 2008; Butler, 1999; Newdick, 2005; Morreim, 1991). The quest for rationing-free efficiency in the health care system is largely a mirage, an unholy Grail that would distract physicians and the rest of us from the many unjust allocations that are part of the US health care system.

At this point, it is possible to offer a couple preliminary conclusions. First, physicians cannot be unconstrained loyal advocates of the unconstrained best interests of each of their patients as Levinsky requires. Physicians cannot escape the need to make bedside rationing decisions (Reuben & Cassel, 2011; American College of Physicians, 2012). If rationing by definition involves denying some patient some medical benefit, no matter how marginal, then rationing by physicians will necessarily involve compromising the best interests of their individual patients. Second, the political and economic realities of the US health care system, and any other health care system, are that patients who are very well insured are least likely to have their immediate best interests as patients compromised by rationing decisions. McAllen, Texas, illustrates this point nicely. The problem with such medical generosity is that it drives up the overall cost of health care in the system with the consequent dumping of health insurance by marginal employers, thereby steadily increasing the pool of uninsured in the United States (Bodenheimer & Grumbach, 2012, ch. 3). Finally, Americans should take no comfort in the fact that many of the uninsured never show up in their physicians' offices when they need medical care (because they are uninsured). It would seem that their absence from the doctor's office leads to the Levinskian implication that these physicians cannot be blamed for bedside rationing since no one is there before them for whom they must be loyal advocates. Yet the ultimate effect is that these individuals have encountered the results of rationing (Wilper et al., 2009). Fortunately, this scenario is not an issue in Europe and should be of diminishing significance as the Affordable Care Act is implemented in the United States.

We are back at our starting point. If physicians cannot avoid the need to make bedside rationing decisions, then how can they make these decisions in ways that are as morally defensible as possible? Some would respond by arguing along with Calabresi and Bobbitt (1978) that what we are faced with is a "tragic choice" situation. In other words, no matter what decision might be made, some deep social value is going to be violated. They call attention to the frequency with which people in the United States invoke the value of the "pricelessness of human life." But the fact of the matter is that resources are always limited relative to need. So various ways are found for hiding or rendering invisible the rationing choices that must be made (Mechanic, 1995; Hall, 1997). Calabresi and Bobbitt endorse such practices as a way of preventing the corrosion of the social bonds of trust. They recognize that there is something fundamentally dishonest about such policies and practices. But that is the tragic choice. I have criticized their arguments thoroughly elsewhere (Fleck, 2009, ch. 3).

▪ RATIONAL DEMOCRATIC DELIBERATION: MAKING RATIONING EXPLICIT

There is an alternative strategy for diminishing the morally problematic features of bedside rationing and avoiding the language of tragic choices. This is the role of rational democratic deliberation in coming to publicly shared understandings of fair and reasonable rationing protocols that will apply to all in the relevantly similar clinical circumstances. Again, I have written extensively on this topic (2009) so I will only highlight some core ideas relevant to this discussion.

We start with the assumption that the most morally relevant consideration with respect to rationing decisions is some conception of justice. This is because health care represents a socially generated good that will never be sufficient to meet everything we would identify as reasonable and morally relevant health care needs. Hence, some sort of distributional judgment needs to be made. I have argued that the two most important features of a fair process of health care rationing are that it be public or visible and that it be self-imposed. Fair rationing decisions and the rationale behind those decisions should be public so that those who see themselves adversely affected by that decision (or who simply see the decision as being morally flawed) have the opportunity to challenge that decision and argue for a more just choice. This is what Rawls (1971, 1993) has identified as the "publicity condition" at the core of our shared conception of justice.

The other element I argue is essential to a fair approach to health care rationing is that rationing decisions be self-imposed *through a democratic deliberative process*. A fair and reasonable democratic deliberative process will be a constructive process of mutual moral education (Gutmann & Thompson, 2004, 1996). We realize that the rationing options available in a health care system will be morally, politically, medically, and economically complex. No simple theories of justice will yield easy or obvious answers to the question of what the fairest rationing choices are. Often there will be multiple rationing options available to us, all of which might be roughly morally equal from the perspective of several different conceptions of health care justice. What would clearly be unfair would be to allow different conceptions of health care justice to be invoked somewhat arbitrarily to yield a "fair" rationing outcome in essentially similar clinical circumstances. In other words, while a variety of perspectives might yield different morally sound answers, we need to employ the same perspective to similar situations to ensure a fair outcome. We need a *certain degree* of moral consistency across an entire health care system in order to protect the justness of the system as a whole. The democratic deliberative process would be the primary mechanism to use to achieve sufficient agreement regarding the mix of broad rationing protocols that would be "fair enough" (non–ideally just) across the entire health care system. I should add, given multiple reasonable "just enough" trade-offs that might be made with regard to more fine-grained rationing protocols, that there could be democratically legitimated differing sets of rationing protocols from one health plan to another, or from one sickness fund to another in Germany, or from one "commissioning group" to another in the United Kingdom. Internal moral consistency would be "just enough" so long as those choices were congruent with the broader considerations of health care justice that applied across the entire health care system of a country.

That democratic agreement would give legitimacy to the mix of rationing protocols articulated through the deliberative process. The understanding would be that this mix of rationing protocols would apply to all who were part of that health care system (or plans within the system) who had the opportunity to be among the democratic deliberators, directly or representatively. It is in this respect that the rationing protocols would be self-imposed. That is, the rationing protocols would not be imposed on the sickest or most vulnerable members of the health care system by those who were well off. This sort of outcome is effectively precluded by the way in which the deliberative process itself is conducted. Readers will recall how Rawls (1971) invoked the "veil of ignorance" to assure that no one group in society could construct the basic structure of society in a way that was favorable to one group rather than another. This veil of ignorance was regarded as an idealization not generally realizable in the real world. However, the "veil of ignorance" is operable in the health care arena because rationing protocols would be articulated by individuals who were essentially healthy and ignorant of their future possible health needs. At any given point in time, the vast majority of us are in precisely this circumstance. Even if we already have some serious chronic illness, only a little thought would remind us that we are vulnerable to other serious medical problems as well; consequently, we would have to choose a mix of rationing protocols from a more objective and impartial point of view.

The practical import of this analysis, so far as the bedside rationing problem is concerned, is that the problem might be substantially resolved. If we have democratic social agreement that no life-sustaining medical efforts would be employed to sustain the life of someone who had been confidently diagnosed to be in a persistent vegetative state [PVS], then a physician could withdraw life-sustaining care from such a patient and could not be fairly judged to have been disloyal to that patient. That patient would have agreed at an earlier point in time to this general rationing protocol, not knowing at the time that he would actually be the object of implementation for this protocol. So this would be a freely chosen, self-imposed rationing protocol that that individual judged to be in his best interest, where "best interest" would be judged from a broader temporal and medical perspective (in the way that David Eddy [1996] has described in his writings). The physician caring for this patient would be loyal to the judgment that patient had made for an indefinite array of future possible selves that patient might become. Of course in the case of a PVS patient, that patient is not in a position to voice an objection in the present to having life-sustaining care withdrawn. Family members might care to voice an objection, but it would be reasonable to ask what the basis for that objection might be if we have societally agreed to the rationing protocol. Invoking some sort of self-interest would not be morally sufficient to defeat a just rationing protocol that was a result of a fair process of democratic deliberation.

We could call attention to an alternate scenario in which we have a conscious, competent patient who is objecting to being denied some form of life-sustaining medical care that had been the object of another rationing protocol. What we might imagine is an extraordinarily expensive "last chance" cancer drug, such as bevacizumab that might be used for lung cancer or colon cancer. The cost of a course of treatment with this drug might be $50,000–$100,000 and the gain in life expectancy might be measurable as no more than a few weeks or a few months. This patient is now in the end stages of his cancer and wants every opportunity to have every additional bit of life that medicine might offer him. What is a loyal patient advocate supposed to do under those circumstances? Can a physician serve as a stone-faced judge and simply deny his request by calling attention to the rationing protocol that is denying him access to that drug as a matter of justice?

The short answer to our question is that this physician ought not to be a stone-faced judge but should be instead a *just and compassionate* patient advocate. But, there are moral limits to being a loyal patient advocate. Those limits are defined by a number of morally relevant considerations besides justice. As we noted earlier, physicians are mostly distributing social resources that have been entrusted to them. Physicians do not have the right to distribute those resources in accord with personal whim or ties of affection. Several years ago Freeman et al. (1999) reported, in a nice piece of empirical survey research, the number of physicians who would lie for their patients in order to obtain some form of needed medical care (with varying degrees of urgency attached to that care) that would otherwise be denied those patients in accord with the rules of their insurance plan. Roughly 58% of physicians in that survey would lie to an insurance plan in order to get bypass surgery for a patient. We can imagine our patient who now wishes to receive bevacizumab being familiar with that research, calling that to the attention of his physician, and expecting his physician to act accordingly. He might argue that both he and the bypass patient see their desired intervention as the only life-prolonging option open to them. However, a strong argument can be made that the two situations are radically different from one another.

The US health care system has been enormously fragmented and controlled by arbitrary rules put in place by private insurers to protect their own profit margins and to reduce costs to their subscribers as a group (large employers especially). This would be in marked contrast to the health care systems in Canada and most European nations. In the United States, substantive considerations of health care justice rarely shape these rules and limits on access to care. More importantly, the patients who are most directly affected by these rules have virtually never autonomously endorsed any of these rules or participated in the construction of these rules. In that sort of situation we can readily see why physicians would rightly wonder whether cooperating with those rules was really congruent with their responsibilities as loyal patient advocates. But in the future possible state of affairs envisioned here, where everyone would be covered by the same relatively comprehensive package of health benefits and costs would be constrained by rationing protocols that had been fairly and rationally and autonomously determined through a process of rational democratic deliberation, physicians would not seem to have any reasonable moral excuse for failing to act in accord with those rationing protocols. (Hall [1997, ch. 6] will argue that patients have given their autonomous consent when they agree to an insurance contract, but I would note that the content of that contract is largely determined by an employer, not the employee.)

A physician would have to remind our patient who seeks bevacizumab that earlier in his cancer care he had been a beneficiary of the rationing protocols that he is now seeking to dodge with the help of his physician. That is, there would have been costly and effective treatments at earlier stages of his cancer that we were able to provide to him that yielded a significant gain in both length of life and quality of life. Perhaps he needs to be reminded that under the "old system" (prior to the passage of the Affordable Care Act in the United States) he would have had no *assured access* to those more effective costly cancer therapies because he could have lost his job and his insurance coverage during a major recession, or he could have been underinsured and expected to pay what for him would have been an unaffordable price for those earlier therapies. He had agreed with all his fellow citizens/future possible patients that it was reasonable and fair to give up the very costly marginal benefits associated with bevacizumab as a "last chance" therapy in order for all future possible colon cancer patients to have secure access to more effective earlier costly cancer therapies. Further, others before him with colon cancer would have faithfully acted in accord with these just rationing protocols (not pressuring their physicians to somehow bypass those protocols), thereby generating the savings that allowed him to have his life prolonged at an earlier stage in the disease process. How could he now unilaterally and unjustifiably abrogate his responsibility to accept those same rationing protocols? Can he give any account for why he should be seen as being morally special, an exception to the rule?

We should add that this patient is not being denied access to bevacizumab absolutely. He is only being denied access to the drug at social expense. If he has the resources to pay out of pocket for access to that drug, then his physician could provide the drug to him. This drug is not something that is absolutely scarce; no other patients are made worse off so far as considerations of justice are concerned if he pays for this drug himself. But if he does not have those resources, then the most that can be said is that it is *unfortunate* that he will be denied access to that drug but *it is not unjust.* And his physician would not be open to any moral criticism because he would have been both a just and loyal patient advocate.

We return to our central question: If we were to embrace a rational, democratic, deliberative approach to the problem of health care rationing, would the need for bedside rationing essentially disappear? The answer to this question must be negative. Any rationing protocols that were a product of this deliberative process would always have a general character to them. This would be true of even very fine-grained rationing protocols. No rationing protocols that are useful for policy purposes could possibly be specific enough to address the complex clinical circumstances of individual patients.

This is a hard empirical reality that reflects the complexity and uncertainty of medicine as well as what Rawls (1971, 1993) has referred to as the "burdens of judgment" (a phrase meant to capture the real-world complexity of making moral judgments, especially with regard to matters of justice). What this point means in practice is that any fair and reasonable approach to health care rationing will have to grant to physicians a degree of flexibility in applying these rationing protocols to the patient they are caring for now. That degree of flexibility creates "moral space" in which the issue of loyal patient advocacy and attentiveness to the best interests of each patient would have to be addressed again. How can that be done fairly, that is, without subverting entirely the presumed justness of the set of rationing protocols as a whole? That is the question to which we next turn.

Some physicians might respond to this last query by saying that they accorded no moral legitimacy to these rationing protocols whatsoever because they were a product of some *democratic* deliberative process. That is, they would be saying that these rationing protocols were uninformed by authoritative medical judgment, and consequently it would be contrary to good medical practice to incorporate them into their care of patients. However, that is not at all how I would imagine such rationing protocols being generated. Physicians would certainly be among the citizen deliberators responsible for the creation of these protocols from the beginning of the deliberative process, as Norheim (2008) has argued. Beyond that, I would imagine that all rationing protocols given a preliminary democratic endorsement would be assessed by a group of expert physicians for their medical reasonableness *and only their medical reasonableness*. That is, this panel of physicians would not have the authority to replace democratically legitimated rationing protocols that were "just enough" with protocols that reflected *their* sense of health care justice. (If that were permitted, we would no longer have a basis for saying these rationing protocols were "self-imposed" with the moral legitimacy conveyed by that notion.) Their sole responsibility would be to correct errors of medical understanding that might have been incorporated into a rationing protocol. And, even in this case, their judgment would have to be well justified in the medical literature (as opposed to reflecting what might be currently indiscriminate uses of medical technology).

Another way in which physicians might respond to the flexibility required for fair and reasonable rationing protocols would be the following: They might want to argue that human life is priceless (in their judgment); and consequently, these rationing protocols would have no moral authority when lives would be shortened by their acting in accord with one of these protocols. Alternatively, they might want to argue that they had a "duty to rescue" patients who were terminally ill but for whom there was some medical intervention that might offer them an extension of life they desired. In other words, they would refuse to carry out a rationing protocol that interfered with what they would judge would be the morally more compelling "duty to rescue" the patient for whom they are caring now. Or they might want to say that rationing protocols that only put statistical lives at risk might be morally acceptable so far as their medical obligations were concerned but not rationing protocols that would result in a "premature" death for their identifiable terminally ill patient. Or they might want to argue that physicians had a moral obligation to avoid being the "cause of death" for a patient by denying that patient the life-sustaining care they needed but was supposed to be denied them by a specific rationing protocol. In other words, these physicians would be claiming that any rationing protocol bringing about the death of a patient sooner than would have occurred with maximal medical effort represented a form of euthanasia to which they might be opposed. Or, finally, physicians might say that they were willing to cooperate in good conscience with rationing protocols that in no way added to the risk of premature death for a patient, but they were certain they were morally obligated to provide "last chance" therapies to their patients as loyal advocates of their patient's best interests.

My response to all these invocations would be the following: There might well be some very limited range of very specific clinical circumstances in which invoking one or another of these moral arguments might be appropriate. But explaining why a particular invocation was appropriate in particular clinical circumstances would require substantial careful moral argument and analysis. If we permitted these types of arguments to be invoked in the perfectly general way they have been presented here to justify exercising "flexible medical moral judgment" in response to some particular rationing protocol, the result would be the entire evisceration of the utility and the justness of these rationing protocols.

Our point can be substantiated by calling attention to the fact that in the United States the 5% of patients who are the costliest patients in any given year will account for 50% of all health expenditures that year (Schoenman, 2012). In 2011 in the United States that 50% figure would have been equal to about $1.3 trillion. We need to emphasize that a substantial portion of these dollars would have been spent on very expensive but very effective medical therapies at relatively early stages of a disease process that might well prove fatal years later. These costs can often be readily seen to be just and cost effective in that they yield substantial improvements in length of life and quality of life. But the same cannot be said for extraordinarily high expenditures in what are predictably the last months of life. These expenditures are for very marginally beneficial cost-ineffective health care.

It is worth noting what have been the moral consequences of misallocations in this regard. In England, the National Institutes for Health and Clinical Excellence (NICE) initially ruled that trastuzumab for metastatic breast cancer cost too much for too little gain in length of life or quality of life. But very strong pressure by pharmaceutical companies through cleverly disguised "public outrage" resulted in NICE reversing itself and permitting coverage for trastuzumab. The British government did not increase allocations to the Primary Care Trusts to cover the costs associated with this drug (and several other very expensive cancer drugs). The expectation was that the Primary Care Trusts would judge what other health services would be given up in order to pay the costs of trastuzumab. In one of these Trusts, funding for medications for young adult patients with ankylosing spondylitis was withdrawn (Hope, 2007). This is not a life-threatening medical problem but it is extremely painful without the medications these patients needed. It is not at all obvious that this was a fair or reasonable judgment to make. But if we permit unregulated invocation of the language of the pricelessness of human life, or insist there is an absolute moral obligation to give top priority to "last chance therapies," denying patients costly drugs that alleviate pain or other quality of life sapping symptoms could be one consequence. One might conclude with respect to our bedside rationing problem that invoking any of these rationales by physicians to justify "flexibility" with respect to enforcing a relevant democratically legitimated rationing protocol is unwarranted. That degree of flexibility would be too broad to protect fairness.

Two objections related to democratic deliberation need to be addressed at this point. First, it seems entirely unrealistic for broad deliberative processes to be used for thousands of potential rationing protocols. This is true as a practical matter. What we need to imagine is that more garden-variety rationing protocols, such as statins, will only be prescribed at 240 total cholesterol rather than 200 and would be determined by a relatively small committee of plan or sickness fund members. Those judgments and their rationales would be widely disseminated among plan members through the Internet. Comments and concerns would always be welcome and could result in modifications after due consideration. In contrast to that, rationing protocols predictably more consequential and controversial would be subject to a much more sustained and widely disseminated process of deliberative engagement, for example with regard to these extraordinarily expensive cancer drugs that yield generally very marginal gains in life expectancy. Presumably, discussions of such matters would be shared across health plans or sickness funds because these issues would arise for all at roughly the same time.

A second objection is that allowing physicians to make bedside rationing decisions seems to be in tension with the point of the deliberative process. This will only occasionally be true. Remember that most of the time in this reformed scenario physicians are carrying out rationing protocols enacted through the deliberative process. The moral tension is with the norms of medicine and the wishes of individual patients being cared for in the present. But all rationing protocols, just like all rules, will have some level of generality attached to them. That means they are not self-interpreting with respect to application in complex clinical circumstances. This is where some degree of medical flexibility in the clinic is essential, both to protect fairness and the role of physicians as patient advocates. Reasonable deliberators will endorse a reasonable degree of such clinical flexibility suitably constrained (as discussed below), again not knowing whether their future possible selves as patients would be advantaged or disadvantaged in specific clinical circumstances.

■ BEDSIDE RATIONING: DEFINING THE LIMITS OF JUST FLEXIBILITY

We next consider some more promising approaches to addressing the clinical flexibility problem in connection with protecting the justness or integrity of publicly legitimated rationing protocols. We will consider a number of individual cases. Our goal is to identify reasonable factors that would justify a degree of medical flexibility that protects fairness in the context of bedside rationing. In effect, we are endorsing a conclusion reached by Baeroe (2008, p. 87) that "even though we assume the legitimacy of macro-level guidelines, this legitimacy is not directly transferable to decisions at the micro-level simply by adherence to the guidelines' recommendations."

The first case is the well known *Wickline* case from California (1987). The clinical aspects of the case occurred in 1977; final adjudication was in 1987. Mrs. Wickline (age 42) had serious vascular problems that affected her legs but were related to an occlusion of her abdominal aorta. Because of various complications associated with the surgery, she had to have a total of three operations. Her primary surgeon, Dr. Polonsky, was very concerned to make sure there were no additional complications. But Mrs. Wickline's hospital care was being paid for by Medi-Cal and was subject to utilization review. At one point Dr. Polonsky was told it was time to discharge her. He was confident this was contrary to what his best medical judgment said she needed. He said she needed an additional 8 days in the hospital. However, after much debate and arguing, he agreed that he would discharge her in 4 days. When that fourth day arrived he again believed she needed 4 additional days in the hospital, but pressure from the hospital administration was such that he discharged her anyway. A few days later, a serious infection set in which required amputation of her right leg.

This amputation might not have been necessary if she had been allowed to remain in the hospital as Dr. Polonsky believed was necessary. Dr. Polonsky ended up being successfully sued for failing in his medical duties to this patient. In effect, the court said that no one but Dr. Polonsky had the right to discharge her from the hospital and he should have stood his ground and demanded those extra days. What we can imagine is that something like one of our rationing protocols (a Medicaid DRG) determined the average length of time that a patient like Mrs. Wickline needed to be hospitalized. But medical judgment needs to be individualized, and in this case Dr. Polonsky had a clear and strong medical rationale for insisting on the extra hospital days. This is a good example of the kind of medical flexibility we want to protect in our health care system. We would have no reason to believe that Dr. Polonsky acted unjustly in demanding those extra days; this was a reasonable exercise of his obligation to be a loyal patient advocate. The bedside rationing he actually engaged in was open to justified moral criticism. (Readers should not overgeneralize from this case. We assume the medical interpretation at the time was accurate. Today we know that extended hospital stays represent an increased risk of hospital-acquired infections.)

We can compare the Wickline case to the case of Mrs. Peake. This was a case reported in 1996 (April 14) on the front page of the *Chicago Tribune*. Mrs. Peake had been in a terrible auto accident that had shattered her leg. Her orthopedic surgeon believed that he could save her leg with a very costly complex surgery. The cost of the surgery would be $80,000–$90,000. The account in the newspaper said nothing about the likelihood of success for this surgery, but we will put that figure at 70% (for the sake of discussion). Her managed care plan required prior approval for this surgery. The orthopedic surgeon was asked by another physician attached to that plan what the least expensive therapeutically effective medical option was available. The surgeon replied that an amputation would cost $8,000 plus another $12,000 for rehabilitation and a prosthetic leg. He was denied the option of doing surgery to save her leg because of the high cost and the chance of failure. He did the surgery anyway and saved her leg.

Is this another example of the sort of moral and medical flexibility that must be permitted if we are to be respectful of the commitment of this surgeon to be a loyal patient advocate? The surgery could have failed. If it had, the additional cost required would have been for the amputation and prosthetic leg. Was this surgeon's choice really an injustice rather than a morally defensible example of commitment to the best interests of his patient? What if the probability of saving that leg were only 30%, or as low as 10%? If we believed the level of flexibility permitted at the 70% level of success was reasonable and just, would we be just as confident of that judgment at the 30% level or lower? Maybe a pragmatic compromise is possible that would be respectful of patient autonomy, protect a desirable level of clinical flexibility, and preserve overall commitments to health care justice. If there were any risk that this complex surgery would fail (and an amputation and rehabilitation would be necessary), the patient would have to agree to bear those latter costs. This might not be unreasonable or unfair. As an aside, this approach would be a good way of creatively circumventing the temptation to invoke the language of tragic choices.

Next, consider the case of Hannah Krauss (Veatch et al., 2009). She is 92 years old in a nursing home. She has suffered a debilitating stroke; she has atherosclerotic heart disease and diabetes. She is semi-mobile but mentally alert. She is complaining of intermittent chest pain, which could probably only be relieved adequately with coronary artery bypass graft (CABG). Note: The average cost of a CABG would be $65,000, but it would likely be a lot more in her case because of a prolonged hospitalization. Her cardiologist is not at all supportive of this idea because of the very serious risks of such surgery for someone of her age with her comorbidities. But she insists that she is perfectly comfortable with those risks. What should a just and loyal patient advocate do under these circumstances?

We might imagine two versions of this scenario. In one version the case arises in the Medicare system as it is now. For our purposes the salient feature of the case is that if the surgery went forward, the hospital would almost certainly lose a substantial sum of money because of likely complications and a prolonged stay. Medicare would also "lose" that money. Are these facts relevant to determining whether or not Mrs. Krauss has a just claim to those resources? The fact of the matter is that nothing in the Medicare legislation would require denying Mrs. Krauss her CABG; it is entirely up to the physician to judge whether that surgery is "medically necessary." So, what should her physician do as a loyal patient advocate? How is this case like or unlike our case with Mrs. Peake or Mrs. Wickline?

The alternate version of this case imagines that there has been the rational democratic deliberative process described earlier. One of the outcomes of that deliberative process was a rationing protocol that said, in effect, patients over age 85 would not be offered a CABG (at social expense) unless they were extraordinarily vigorous for their age and were afflicted with no more than minor comorbidities. What should a loyal patient advocate do under these circumstances? Could a physician in this situation justifiably argue that this rationing protocol was badly morally flawed, that it represented unjust discrimination against older persons with disabilities, and consequently he would vigorously lobby for the surgery (even if he had concerns about the outcome of the surgery)?

Here is another situation reported a few years ago that might be construed as morally objectionable age-based discrimination (Levinsky, 1998). The CEO of a large hospital requested that all orthopedic surgeons use a much less expensive hip prosthesis in patients who were more than 80 years old who had a likely life expectancy of less than 10 years. The prosthesis was likely to be good for 10 years but not much more than that; apart from durability the device the CEO was recommending was as good as the more expensive device he wished to give up. Should good doctors who were loyal patient advocates cooperate with this request? Or should this request be regarded as a morally objectionable form of bedside rationing? We argued above that rationing decisions ought to be visible and explicit, not hidden, especially from patients whose well-being might be directly affected by those decisions. Would the moral objection to bedside rationing be obviated if the physician informed patients that the less expensive and less durable device was going to be used in them (because they were not likely to live another 10 years in the judgment of their primary physician)? If patients objected to the use of the less expensive device, would that physician have to comply with their request in order to remain a loyal patient advocate? [Note: It may be the case that Medicare rules do not allow hospitals the option of charging patients the cost difference if they insist on receiving the more expensive device.] How is this case like or unlike the case of Mrs. Peake or Mrs. Wickline?

Next, consider the case of JW, a 54-year old male involved in a serious automobile accident. Without surgery and a blood transfusion, he will bleed to death. But he is refusing any transfusions because he is committed to being a Jehovah's Witness. However, he is not ready to die. He has read about a drug called recombinant Factor VIIa used with hemophiliacs to bring about rapid clotting. He wants to be given that drug to save his life. The cost of giving him that drug could be as high as $100,000, and the modest health insurance coverage he has will not pay for it. Nor does he have the resources to pay even a small portion of the cost of that drug. Would his surgeon be open to justified moral criticism if she were to provide the drug to him with the expectation that the hospital would absorb those costs as a charity care expense? Or is this something she is morally obligated to do as a loyal patient advocate? Is this a legitimate part of the range of clinical flexibility that physicians must have in order to meet fairly the distinctive health care needs of their patients? How is this case like or unlike the case of Mrs. Peake or Mrs. Krauss or Mrs. Wickline?

Then there is the case of Nataline Sarkisyan that grabbed newspaper headlines in 2007. The case occurred in Los Angeles. Nataline was 17 years old; she had been suffering from a very aggressive leukemia. She had failed two earlier efforts to defeat her cancer. She had received a bone marrow transplant from her brother, which she was now rejecting (the cost of which was $250,000). She was in multiorgan failure with severe neurological complications. Her surgeon was proposing doing a liver transplant, which he believed offered her a 65% chance of 6 extra months of life (Hennessy-Fiske, 2007; Burling, 2007). Other surgeons believed even that very marginal measure of success was excessively optimistic; too many things were going wrong too quickly. Nataline was doomed to die in a brief period no matter what was attempted medically or surgically. Her HMO refused to authorize payment for the liver transplant, which is what precipitated the newspaper headlines. Given this case description, would a surgeon who was a loyal patient advocate be open to justified moral criticism if he failed to do everything possible to secure that liver transplant? That is, should we think of this option as being "in bounds" so far as morally legitimate clinical flexibility is concerned when we are trying to distinguish morally permissible from morally impermissible acts of bedside rationing?

It might be useful to compare the Sarkisyan case to a broader array of cancer cases. One author writes: "Many patients with cancer want aggressive treatment until the very end, no matter how small the benefit or how great the toxicity" (Wilson, 2009, p. 573; Lakdawalla et al., 2012). Wilson cites a study in which it was found that 20% of Medicare patients with metastatic cancer started a new chemotherapy regimen within 2 weeks of death (Earle et al., 2004). Lakdawalla and coauthors (2012) found that 77% of surveyed cancer patients with solid tumors preferred hopeful gambles to safe bets, concluding that a higher threshold of cost-effectiveness needs to be set in an end-of-life context. Again, Wilson also calls attention to the work of Deborah Schrag, a medical oncologist who looked at pancreatic cancer patients who were treated with gemcitabine alone compared to those patients when erlotinib was added to the regimen. The addition of that drug added just 12 days to survival and it "increased the risk for such toxicities as diarrhea, interstitial lung disease, and treatment-related death" (Wilson, 2009, p. 574). That added about $15,000 to the cost of treating those patients, or $410,000 per added year of life. I should add that if we translated this into a Quality-Adjusted Life Year QALY measure (See ch. 17 this volume), the cost would be far in excess of a million dollars per QALY. The medical oncologists providing this care believed either that they were morally obligated to provide such care or that it was morally permissible that they do so. A recent survey of terminally ill cancer patients found that such patients believed we ought to be willing to spend $282,000 to gain an extra year of life for a cancer patient (Seabury et al., 2012). Given these survey results, our question is this: If these oncologists refused to go along with patient or family requests for this aggressive care, could they have been justifiably judged to have engaged in morally objectionable bedside rationing? How are such cases like or unlike the Sarkisyan case, or the case of Mrs. Peake or the case of Mrs. Krauss?

In England, the case of Leslie Burke garnered considerable media attention. He had been diagnosed with cerebellar ataxia at age 23. He was 41 years old in 2007. The disease process had advanced to the point where he was completely paralyzed from the neck down. Eventually, the paralysis would be total. He was still mentally quite alert, though severely debilitated. He was mindful of the Schiavo case in the United States. He knew that he would become incompetent in the near future and that his life would be sustained via feeding tubes. What he wanted from the NHS and his physicians was an ironclad guarantee that everything medically possible would be done to sustain his life for as long as possible no matter what the quality of his life might become. The question we raise is whether this is a demand that his physicians were morally obligated to fulfill, given the persistent shortage of hospital beds in the United Kingdom and the general shortage of resources for the NHS. His physicians made clear to him that they would not accede to his demands for reasons of both justice and compassion. This case was adjudicated, and the British courts ultimately sided with the physicians (Cruz, 2007). What do we see as the considerations of health care justice that would speak for or against this legal decision?

Another case for consideration would be that of Angel Diaz. This case was first reported on the front page of the *Wall Street Journal* (Anand, 2003). Angel was then (2003) 69 years old and in the very advanced stages of Alzheimer's. He had exhibited early signs of the disease in the early 1990s. In May of 2002 he had choked on some food, perhaps causing additional brain injury, which resulted in his being placed in a long-term care facility supported by a ventilator and feeding tubes. One year later he acquired pneumonia and began to bleed from his intestines for medically unknown reasons. His physicians were unable to stop the bleeding. He spent a total of 140 days in the hospital before dying at a cost somewhere in excess of $280,000. Apparently no bedside rationing decisions were made, but there could have been. So in our alternate scenario, we want to imagine that his physicians conclude they are very unlikely to be able to stop the bleeding. Would they then have been warranted (knowing that he could occupy that hospital bed for several additional months) in making a bedside rationing decision to discontinue all life-sustaining care, just as the physicians in the Burke case were prepared to do? If so, what would we see as the morally relevant considerations of health care justice that would have justified that decision?

There are also some issues around the implantable cardiac defibrillator [ICD]. The matter has not come to a head in the United States, but it has received considerable attention in Canada. The core issue is this. These devices cost about $40,000 each. They are intended to reverse what would otherwise be a fatal arrhythmia. According to recent research, however, 81% of these devices never fire over a 5-year period of time, at which point their battery needs to be replaced at a cost of about $20,000. Another 10% of these devices get implanted in individuals with advanced heart disease who have had serious heart attacks (Pauker et al., 2005; Goldberger & Lampert, 2006). These individuals often live less than a year after ICD implantation, and the device can do nothing to reverse a heart attack related to an arterial blockage. This situation looks very wasteful so far as use of social resources is concerned.

In the United States, about 200,000 of these implantations are performed per year at a cost of about $8 billion. That number can be reduced by 33% if a test called the "T-wave alternans test" were used to identify patients who were 98.8% unlikely to have an arrhythmic event in the next 2 years. The number of "mistakes" or falsely negative test results yielded by the test equals about 800 individuals who would die as a result of a fatal arrhythmia that would likely have been reversed if they had an ICD in them. But use of such a test on that scale would save almost $3 billion. Canada has actually put in place limitations on access to the ICD at the provincial level, which in turn put in place limits at the hospital level. But the actual decision as to which patients receive one of these devices and which are denied them has been left to the discretion of physicians (Simpson et al., 2005). In Europe generally, ICD implantation is only 25%–33% of the US rate with large variations among countries mostly related to economic circumstances (Camm & Nisam, 2010). The European Society of Cardiology is currently struggling to articulate guidelines for the cost-effective use of ICDs, especially in connection with the primary prevention of sudden cardiac death (Lubinski et al., 2011). Their goal is to convince policymakers that expanded access to ICDs should have much higher priority for health care resources (European Society of Cardiology, 2012). In both Canada and Europe restricted funding for ICDs is increasing the need for bedside rationing. In such circumstances how can physicians know whether or not they have made a morally defensible choice with regard to any individual patient if they are supposed to be a loyal advocate for the best interests of each of the patients before them? Should they be morally comfortable with just using the results of the T-wave alternans test to determine their clinical judgment? (For the sake of accuracy, we will note that there is continued debate in the medical literature regarding the utility of the T-wave alternans test as a stratification method.) How is this like or unlike the case of Mrs. Wickline or Mrs. Peake? Does it matter (morally speaking) that this limitation has been widely publicized in the Canadian Medicare system, including the fact that individual physicians ultimately decide? Does it matter (morally speaking) that this limitation is not widely publicized in Europe?

Our last case will be that of Hunter syndrome. This is an X-linked recessive genetic disorder. Individuals with this disorder have a severe deficiency of the lysosomal enzyme iduronate-2-sulphatase. This leads to a progressive accumulation of glycosaminoglycans in nearly all cell types, tissues, and organs (Wraith et al., 2008). Death usually occurs in the second decade of life, though some patients will have a less severe form of the disease and may survive until the fifth or sixth decade. There is now a drug, idursulfase, a form of enzyme replacement therapy that can partially correct for the deficiencies of this disease. That is, it can minimize the problem of organ enlargement. But this drug cannot reverse the adverse effects of this disease on the central nervous system, and this is where the worst effects of Hunter syndrome will be noticed.

The rationing issue is this: The drug costs about $300,000 per year. This drug can make a significant difference in length of life and quality of life for the relatively small fraction of these patients who do not have CNS involvement.

For those with CNS involvement, the effects on the clinical course of the disease will be marginal. Consequently, the clinical recommendation is that patients be started on the drug for 12–18 months with neurobehavioral testing aimed at determining whether there is CNS involvement. If there is evidence of neurobehavioral deterioration during this period (and this can be a challenging judgment call for those who do this testing), then the recommendation is that the drug be stopped (which means that the enlargement of organs will occur again). If there were no neurobehavioral testing done and the drug were simply given for, say, 10 years, that would be a cost per child of $3 million. That expenditure would not alter the fact that these children would still die in the second decade of life. The implicit moral argument behind these recommendations is that the drug should certainly be available to those patients without CNS involvement who would have a much longer life expectancy and improved quality of life with the drug. To make these resources available, we should deny them to those children who (after that trial period) are unlikely to benefit more than marginally from having continuing access to that drug. This is a sort of utilitarian argument aimed at maximizing the saving of the most high-quality life years. Should physicians caring for such children (who wish to see themselves as loyal patient advocates) cooperate with what I will call these rationing protocols/clinical recommendations, especially if the results of neurobehavioral testing after 18 months yield less than clear and convincing evidence of CNS deterioration?

We now have a rich collection of clinical cases that raise in different ways the problem of bedside rationing and how we might formulate a strategy for addressing that challenge that was just and compassionate and protective of the role of physicians as loyal patient advocates. What lessons might we draw from these cases? We should begin with a quick summary of our argument up to this point.

First, there is no "purely principled" way of addressing the bedside rationing problem. The "burdens of judgment" (moral and clinical) are too complex; the relevant reasonable conceptions of justice pertinent to health care are irreducibly pluralistic. The best judgments we will be able to make will be non-ideal.

Second, it would be wrong to draw from our first point that we are faced with a "tragic choice" situation that would warrant using implicit or invisible approaches to addressing specific bedside rationing challenges. This is a point that Syrett (2007, and in this volume) would agree with. Any just judgment in these circumstances will need to be public and visible, especially to those whose welfare is most directly affected by any bedside rationing decision. Further, ultimate legitimating of these judgments requires public conversation aimed in part at critically assessing these prior judgments. This is how we develop broad capacities for public moral reason, a process that would be severely attenuated if we invoked a "tragic choice" strategy.

Third, the claim that bedside rationing is always morally wrong is mistaken. The need for bedside rationing judgments by clinicians is inescapable; it would be an abdication of professional moral responsibility for such judgments to be delegated to administrators or bureaucrats.

Fourth, a more just approach to health care rationing would involve the construction of rationing protocols and practices through a process of rational democratic deliberation so that such protocols would be public and self-imposed. This would minimize the moral tension physicians otherwise experience who must implement rationing protocols and still be loyal patient advocates (since they would be implementing the rationing choices their patients had freely accepted for themselves).

Fifth, physicians will still need some degree of clinical flexibility in applying these rationing protocols in individualized patient circumstances, and we have to have some way of knowing that this flexibility does not undermine the justness of the rationing protocol. In the remainder of this essay we will try to tease out some guidelines for constraining that flexibility justly.

We should begin by noting that we agree with Strech et al. (2009) that this entire discussion needs to be situated within a certain understanding of the empirical realities of physicians' current attitudes toward bedside rationing. This does not mean that we should accept those empirical realities as immoveable. Rather, these represent the starting points for moral education. The analysis by Strech and colleagues of a large number of surveys of physician attitudes regarding rationing shows that physicians prefer (for the most part) *implicit* rationing to *explicit* approaches to rationing. The authors identify *explicit* forms of rationing with rules or protocols or guidelines that are imposed by *external authorities*, whether governmental or nongovernmental. In contrast, *implicit* forms of rationing are a product of clinical judgment by an individual physician in relation to an individual patient.

A reasonable interpretation of this preference by physicians is that these external authorities usually have no license to practice medicine and are completely unfamiliar with the patient for whom the physicians are caring. It would be a complete abrogation of the physicians' professional obligations if they were to carry out these rationing protocols nonreflectively. The obvious question we can ask is whether their response to rationing protocols would be more accepting if those rationing protocols were entirely a product of the work of a group comprised primarily of physicians (and other relevant experts) and based on the soundest possible medical evidence. This would address one major aspect of resistance to rationing protocols from "external authorities." That is, it would at least be *medical* authority whose judgments reflected medical knowledge and the values of medicine in general, and this does garnish support for such guidelines from many physicians (Hurst et al., 2006). However, these protocols or guidelines still would have been constructed apart from the medical circumstances of the patient before a particular physician right now. This is where the need for clinical flexibility and judgment is needed. However, the *implicit* quality of this judgment can be morally problematic, especially if this implies that bedside rationing decisions are not explicitly shared with the patients who are directly affected by those choices.

It is not unreasonable to expect that physicians would be able to explain and justify their clinical judgments, which I assume most physicians are willing and able to do. What is more difficult, however, is getting physicians to explain and justify bedside rationing judgments with clear and careful reasoning that makes explicit the justice-relevant considerations supporting their judgment. Hurst and Danis (2007) as well as Strech et al. (2009) point out that physicians are not well educated with respect to the language of justice as it applies in a clinical context. Most physicians today have taken up the central concepts that define contemporary medical ethics. That is, for example, they understand the need to be respectful of patient autonomy, they understand there are limits to that respect, and they have the capacity to explain what those limits are and why they are reasonable. We cannot say the same thing when it comes to matters related to health care justice. This may be a deficiency in medical education. Or it might reflect the view that there is something too political and too ideological associated with the language of justice that is not associated with the medical practice of respect for patient autonomy. In either case, the justice-based directive that rationing decisions ought to be public and transparent is not something to which physicians will generally be able to be responsive if they lack the language and concepts related to health care justice.

With regard to this last point, the practical proposal by Hurst and Danis (2007) is one clearly worthy of implementation as a starting point for clinician education. Specifically, they note that bedside rationing decisions of many kinds are a common occurrence within an ICU. Physicians should be expected to identify explicitly in a medical chart (or comparable document) that such a decision has been made and what they see as the morally relevant reasons that would justify that decision. That is, they should be able to make clear why that decision does not represent a failure to be a loyal patient advocate. This is not something that has to be long and complex. But it is something that would be reviewed and discussed in some formal educational setting by the physicians who are the staff for that ICU.

The goal of the discussions would be to gradually articulate a complex set of shared understandings regarding what would represent reasonable grounds for making various bedside rationing decisions. In all likelihood, there would be a realization (after the fact) in some cases that a moral mistake had been made. Such mistakes will be regrettable, but this is the best that is reasonable when non–ideally just (or sufficiently just) outcomes are all that we can hope for. Such a process is public, which is one way of bringing to light and remedying (in the future) very unjust decisions that might have been made. Further, this is a way of making such bedside rationing judgments transparent (as to the reasoning that would support them) as well as more consistent across clinicians in that ICU. What you ultimately have as a result of this process are *explicit* rationing protocols that are not vulnerable to the criticism that these protocols were generated by nonclinician outsiders serving interests that were not necessarily the interests of patients.

What we may derive from our analysis up to this point is a series of Take Home Messages (THMs).

THM #1: **Physician involvement.** Physicians need to be intimately involved in the creation of bedside rationing protocols, including the defining of their scope and limits, for moral reasons and reasons of professional integrity. This means that they need to be willing to invest the time and energy needed to create these shared moral understandings. If physicians needed some motivation for investing in this task, then it might be good to ask them as future possible patients in an ICU (as opposed to being attendings in an ICU) whether they would simply acquiesce to a bedside rationing decision that had been made regarding their own care without any explanation or justification for that decision. Instead, a decision would simply be made by whatever attending was caring for them for whatever private internal reasons that attending might have. It is difficult to imagine any physician-patients who would be perfectly comfortable with such a state of affairs. Again, the option physicians do not have in this scenario is rejecting all bedside rationing. This is very much like finding it morally objectionable that it will rain today; bedside rationing decisions are ubiquitous.

THM #2: **Collaborative physician involvement.** It is "groups of physicians" who must take responsibility for articulating the shared moral understandings regarding the scope and limits of bedside rationing. This is how idiosyncratic judgments by individual physicians would get identified and critically assessed. Physicians are accustomed to having considerable discretion in their making of clinical judgments. But the understanding is always there that they must be able to explain and defend medical judgments that deviate widely from established clinical norms. This same approach needs to be taken with regard to the range of flexibility seen as morally legitimate for bedside rationing. We should also note a significant side benefit associated with this second Take Home Message. Bedside rationing decisions (making or resisting them in a specific case) will be more likely to be accepted as socially legitimate if such judgments are endorsed by large groups of physicians (along with the moral rationale that justifies those judgments). Dr. Polonsky made the right decision initially in the Wickline case when he judged that she really needed a total of 8 extra days of hospital care. He should not have been cowed by the hospital administration into sacrificing 4 of those days at the expense of

Mrs. Wickline. If Dr. Polonsky had broader medical and moral support for his judgment, he might have been more able to stand his ground.

THM #3: **Identify and reduce excessive care.** If physicians have a fundamental objection to doing bedside rationing because their patients are being denied benefits for the sake of meeting the cost-cutting or profit-enhancing interests of some third party, then these same reasons speak against physicians providing "excessive care" to their patients that puts their patients at some risk of harm in order to enhance their own economic interests. Very aggressive end-of-life cancer care would be one example of a concern that requires reflective moral attention by physicians. Some number of patients may "want" that care, but this does not mean that physicians as loyal patient advocates concerned about the best interests of those patients ought to acquiesce to those wants, especially if those patients have a very distorted or excessively optimistic belief regarding what might be accomplished by such care and a very poor understanding of the medical risks to which they will be exposed (see Gawande, 2010). Further, invoking a commitment to the "pricelessness of human life" to justify providing such cancer care when a more objective medical assessment would question the appropriateness of that care is both morally and medically disingenuous. The same reasoning in less dramatic medical circumstances applies as well, such as excessive use of imaging, or mammograms, or PSA tests, or use of statins. Welch et al. (2011) have provided compelling examples and analyses regarding the harmful consequences to patients of overuse of all these medical interventions. That brings us to our fourth point.

THM #4: **Congruence of social and bedside rationing judgments.** Just bedside rationing judgments need to be congruent with broader just rationing policies and protocols at the social level. This is another way in which the clinical flexibility integral to fair and reasonable bedside rationing can be constrained. Again, the health care resources being distributed in accord with medical judgment are *social* resources in the vast majority of cases. These are not resources that either individual patients or physicians own to do with as they please.

Some might argue that there are no "broad just rationing understandings" in our society with which bedside rationing judgments can be congruent. This is a half-truth at best. We have largely failed to have the public, deliberative conversations necessary to articulate those broad rationing understandings. However, there are numerous such understandings that are widely agreed upon and implicit in our moral practices. For example, although the United States is very much a capitalistic society, virtually no one in the United States would accept as fair or just auctioning off the last bed in the ICU to the highest bidder. And the same would be true for transplantable organs (see Barilan, chapter 9).

We have in our society broad sympathy for those who are "medically least well off," especially if they might be faced with imminent death. We believe something needs to be done for them, something that might prolong their life a bit. But if the medical options available are extremely unlikely to alter their fate, if those options are extremely costly, and if we appreciate what it means to be morally consistent in matters of justice (the same commitment to all who are "medically least well off"), then we might pause to consider whether some form of palliative care might be both more just and more compassionate than costly, ineffective life-prolonging care. This is a complex judgment, but it can be refined considerably through the use of a large number of concrete cases that most laypersons could understand.

One strategic move aimed at achieving the social understandings of justice we need might begin in this way: You (just and caring citizens) want to be responsive to the health care needs of those who are medically least well off, which is a morally reasonable commitment. But there are many sorts of patients that might fit under the rubric of those who are medically least well off. Some of them have chronic degenerative conditions that end in death. The course of these diseases is often very predictable, especially near the end when there is little medicine can do to delay or prevent imminent death. But other individuals may be among the medically least well off because their diseases very adversely affect their quality of life and will adversely affect length of life if little is done for them medically. This latter group has medical conditions that may be very expensive to treat, but medicine in these cases is quite effective, at least in improving significantly quality of life and length of life. (Think of patients with ankylosing spondylitis.) Would you judge it more morally appropriate that we allocate much more in the way of life-prolonging medical resources to this latter group rather than the former group? Would you see such a choice as being fair and reasonable, especially if it were clear that we were not abandoning the first group since we would be certain to provide them with effective palliative care rather than minimally effective life-prolonging care? In this way, we meet what we see as our moral obligation to be responsive to the health needs of the medically least well *who are capable of benefiting from expensive life-prolonging or quality of life–maintaining medical care* while at the same time preserving needed medical resources for all other medical needs not attached to those who are medically least well (See Fleck, 2011).

This somewhat general approach might be concretized by going back to some of the cases we introduced earlier. Thus the Nataline Sarkisyan case is very unfortunate, but she has no just claim to a liver transplant that will make virtually no difference to her fate. She was provided with three expensive prior efforts to save her life that all failed. Her physicians could have denied her the liver transplant in good conscience as a morally legitimate bedside rationing decision. The same will hold true in the Leslie Burke case. Again, Burke had been provided with all the care that was medically effective and medically reasonable in earlier stages of his disease process over almost a 20-year period of time. Consequently, he has no just claim to occupy a scarce ICU bed and incur very substantial other medical costs to have his life sustained for months or longer in a completely nonfunctional state that he himself could not appreciate. This too is a reasonable bedside rationing decision, which does not represent any threat to the just claims of persons with disabilities such as a vent-dependent quadriplegic, since such individuals can be quite functional and quite capable of appreciating the life that they have. What this last point represents for our Hunter syndrome cases is that we should make the social commitment to sustain the lives of these patients at $300,000 per year for idulsulfase if the disease has not attacked the CNS. Otherwise, the 18-month trial of support is a reasonable limit given that additional use of the drug is unlikely to alter the fate of those individuals.

To return to our main point, bedside rationing decisions need to be congruent with broader social understandings of what health care justice requires. What needs to be noticed in the examples explicated above is that no self-serving, third-party interests are being directly advanced by these bedside rationing decisions. These are not judgments that come from bureaucrats or administrators who are far removed from the concerns of patients. These are judgments that physicians as physicians can endorse, unless they are prepared to argue that society is morally obligated to pour unlimited resources into medical care.

THM #5: **Medical gaming is morally problematic.** If we have "sufficiently just" rationing policies and practices at the social level, then physicians have no moral justification for gaming the system in order to gain special advantages for "their" patients. Further, physicians would have no moral justification for corrupting their own medical judgment in order to gain special advantages for "their" patients. Thus, in the case of Mrs. Krauss the physician's best medical judgment is that a CABG for her at age 92 with her medical history would be a very bad medical choice (more likely than not contrary to her medical best interests). He would be open to justified moral criticism from the perspectives of both justice and medical integrity if he were to ignore his own medical judgment and advocate for her receiving the CABG. This would clearly be an exercise of medical flexibility aimed at avoiding a bedside rationing judgment that would be unwarranted. Again, this would be in contrast to the Wickline case where that physician could have (and should have) exercised his right to make the medical judgment he initially made contrary to the rationing expectations of the hospital. The case of Mrs. Peake is more complex. The facts make a difference there. Mrs. Peake could likely have adapted to having an artificial leg, but it would be wrong to characterize saving her leg as a cosmetic procedure. The surgery might have failed, thereby risking a substantial increase in "unnecessary" costs. But this was a very skilled surgeon with a 70% (hypothetical) likelihood this would work. So maybe this surgeon was justified in acting as a loyal patient advocate, which would not be true in a Hunter syndrome case where neurobehavioral testing indicated likely CNS involvement and the physician still wanted to continue idursulfase indefinitely. But if that prior likelihood of success dropped to 20%, it would be much harder to justify the surgeon's decision as a just and reasonable invocation of flexible medical judgment.

THM #6: **Transparency about rationing protocols is essential.** Respect for patients and respect for justice require that bedside rationing decisions (and the rationale that would justify them) not be hidden from patients. This is an essential part of the "publicity condition" at the core of our socially shared understanding of justice. Complying with this expectation may require some uncomfortable and difficult conversations with patients or their families, but this is part of the cost of creating and maintaining "just understandings" regarding the scope and limits of bedside rationing. Social research seems to indicate that this is something the vast majority of patients want (Schwappach & Koeck, 2004). Thus, in the ICD example in Canada, patients would have a moral right to know that they had been denied one of these devices and the reasons why this denial was fair and reasonable. If clinicians had collaborated with one another to develop clinical guidelines and clinical tests for determining who was or was not a candidate for an ICD, then this would make it easier to have these conversations with patients without being at risk of an accusation of disloyalty. The justness of the rationing decision at the patient level could be further understood by the patient if the physician were also able to explain the larger social justification for the social policy regarding these ICDs. This helps to build social trust and social stability regarding rationing policies at the societal level.

Another example of an apparently successful real-world rationing policy worked out collaboratively among clinicians in the NHS regarded a drug called *palivizumab*, used to treat bronchiolitis (Teale, 2009). This is an expensive drug whose cost can be justified so long as its use is restricted to those types of infants who are most likely to benefit substantially from the drug because they are most of risk of developing complications if denied the drug. Other children could be treated with much cheaper therapies that were very likely to be effective. If use of the drug were somewhat indiscriminate, then the cost of the drug would rise to almost $1 million per quality-adjusted life year. Achieving these clinical moral understandings preserves a commitment to fairness in the use of this drug and limits considerably any arbitrary uses of clinical flexibility regarding its use.

THM #7: **Public reasons must justify bedside rationing.** Bedside rationing (or decisions to avoid rationing in specific clinical circumstances) can only be justified by invoking "public reasons," the kinds of reasons that are reasonable no matter what one's deep religious or philosophic commitments might be. Thus, in our Jehovah Witness case above, this patient has no moral right to demand the drug recombinant Factor VIIa to stop his bleeding (and save his life) at a potential cost of $100,000 in order to remain compliant with his religious beliefs. Nor may a physician justly make available this drug to such a patient for what are essentially religious reasons. In a pluralistic society, reasons such as that would threaten to undermine any commitment to just rationing policies and protocols. The reader can imagine a physician committed to a strong "sanctity of life" view who would avoid virtually all bedside rationing protocols if their consequence would be to shorten a patient's life by as little as a day. If we permitted that as a reasonable exercise of clinical flexibility in relation to bedside rationing, the result would be the extravagant allocation of limited resources to patients of that physician at the expense of the just claims of other patients (most of whom might not endorse the religious views that motivated his noncompliance with otherwise socially endorsed fair rationing protocols). In short, (1) patients do not have any "special" claims to additional health care resources, over and above what similarly situated patients might have, just because they wish to invoke a religious argument in support of those claims; and (2) patients do not have a "liberally legitimate" just claim to additional health care resources if the only arguments they can give in support of those claims are religiously grounded arguments.

We conclude with a few quick points regarding establishing the legitimacy of bedside rationing decisions. Hurst and Danis (2007) call attention to the useful clinical fact that bedside rationing decisions are ubiquitous and largely unnoticed in daily clinical practice today. Their useful practical suggestion is that a broad array of these commonplace bedside rationing decisions should be identified, and the reasons why they are quietly accepted should be articulated. This would provide a rich base for establishing the morally defensible scope and limits of flexibility with regard to bedside rationing. That is, we would then have a rich mix of considered moral judgments related to bedside rationing that could be used to judge the more complex and contentious cases that grab our moral attention, such as the ones I identified earlier. What we seek to achieve among these judgments is what Rawls (1971, 1993) refers to as a *reflective equilibrium*, a kind of careful, complex balancing of morally relevant considerations, the goal being to avoid creating additional ethical problems as a result of a too narrowly focused effort to resolve a current ethical problem.

Next, there is a lot of discussion in the press and in medical circles about patients needing to take more personal responsibility for their health. There are numerous things physicians might do to facilitate patients in making better choices related to their health. But one of the things that would be out of bounds would be invoking this rationale as a fair and reasonable basis for certain bedside rationing decisions that would in some cases deny patients expensive life-prolonging medical care because their physician judged their health problems were related to poor health choices they had made. In general, these patient circumstances are so complex and opportunities for very arbitrary denial judgments so readily available that the result would be very unfair instances of bedside rationing (See Fleck, 2012).

Finally, Strech et al. (2009) call attention to the empirical fact that the vast majority of physicians are reluctant to make bedside rationing decisions that are related to or justified by judgments of cost-effectiveness. There may be multiple sources of this reluctance. Many physicians might have an unreflective commitment to the belief that human life is priceless. Or they might feel that economic judgments should not shape the practice of medicine, that this was an unseemly kind of authority. Or they might believe that the methodology for generating these judgments is too arbitrary and too controversial to be incorporated into the making of weighty medico-moral bedside rationing judgments, such as in connection with last-chance therapies. Or, physicians may simply have little understanding of cost-effectiveness analysis, which seems also to be true with regard to the language of justice. But to my mind these are all deficiencies to be remedied rather than empirical realities to be accepted. The largest aspect of the rationing problem in health care is not about absolutely scarce medical resources, such as transplantable organs, but fiscal resources and opportunity costs. What cost-effectiveness analysis permits is making reasonable comparisons about the relative value of various medical interventions across the whole field of medicine. As Peter Ubel (2000) has pointed out, cost-effectiveness analysis is not the ultimate determinant of just and right bedside rationing decisions. But it does provide useful data for making more informed judgments about how to use health care resources wisely and justly when we have only limited resources to meet virtually unlimited health care needs. A utilitarian framework is at the base of cost-effectiveness analysis. Utilitarianism is one reasonable conception of justice among a plurality of conceptions of justice we employ in thinking through specific problems of health care justice. Sometimes that conception will yield the most morally defensible approach to a specific health care rationing problem. At other times it will be subordinated to another more relevant conception of justice. Making such relativized judgments will be another part of the public and professional conversations we need to have regarding the challenges of rationing health care fairly.

REFERENCES

Aaron, H., & Schwartz, W. (1984). *The Painful Prescription: Rationing Hospital Care.* Washington, D.C.: The Brookings Institution.

Abrams, F. (1986). Patient advocate or secret agent? *Journal of the American Medical Association*, 256, 1784–1785.

American College of Physicians. (2012). Ethics Manual. *Annals of Internal Medicine*, 156, 73–104.

Anand, G. (2003). "Who gets health care? Rationing in an age of rising costs." *Wall Street Journal* (Sept. 12), p. A1.

Baeroe, K. (2008). Priority-setting in health care: on the relation between reasonable choices on the micro-level and the macro-level. *Theoretical Medicine and Bioethics*, 29, 87–102.

Bodenheimer, T., & Grumbach, K. (2012). *Understanding Health Policy: A Clinical Approach*, 6th ed. New York: McGraw Hill.

Burling, S. (2007). "Cigna's experts say liver transplant would not have saved teen." *Philadelphia Inquirer* (Dec. 24), Business News.

Butler, J. (1999). *The Ethics of Health Care Rationing: Principles and Practices*. London: Cassell.

Calabresi, G., & Bobbitt, P. (1978). *Tragic Choices*. New York: W.W. Norton.

Camm, A., & Nisam, S. (2010). European utilization of the implantable defibrillator: has 10 years changed the 'enigma'? *Europace*, 12, 1063–1069.

Cruz, P. (2007). The *Burke* case: the terminally ill patient and the right to life. *The Modern Law Review*, 70 (2), 306–317.

Daniels, N. (1986). Why saying 'no' to patients in the United States is so hard: cost containment, justice, and provider autonomy. *New England Journal of Medicine*, 314, 1381–1383.

Daniels, N., & Sabin, J. (2008). *Setting Limits Fairly: Learning to Share Resources For Health*, 2nd ed. Oxford: Oxford University Press.

Daschle, T. (2008). *Critical: What We Can Do About the Health-Care Crisis*. New York: St. Martin's Press.

Earle, C., Neville, B., Landrum, M., et al. (2004). Trends in the aggressiveness of cancer care at the end of life. *Journal of Clinical Oncology*, 22, 315–321.

Eddy, D. (1996). *Clinical Decision Making: From Theory to Practice (A Collection of Essays from the Journal of the American Medical Association)*. New York: Jones and Bartlett.

Emanuel, E. (2008). *Health Care Guaranteed: A Simple, Secure Solution for America*. New York: Public Affairs Press.

European Society of Cardiology. (2012). "EHRA ICD for Life Initiative Summit— Belgrade 19-20 October 2012." Retrieved August 25, 2012 from http://www. escardio.org/communities/EHRA/icd-for-life/Pages/summit-belgrade.aspx#. UDqNiRHTFrs.email.

"SCD Awareness Day—December 2012." Retrieved August 25, 2012 from http://www. escardio.org/communities/EHRA/icd-for-life/Pages/scd-awareness-day.aspx#. UDqOcUjDCX0.email.

Fleck, L. (2012). Whoopie pies, super-sized fries: 'just' snacking? 'Just' des(s)erts? *Cambridge Quarterly of Healthcare Ethics 21*, 5–19.

Fleck, L. (2011). Just caring: health care rationing, terminal illness, and the medically least well off. *Journal of Law, Medicine, and Ethics*, 39, 156–171.

Fleck, L. (2009). *Just Caring: Health Care Rationing and Democratic Deliberation*. Oxford: Oxford University Press.

Fleck, L. (2006). Just caring: Who pays? Who profits? Who panders? *Hastings Center Report, 36* (3), 13–17.

Freeman, V., Rathore, S., Weinfurt, K., et al. (1999). Lying for patients: physician deception of third-party payers. *Archives of Internal Medicine, 159,* 2263–2270.

Gawande, A. (2010). Letting go: what should medicine do when it can't save your life? *The New Yorker, 86* (August 2), pp. 36–50.

Gawande, A. (2009). The cost conundrum: what a Texas town can teach us about health care. *The New Yorker, 85* (June 1), pp. 36–44.

Goldberger, Z. & Lampert, R. 2006. "Implantable cardioverter defibrillators: expanding indications and technologies." *Journal of the American Medical Association, 295,* 809–818.

Gutmann, A., & Thompson, D. (2004). *Why Deliberative Democracy?* Princeton, NJ: Princeton University Press.

Gutmann, A., & Thompson, D. (1996). *Democracy and Disagreement.* Cambridge, MA: Harvard University Press.

Hall, M. (1997). *Making Medical Spending Decisions: The Law, Ethics, and Economics of Rationing Mechanisms.* Oxford: Oxford University Press.

Hennessy-Fiske, M. (2007). Tough Calls in Transplant Case: A Northridge Teen Dies Shortly After her Insurer Reverses its Refusal to Pay for a Treatment it Called Experimental. *Los Angeles Times* (December 22), p. A1.

Hiatt, H. (1975). Protecting the medical commons: who is responsible? *New England Journal of Medicine, 293,* 235–241.

Hope, J. (2007). "Arthritis patients 'face a life of pain' from drug rationing." *Daily Mail* (Nov. 11). Accessed June 9, 2009 from http://www.dailymail.co.uk/news/article-493071/Arthritis-patients-face-life-pain-drug-rationing.html.

Hurst, S., & Danis, M. (2007). A framework for rationing by clinical judgment. *Kennedy Institute of Ethics Journal, 17,* 247–266.

Hurst, S., Slowther, A., Forde, R., et al. (2006). Prevalence and determinants of physician bedside rationing: data from Europe. *Journal of General Internal Medicine, 21,* 1138–1143.

Hurst, S., Forde, R., Reiter-Theil, S., et al. (2007). Physicians' views on resource availability and equity in four European health care systems." *BMC Health Services Research, 7,* 137–145.

Lakdawalla, D., Romley, J., Sanchez, Y., Maclean, J., Penrod, J., & Philipson, T. (2012). How cancer patients value hope and the implications for cost-effectiveness assessments of high-cost cancer therapies. *Health Affairs, 31,* 676–682.

Levinsky, N. (1998). Truth or consequences. *New England Journal of Medicine, 338,* 913–915.

Levinsky, N. (1984). The doctor's master. *New England Journal of Medicine, 311,* 1573–1575.

Lubinski, A., Bissinger, A., Boersma, L., Leenhardt, A., Merkeley, B., Oto, A., et al. (2011). Determinants of geographic variations in implantation of cardiac defibrillators in the european society of cardiology member countries—data from the European Heart Rhythm Association white book. *Europace, 13,* 654–662.

Luft, H. (2009). Beyond the public plan debate: a pathway to transform the delivery system. Available in draft form at: http://securechoice.info/storage/Beyond%20the%20Public%20Plan%20Debate.pdf

Luft, H. (2008). *Total Cure: The Antidote to the Health Care Crisis.* Cambridge, MA: Harvard University Press.

Mechanic, D. (1995). Dilemmas in rationing health care services: the case for implicit rationing. *British Medical Journal, 310*, 1655–1659.

Morreim, H. (1991)_. *Balancing Act: The New Medical Ethics of Medicine's New Economics.* Dordrecht, Holland: Kluwer Academic Publishers.

Morreim, H. (1989). Fiscal scarcity and the inevitability of bedside budget balancing. *Archives of Internal Medicine, 149*, 1012–1015.

Newdick, C. (2005). *Who Should We Treat? Rights, Rationing, and Resources in the NHS.* Oxford: Oxford University Press.

Norheim, O. (2008). Clinical priority setting. *British Medical Journal, 337*, 1846–1848.

Orentlicher, D. (2010). Rationing health care: It's a matter of the health care system's structure. *Annals of Health Law, 19*, 449–465.

Pauker, S., Ester, N., Salem, D. (2005). Preventing sudden cardiac death: can we afford the benefit? *Annals of Internal Medicine, 142*, 664–666.

Rawls, J. (1993). *Political Liberalism.* New York: Columbia University Press.

Rawls, J. (1971). *A Theory of Justice.* Cambridge, MA: Harvard University Press.

Reuben, D., & Cassel C. (2011). Physician stewardship of health care in an era of finite resources. *Journal of the American Medical Association, 306*, 430–431.

Schoenman, J. (2012). The concentration of health care spending. NIHCM Foundation Data Brief (July). Available at: http://www.nihcm.org/pdf/DataBrief3%20Final.pdf.

Schwappach, D., & Koeck, C. (2004). Preferences for disclosure: the case of bedside rationing. *Social Science and Medicine, 59*, 1891–1897.

Seabury, S., Goldma, D., Maclean, J., Penrod, J., & Lakdawalla, D. (2012). Patients value metastatic cancer therapy more highly than is typically shown through traditional estimates. *Health Affairs, 31*, 691–699.

Simpson, C., Hoffmaster, B., & Dorian, P. (2005). Downward delegation of implantable cardioverter defibrillator decision making in a restricted-resource environment: the pitfalls of bedside rationing. *Canadian Journal of Cardiology, 21*(7), 595–599.

Strech, D., Synofzik, M., & Marckmann, G. (2008). How physicians allocate resources at the bedside: a systematic review of qualitative studies. *Journal of Medicine and Philosophy, 33*, 80–99.

Strech, D., Persad, G., Marckmann, G., & Danis, M. (2009). Are physicians willing to ration health care? Conflicting findings in a systematic review of survey research. *Health Policy, 90*, 113–124.

Syrett, K. (2007). *Law, Legitimacy and the Rationing of Health Care: A Contextual and Comparative Perspective.* Cambridge: Cambridge University Press.

Teale, A. (2009). Palivizumab and the importance of cost effectiveness. *British Medical Journal*, 1935–1938.

Ubel, P. (2000). *Pricing Human Life: Why It's Time for Health Care Rationing.* Cambridge, MA: MIT Press.

Veatch, R., Haddad, A., & English, D. (2009). *Case Studies in Biomedical Ethics.* Oxford: Oxford University Press.

Veatch, R. (1986). DRGs and the ethical re-allocation of resources. *Hastings Center Report, 16*, 32–40.

Welch, H., Schwartz, L., & Woloshin, S. (2011). *Over-Diagnosis: Making People Sick in the Pursuit of Health.* New York: Beacon Press.

Wilper, A., Woolhandler, S., Lasser, K., McCormick, D., Bor, D., & Himmelstein, D. (2009). Health insurance and mortality in US adults. *American Journal of Public Health*, 99, 2289–2295.

Wilson, J. (2009). Cancer care: a microcosm of the problems facing all of health care. *Annals of Internal Medicine*, 150, 573–576.

Wraith, J., Scarpa, M., Beck, M., et al. (2008). Mucupolysaccharidosis type II (Hunter syndrome): a clinical review and recommendation for treatment in the era of enzyme replacement therapy. *European Journal of Pediatrics*, 167, 267–277.

LEGAL CASES

Wickline v State of California. Court of Appeals of California, Second Appellate District

11 Overdiagnosis and Overtreatment

Implications for Bedside Rationing

■ HOWARD BRODY

Over the past several decades, those involved in the ethical debate over health care rationing have tended to agree on a basic assumption—that there is little to be gained by addressing frank waste in the health care system and that talking about "waste, fraud, and abuse," as politicians are prone to do, counts as a serious distraction from the real issues. Schwartz, in a classic paper, argued that any reduction in wasteful spending would be a small, one-time-only solution that would leave the fundamental drivers of cost increases unaffected (Schwartz, 1987).

Why, then, are some policy analysts returning to waste avoidance as a central theme in cost containment (Brody, 2012)?

Avoiding waste through overdiagnosis and overtreatment has important ethical implications in its own right, as well as shedding further light on the ethics of rationing. As a case study in waste avoidance and ethics, we may focus on the Choosing Wisely campaign launched by the American Board of Internal Medicine Foundation (Cassel & Guest, 2012). In its initial phase, Choosing Wisely enrolled nine medical specialty societies each to identify their "top five" interventions that provided no benefit and caused substantial costs, yielding a list of 45 such interventions (Brody, 2010). Choosing Wisely did not, however, recommend any further action on the part of those specialty societies or suggest that any third-party payers cease reimbursement. Instead they proposed that the list be addressed via shared decision making—that physicians and patients should discuss in each such case why the modality offered no benefit, and consider any evidence that this patient might be an exception to the rule and that some benefit might be likely. Consumer organizations like Consumers Union were brought on board to assist in developing patient-friendly decision aids, and patients were encouraged to become a force in questioning their physicians if such interventions were recommended to them.

■ CONTINUUM AND DISCONTINUUM MODELS

The extensive literature on the ethics of rationing in health care appears largely to have relied on a continuum model. At one end of a spectrum lie medical interventions that have the lowest predicted benefit and the highest cost. At the other end are treatments that have lower cost and considerable predicted benefit. It is assumed that where an intervention lies on the spectrum has a lot to do with the ethical justification of restricting access to that modality by means of rationing, and the ability of the rationing program accurately to locate any medical treatment for any given patient along that continuum has a lot to do with the fairness of that rationing approach.

To illustrate the continuum idea, let's briefly recall the days before it was realized that autologous bone marrow transplant following high-dose chemotherapy for advanced breast cancer was probably useless and harmful, and when it was thought that such patients might have a 10% chance of prolonged survival with such therapy (which, in the mid-1990s, cost in the range of $150,000 per patient). Many were outraged when American managed care plans denied this treatment to patients, claiming that the therapy was experimental and hence not a covered benefit. Patients and their supporters commonly went to court to demand that plans pay for the treatment. Yet among those so outraged, I doubt if any would have agreed that a patient deserves access to a hypothetical modality that would extend life by 10 minutes at a cost of $10 million. At some point, most would agree that a line is crossed and that shrinking benefits are simply not worth the exorbitant costs—even if the benefits never quite reach zero.

In the past few years, increased attention has been paid to the phenomena of overdiagnosis and overtreatment, particularly in the United States (Brownlee, 2008; Welch et al., 2011). These issues raise a possibility that appears to challenge the traditional continuum model of rationing. Some indeed have proposed a discontinuum model, according to which there are two distinct areas requiring policy attention. One area represents the traditional rationing continuum—variable degrees of patient benefit associated with varying costs. The other area represents medical interventions that can be reliably categorized as effectively having zero patient benefit (Brody, 2010, 2012). (It makes no sense to call such modalities "treatments" or "care," so the more awkward term "interventions" is required.)

Two factors make it tempting to adopt a discontinuum model, one fiscal and the other ethical. The fiscal factor arises from recent research into the percentage of the US health budget now devoted to interventions arguably in the no-benefit category. One very conservative estimate put the figure for waste due to overtreatment at around $191 billion (Berwick & Hackbarth, 2012), but we more commonly see estimates in the range of $600–$750 billion annually (e.g., Fuchs & Milstein, 2011). Many experts appear to agree that as much as one-third of the US health budget buys interventions that fail to benefit patients, according to the best available scientific evidence. Hardly any other category of health costs offer anything near these potential savings, so in an era dominated by concerns about cost containment the possibility of identifying no-benefit interventions offers policymakers a tempting target.

The ethical factors could be crudely labeled as "ethically clean" and "ethically mandatory." Saving money by discontinuing zero-benefit interventions is *ethically clean* in the sense that no patient is deprived of any health benefit as a result, so the usual arguments against any form of rationing seem not to apply. Going further, eliminating such interventions appears *ethically mandatory*, not merely desirable. It is seldom the case that a medical intervention, even one that offers no benefit, is free of risks of harm. Nonbeneficial drugs and surgery can cause adverse reactions, even fatal ones. (It has been estimated that more than 100,000 people die in the United States every year as a result of taking prescription drugs, not counting errors or overdoses; see Light, 2010). Unnecessary diagnostic and screening tests can produce false-positive results and overdiagnoses, which in turn prompt further invasive procedures. Since the only justification for exposing a patient to potential harm in medicine is the chance of securing a benefit, something that predictably offers no chance of benefit has no justification whatever for being administered to any patient.

■ ETHICAL CONCERNS

When the possibility of a discontinuum model is raised, at least four sets of ethical questions follow. The first is one of policy priorities. If huge sums are now spent on useless interventions, what is the justification for devoting powder and shot to the more usual rationing continuum? Why even talk about depriving any patient of a low-benefit but high-cost treatment if we are wasting billions on predictably no-benefit treatments? Do we not have an overriding moral duty to do everything practically possible to eliminate the first area, that of waste due to overdiagnosis and overtreatment, before we turn to *any* potential cost savings that eliminate even small degrees of patient benefit?

The second set of questions has to do with empirical research and its implications. If we have an overriding moral duty to eliminate no-benefit interventions before undertaking the more usual types of rationing, we also seem to have an overriding moral duty to prioritize the types of research that will best help us confidently identify those interventions. That in turn assumes that such interventions can indeed be identified with sufficient confidence to justify policy choices. Questions of the necessary evidentiary threshold become paramount. One likely argument is that we can dismiss zero-benefit interventions as an area of policy concern, simply because no evidentiary threshold that can be achieved in the real world will reliably conclude that an intervention has absolutely zero benefit for any specified category of patients (let alone for any individual patient). An opposing argument is that everyday medical practice gives us numerous examples of reasonable certainty that a given intervention offers no benefit for a given patient group, and we simply need better to understand how those practical decisions are made and justified. It is possible that this debate will mirror at least to some extent the extensive ethical debate over the notion of medical futility, with which it clearly has overlap (Brody, 2012).

A third set of questions has to do with proper terminology and definitions. Language has a lot to do with how any policy proposal is accepted by the public in politically divisive times. For example, early in 2012 the media suddenly took note of a word that had been in the ethics manual published by the American College of Physicians (ACP) since 1998 but had never previously attracted attention—*parsimonious*. Somehow it now seemed ominous that the ACP ethics manual urged physicians to be "parsimonious" and "efficient," "to use resources wisely and to help ensure that resources are equitably available" (American College of Physicians, 2012; Anonymous, 2012). Some commentators seemed worried, despite the fact that if one read the entire ethics manual one could find lots of support for the idea that the well-being of the individual patient ought to be the physician's first priority, so that any call for "parsimony" had to be interpreted in that light.

Just three months later, the first Choosing Wisely list was released (Cassel & Guest, 2012). The media, in general, responded very positively to the Choosing Wisely initiative. Partly this was due to how the recommendations were framed. First, Choosing Wisely took pains to argue that their real goal was improving the quality of care and not merely slashing costs. Second, Choosing Wisely carefully avoided any suggestion that insurers and other payers ought not cover these procedures. Instead they called for shared decision making, with physicians and patients discussing the pros and cons of these procedures in individual cases. Finally, Choosing Wisely stressed its partnership with consumer organizations such as the Consumers Union and the American Association of Retired Persons.

In short, the public through the media appeared to react negatively when it seemed that somebody was calling for health care *rationing*, and positively when a campaign was able to distance itself from the "rationing" taint.

Is it proper to speak of *rationing* in relation to restricting access to zero-benefit interventions? Menzel, in this volume, recommends a more restricted use of the word *rationing* than is generally accepted, based in part on the desire not to hand irrational opponents of sound policy more ammunition. By similar logic, one could examine a number of definitions offered for "rationing" in health care and note that most either require, or imply, that the treatment under review be potentially beneficial—so that denying a patient a zero-benefit intervention is by definition *not* rationing. A counterargument is that rationing, when done transparently and in accord with a fair system, is ethically justified even if the "R word" is politically unpopular. If we shy away from calling something "rationing," because we fear the popular or political fallout, we merely perpetuate the impression that rationing is ethically intolerable and hence postpone the day when our society can have a reasonable discussion of these issues. Avoiding the "R word" may win the battle in the short term but risk losing the war.

■ BEDSIDE RATIONING IMPLICATIONS

The fourth set of questions relates directly to the clinician at the bedside. What is the role of the individual practitioner with regard to zero-benefit interventions? Since virtually all such modalities have to be ordered for patients by physicians, it is intriguing to note that in theory these incredible sums of money could be saved immediately without the government, or any third-party payer, doing anything at all. Of course in the real world, physicians today order all these interventions—and we have to ask why, what incentives drive this, and what might be done at all various levels to change this behavior.

As an example of the ethical questions that then arise, consider again the Choosing Wisely campaign. One might have imagined that consumer representatives would welcome the call for shared decision making, which would also delight any defenders of respect for patient autonomy. Presumably these organizations would be delighted that no one was recommending denying patients access to these interventions by relocating the critical decisions elsewhere in the health system. I was therefore intrigued, in attending a meeting on the overuse issue late in 2012, to hear the consumer representatives in the room loudest in their criticism of Choosing Wisely. In their view, this program was a way for physicians to dodge all the responsibility and instead to place an unreasonable burden upon the patient. How many patients, they asked, had the knowledge and time to first master the list of 45 nonrecommended interventions and then the gumption to confront their own physicians and dispute the wisdom of ordering one of those interventions?

Generally, "patient-centered care" has been accepted by physicians and health managers as an ethically desirable descriptor (Duggan et al., 2006). These consumer representatives, however, took a dim view of this mantra. It appeared to them that the health care system was using "patient-centered care" to shift too much responsibility onto relatively powerless patients. Choosing Wisely seemed to them a further step in that direction. If these interventions were costly, without benefit, and potentially harmful, why was it the patient's responsibility to raise questions about them? Why was it not the system's responsibility to weed out such interventions?

■ CONCLUSION

In sum, the role of the physician at the bedside in dealing with any defined category of zero-benefit interventions has yet to be worked out satisfactorily. This physician's role presupposes that other players in the system—payers, investigators, medical organizations, the tort system—are also doing what they need to do, whatever that might be. But no matter what roles are assigned to these other players, there will certainly be a necessary role for the individual physician. The ethical ramifications of that role have yet to be fully explored.

Some, perhaps impressed by the initial public-relations success of Choosing Wisely, might propose that we strive to separate efforts to avoid overdiagnosis and overtreatment from the stigma of "bedside rationing." While I admire many features of Choosing Wisely, I believe such advice ultimately to be short-sighted. Physicians caring for individual patients will ultimately have to make many of the decisions needed to implement any meaningful scheme of cost containment. It seems fully reasonable to ask these physicians to strive to put patient benefits and harm avoidance first, and to relegate cost containment to a secondary status. But it seems both unrealistic and irresponsible to imagine that these physicians ought simply to ignore cost considerations entirely. So bedside rationing, or something that looks enough like it to raise many of the same ethical concerns, seems to be in the equation regardless of whether we ultimately employ a continuum or a discontinuum model.

REFERENCES

Anonymous. (2012). Do no harm—and keep an eye on costs. *Kaiser Health News*, January 11. Available at: http://www.kaiserhealthnews.org/stories/2012/january/11/parsimonious-care.aspx.

American College of Physicians. (2012). *Ethics Manual*. 6th ed. Available at: http://www.acponline.org/running_practice/ethics/manual/manual6th.htm

Berwick, D. M., & Hackbarth, A. D. (2012). Eliminating waste in US health care. *Journal of the American Medical Association, 307*, 1513–1516.

Brody, H. (2010). Medicine's ethical responsibility for health care reform—the Top Five list. *New England Journal of Medicine, 362*, 283–285.

Brody, H. (2012). From an ethics of rationing to an ethics of waste avoidance. *New England Journal of Medicine, 366*, 1949–1951.

Brownlee, S. (2008). *Overtreated: Why too much medicine is making us sicker and poorer*. New York: Bloomsbury USA.

Cassel, C. K., Guest, J. A. (2012). Choosing wisely: helping physicians and patients make smart decisions about their care. *Journal of the American Medical Association, 307*, 1801–1802.

Duggan, P. S., Geller, G., Cooper, L. A., & Beach, M. C. (2006). The moral nature of patient-centeredness: is it 'just the right thing to do?'" *Patient Education and Counseling, 62*, 271–276.

Fuchs, V. R., & Milstein, A. (2011). The $640 billion question—why does cost-effective care diffuse so slowly? *New England Journal of Medicine, 364*, 1985–1987.

Light, D. W. ed. (2010). *The Risks of Prescription Drugs*. New York: Columbia University Press/SSRC.

Schwartz, W. B. (1987). The inevitable failure of current cost-containment strategies. Why they can provide only temporary relief. *Journal of the American Medical Association, 257*, 220–224.

Welch, H. G., Schwartz, L. M, & Woloshin, S. (2011). *Overdiagnosed: Making people sick in the pursuit of health.* Boston: Beacon Press.

12 How Can Bedside Rationing Be Justified Despite Coexisting Inefficiency?

The Need for "Benchmarks of Efficiency"

■ DANIEL STRECH AND MARION DANIS

No health care system can provide all patients with all treatments that may have the potential for benefit.(Fojo & Grady, 2009; Kent 2010) Reasons given for this claim include a demographic shift to a more elderly and chronically ill population, the growing gap between what is technically possible and what can be afforded, the rising cost of medical goods and services, and the competition for public funds from other sectors. The claim is underscored by evidence from surveys of doctors in a number of countries indicating that they are currently making rationing decisions in both outpatient and inpatient medicine (Hurst et al., 2006; Ward et al., 2008; Strech et al., 2009). Rationing is defined here and most widely understood internationally as the withholding, for reasons of cost, of medical interventions that are expected to have net additional benefit for the patient (Ubel & Goold, 1998). Indirect evidence about the practical relevance of bedside rationing has been gathered also for the US health care system in several surveys about physicians' willingness to ration healthcare (Holloway et al., 2000; Shrank et al., 2006; Strech et al., 2009).

In response, various normative frameworks have been developed in the last 10 to 15 years to encourage or ensure ethically appropriate implementation of unavoidable rationing (Emanuel, 2000; Hurst & Danis, 2007; NICE, 2007; Daniels, 2008; NICE, 2008; Strech et al., 2010). These frameworks involve the application of a number of theories of distributive justice—in particular utilitarian, egalitarian, prioritarian, and social contractarian theories. In the face of these competing theories, procedures to guarantee due process have been developed. While debate continues about precisely how to prioritize and ration care in the most equitable manner, there is general consensus that when resources are constrained rationing is unavoidable and justifiable and should be implemented fairly.

A particular challenge to the justifiability of rationing (independent of the fairness of its implementation) is the worry that it might be possible to reduce the need to ration and still control costs simply by eliminating inefficiencies in health care delivery. We face substantial evidence of inefficient health care delivery (Emanuel & Fuchs, 2008; WHO, 2010; The Good Stewardship Working Group, 2011; Korenstein et al., 2012), and this evidence is often given as a justification for refusing to talk about or explicitly address the need for rationing (Truog 2009; Storz & Egger, 2010). Thus this chapter aims to clarify under what conditions rationing by clinical practitioners can be more or less justified despite coexistent inefficiency.

At the outset we acknowledge that inefficiency is caused by many factors that are the result of both organizational and individual behavior, and both health care organizations and individual practitioners should be held accountable for pursuing efficient delivery of health care services (Chisholm & Evans, 2010; Haas et al., 2005). Thus the ethical arguments we make here about the relationship between inefficiency and justifiable rationing pertain both to organizations and individuals. We believe that individual clinicians will not be able to practice the most efficient care if they do so in the absence of a supportive health care organization. Health care organizations need to provide the guidelines that individual clinicians follow. Otherwise, efforts to be efficient will be carried out inconsistently. In particular, in the absence of an organizational set of guidelines there will be no mechanism for monitoring and reprimanding the noncooperative clinician who takes advantage of the system for his patients while all other clinicians comply. Having said that, we focus the remainder of the paper on the requirement for efficiency among individual clinicians, for two reasons. First, because we think this demand for clinicians to pursue efficiency is sufficiently important and complicated to warrant exclusive attention. Second, the causes of organizational inefficiency are extremely complicated and require a multitude of solutions that are not germane to the individual clinician. Note, for example, that Parker and Newbrander wrote in 1994 about strategies for addressing waste and inefficiency in the health care sector. They argued that waste in health care is caused by limited information and accountability for decisions about the use of resources. Conflicts of interest and limited accountability are likely to cause corruption and fraud. Proposed solutions require changes in information management, policy, management and technical procedures that are crucial for building organizational efficiency but not necessarily pertinent to the individual clinician (Chisholm & Evans, 2010; Haas et al., 2005).

■ DEFINITION OF CLINICAL INEFFICIENCY

There is a variety of definitions of efficiency (and inefficiency respectively) currently in use. For a selection of definitions of efficiency see, for example, the report of the Agency of Healthcare Research and Quality (AHRQ) on health care efficiency measures (http://www.ahrq.gov/qual/efficiency/hcemch1.

htm). The AHRQ defines efficiency as the relationship between a specific product (output) of the health care system and the resources (inputs) used to create the product (Haas et al., 2005; Chisholm & Evans, 2010).

Ideally, clinicians use only those preventive, diagnostic, and therapeutic measures for the management of medical conditions (input) that lead to the improvement of patient relevant outcomes (output). In such circumstances physicians practice effective health care (from a clinical perspective that focuses on patient-centered outcomes; see ABIM Foundation et al., 2002) The effectiveness of a specific medical intervention, however, does not indicate whether its application is efficient in comparison to alternative effective interventions.

For illustrative and didactic purposes this paper focuses on two broad types of "clinical inefficiency" that are consistent with the definition used by AHRQ:

A) The provision of health-related interventions with *no net benefit* for the individual patient.
B) The provision of health-related interventions with *higher costs but equal benefit compared to alternative interventions* for the individual patient.

An example of a type A inefficiency is cancer screening among patients with advanced cancer. Sima et al. demonstrated that a sizeable proportion of patients with advanced cancer continue to undergo cancer screening tests that do have side effects (like every medical intervention) but do not have a meaningful likelihood of providing benefit by altering a patient outcome in any useful way (Sima et al., 2010). Other examples are annual electrocardiograms (ECGs) or any other cardiac screening for asymptomatic, low-risk patients (The Good Stewardship Working Group, 2011).

An example of a type B inefficiency is the prescription of ranibizumab for the treatment of neovascular age-related macular degeneration (AMD) that has equivalent effects to bevacizumab but costs much more (CATT Research Group, 2011). Another example of type B inefficiency is imaging for low back pain within the first 6 weeks of developing symptoms (Bigos et al., 2011; The Good Stewardship Working Group, 2011).

In the following we briefly introduce four assumptions relevant to our analysis below.

Assumption 1: The Determination of Inefficiency Requires Value Judgments

When deciding whether an intervention has proven health-related benefits and harms and whether the benefits outweigh the harms (net benefit), value judgments come into play at several levels (Strech & Tilburt, 2008). One needs to decide, for example, whether the quality of the data regarding effectiveness or inefficiency is "sufficient" or "acceptable" (Kramer, 2009). The need for value judgments, however, does not preclude any reasonable decision about whether or not a medical intervention has a proven net benefit (The Good Stewardship Working Group, 2011). For example, comorbidity or a history of an adverse reaction to a specific active pharmaceutical agent can exclude the patient from a gold-standard treatment option. In these cases the physician may be acting efficiently when prescribing another reasonable medication that has otherwise been proven to be equally beneficial but costs more than the gold standard. However, not every deviation from evidence-based clinical guidelines can be reasonably justified by the specific circumstances of individual patients. Inefficiency is verifiable when the reasons for deviation from gold standards are inappropriate.

Assumption 2: Categorization of Marginal Benefits

Value judgments also play a role in defining "marginal benefits" and in deciding whether interventions with "marginal benefits" should be understood and treated in the same way as interventions that have "no net benefit" (Buyx et al., 2011). One might argue that when broad consensus has been reached among physicians and other stakeholders through fair and transparent discussion as to whether a marginally beneficial intervention counts as clinically valuable or not, it then follows whether it can be considered as an instance of rationing or as an instance of reducing inefficiency. If it is judged to be clinically valuable, then a decision to withhold it would count as an instance of rationing. If a marginal benefit is not considered clinically valuable then a decision to withhold it would count as an instance of increasing efficiency.

A question remains as to how to categorize marginal benefits that have been judged to be of insignificant value in a consensus process but are considered valuable nonetheless by a patient or family. We would suggest that to the extent that someone considers a marginal benefit valuable and it is withheld despite their desire for it, this is an instance of rationing. Whether this instance of rationing is justifiable is a separate question that remains to be determined by examining how equitably the decision to withhold the intervention was taken.

Assumption 3: Ethical Implications of Clinical Inefficiency

Both types of clinical inefficiency decrease the possible aggregate extent of health care in a society and/or the possibility of achieving other goods by diverting funds that could be used for other effective interventions. In so doing, inefficiencies harm people indirectly by wasting resources that subsequently necessitate rationing. This act of rationing (with its inherent health-related harm, see the definition above) would otherwise not be required. Type

A inefficiency harms in a second way as well, by leading to additional fruitless medical evaluations that would otherwise have been unnecessary and can lead to iatrogenic complications. To the extent that both types of inefficiency are avoidable and lead indirectly to forgone benefits, inefficient provision of medical services poses an ethical problem.

Assumption 4: Efficiency Can Be Further Improved but Will Always Be Imperfect

At present, all health care systems have the potential to decrease inefficiency (though not ad infinitum). For example, one study concluded that 447,000 life years could be saved in the US population over the next 20 years if physicians at the micro level simply follow existing protocols for the use of low-cost β blockers (Phillips et al., 2000). Many other micro-level decisions also bear the potential to decrease inefficiency (O'Connor et al., 2004; Garber & Skinner, 2008; The Good Stewardship Working Group, 2011). Although we lack sound empirical data (in a positive or negative direction) that could support this presumption, we think that there is at least some face validity for the claim that efficiency in health care delivery will always be imperfect.

▪ ANALYSIS

Whether an act of rationing is ethically justifiable despite coexisting inefficiency depends on the relationship between the individual or party who makes an inefficient medical decision (resulting in scarce resources) and the individual or party who has to ration health care (because of scarce resources). Most problematic is a situation where the individual who makes inefficient clinical decisions is the same individual who rations health care. If we assume that bedside inefficiency leads to various harms for patients (see assumption 3) and that bedside rationing is avoidable (at least to some degree) through decreased inefficiency (see assumption 4) then bedside rationing cannot be justified under the following conditions:

A) the relevant physician is aware of budget limitations that have precipitated a scarcity of medical supplies or services in the institution where she practices, and

B) this physician consciously continues to prescribe a nonbeneficial medication (type A inefficiency) or medications that are more expensive than other medications with equal net benefits (type B inefficiency).

Bedside rationing on the part of this physician cannot be fully justified if both conditions are fulfilled because the specific physician has consciously contributed to the need to ration, which would otherwise have been less necessary.

More complex are those situations where physicians or health care managers are not aware of their inefficiency. In these cases, it seems important to determine whether the specific physician or health care manager could and should be aware of specific opportunities to reduce inefficiency. For example, a physician who often prescribes off-label medications or costly interventions as their initial choice, although clinical guidelines only recommend them as secondary treatment options (following a trial of equally effective but less expensive options), could know better. It would not be sufficient to argue that the physician was not aware of the inefficiency when easily accessible, evidence-based clinical guidelines (developed by a representative professional society) highlight the ineffectiveness or inefficiency and recommend more efficient alternatives (The Good Stewardship Working Group, 2011). Physicians bear a certain responsibility to learn more about the consequences of inefficient use of scarce health care resources (ABIM Foundation et al., 2002; Brody, 2010). In any case, this specific physician should be expected to justify the deviation from the current standard of care. Deviating from clinical guidelines can be more or less justifiable (Cabana et al., 1999).

Sufficient Efforts to Decrease Inefficiency Make Rationing More Legitimate

Based on our preceding assumptions and analysis, we argue that unavoidable but fair rationing is more legitimate if sufficient efforts are simultaneously undertaken to decrease inefficiency. There is a strong moral imperative underscoring this demand, because inefficiency can harm twice: first by the provision of nonbeneficial but sometimes harmful interventions, and second by the subsequent need for rationing beneficial health care in other situations. It follows that decision makers who manage, fund, or advise a group of physicians (e.g., managers in insurance companies, health funds, hospitals, or health care organizations) need to encourage improved efficiency among physicians as much as possible (ABIM Foundation et al., 2002; The Good Stewardship Working Group, 2011). The term "as much as possible" takes into account the widely shared assumption that perfect efficiency is unrealistic and that thresholds for both "sufficient efficiency" and "sufficient efforts to improve efficiency" can be determined. It is clearly not sufficient when health care managers and health policy decision makers argue that every improvement of efficiency is unrealistic or if they only profess (without explicit actions) that they will improve efficiency in their area of accountability. The need for improved efficiency becomes more urgent when rationing decisions already occur (Strech et al., 2009).[1]

"Benchmarks of Efficiency"

If clinicians need to ration health care, these activities become more (though not completely) acceptable when the same actors simultaneously try to reach benchmarks that reflect "sufficient" efficiency. This paragraph aims to introduce the basic concept of "benchmarks of efficiency" with respect to the two types of clinical inefficiency.

"Benchmarks of efficiency" need to address specific health care activities where inefficiency can be reasonably decreased (Qaseem et al., 2012). As we outlined in the previous paragraphs, various value judgments come into play when determining where and how much inefficiency can be reasonably decreased. Because of the influence of value judgments, reasonable disagreement is to be expected (unavoidably). However, reasonable disagreement on where and how much inefficiency can be reasonably decreased should not result in the reluctance to determine benchmarks. As with other decision making that includes reasonable disagreement due to differing value judgments, rational and fair processes should be applied to reach rational and fair decisions. As we also argued above, broad consent in determining benchmarks of efficiency can and should be expected from physician groups. Recently, some physician groups have outlined health care activities where inefficiency can be reasonably decreased (The Good Stewardship Working Group, 2011; Qaseem et al., 2012). For example, the ABIM Foundation has initiated a campaign (*Choosing Wisely*) to reduce inefficiency (http://choosingwisely.org). Each of the participating specialty societies has identified a list of five common tests or procedures whose use in their profession should be discussed or questioned. Criteria for the chosen interventions were that: (a) the item should be within the specialty's purview and control; (b) it should be used frequently and/or carry a significant cost; and, (c) there is evidence to support each recommendation. The Consumers Union has partnered in this effort by creating consumer education materials for each item, intended for patients and their families.

If one were to apply the concept of "benchmarks of efficiency" to the efforts of physician groups (such as the ABIM Foundation and collaborating specialty groups) and activities (such as Choosing Wisely) one would explicitly set goals regarding how much inefficiency is to be reduced in a reasonable time frame and when the efforts of various individuals and organizations undertaken to fulfill these benchmarks can be called "sufficient." The more specific and transparent those benchmarks are and the more they are realized in the given time frame, the more legitimate are rationing decisions despite coexistent inefficiency.

Take the example of type A inefficiency that we described above: cancer screening among patients with advanced cancer (Sima et al., 2010). A benchmark could define that the ineffective use of cancer screening shall be reduced by increasing adherence to screening guidelines by at least 50% within the next 3–5 years in a specific region or group of health care providers. If the benchmark of efficiency has not been fulfilled within the given time period while rationing of any kind of health care by the same group of physicians has continued, one could question whether "sufficient efforts" have been undertaken to reduce coexistent inefficiency.

To fulfill these benchmarks, several well-developed policy tools could be used by physician groups and health care organizations, including practice guidelines, utilization review, medical practice profiling, and feedback to providers (Liu, 2003; Hughes, 2008; Chisholm & Evans, 2010).

Apart from defining the accountability of specific parties, setting efficiency benchmarks demands a stepwise process. Setting benchmarks for the more efficient use of specific condition–treatment pairs involves:

A) Deliberation about and selection of a set of specific insufficiently efficient health care practices. As exemplary first steps in this direction, see The Good Stewardship Working Group (2011) and Qaseem et al. (2012). This process should acknowledge criteria of procedural justice (e.g., transparency, justification of weightings and trade-offs, minimizing conflicts of interest; see Emanuel, 2000; Daniels, 2008; IOM, 2009). Such procedural criteria help to foster understanding and trust in the application of the more substantial criteria for choosing specific condition–treatment pairs. The Good Stewardship Working Group chose the following more substantial criteria to discuss and justify the selection of specific condition-treatment pairs:
   1) frequency with which physicians engaged in a specific activity in their practice;
   2) potential impact of the activity on quality of care;
   3) potential impact of the activity on cost of care;
   4) strength of the evidence supporting the activity; and
   5) ease or difficulty of implementing the activity in their own practice.

Further research and pilot testing should evaluate whether these criteria result in a fair selection of inefficient health care practices.

B) Determination of how far efficiency can be reasonably improved over a certain time and what counts as "sufficient."
C) Plan and agree how to implement and adapt strategies to fulfill the benchmark requirements and when these efforts would count as "sufficient."

One might ask whether the benchmark approach we have suggested adequately addresses the concern we raised at the outset. Will there be a tight enough correlation between compliance with efficiency demands and legitimacy of rationing? Shouldn't we specify that if a clinician does not follow guidelines regarding the proper indications for a particular procedure, rationing of that procedure by that clinician is not as justifiable as it would be had he followed the guidelines? For example, if a clinician does not follow guidelines regarding the proper indications for MRI studies, any rationing of MRIs by that clinician should be considered unjustified. Some might argue for such a tight correlation. Others might endorse a broader understanding of "correlation" between sufficient efforts to reduce inefficiency on the one hand and more legitimate bedside rationing on the other hand. According to this broader understanding, the crucial point is that a physician tries to decrease inefficiency sufficiently (in different situations). If the physician does so, his efforts to ration health care are more legitimate. We would acknowledge that the approach we have outlined here is most consistent with the broader view and does not offer a tight correlation at this point. For those who endorse a tighter correlation, additional steps (benchmarks) must be set.

Adherence to Benchmarks: Governing the Commons

Several questions concerning the practicability of this benchmark-based approach might be raised that we briefly address here; namely: How should an organization ensure that its doctors are efficient? How might one address the possibility that if the strategy we suggest is not uniformly adopted, this could exaggerate disparity in care received by patients seeing differing physicians?

We offer two suggestions regarding cooperation. One is that the benchmark approach we outlined above could also consider issues of justice. It is likely that health care rationing, if not carried out fairly, would harm lower socioeconomic classes more because they are less able to buy in the private sector what has been rationed in the publicly financed sector. Population-based research is needed to assess the distribution of harms related to inefficiency and rationing among more or less vulnerable populations. If the best available evidence demonstrates the existence of an unjust distribution of rationing-related harms, benchmarks of "sufficient efforts" to decrease this type of injustice can further increase the ethical legitimacy of the unavoidable rationing of health care. See the NICE equality schemes and the NICE annual equality report that take first steps in this direction (NICE 2009; NICE 2010).

A useful possibility to address the problems of inconsistency and noncompliance is to learn from successful strategies for addressing these problems in dealing with historic cases of common resource problems. Elinor Ostrom, for example, describes how the tragedy of the commons encountered in circumstances of limited natural resources such as limited water supplies are sustainably addressed by groups that regulate themselves (Ostrom, 1990). In regulating themselves they foster consistent compliance. Several characteristics that distinguish such successful groups could also be applied to groups of clinicians in the health care sector: clearly defined boundaries, congruence between rules and local conditions, participation in rulemaking by those who are affected, monitoring of behavior by those who must follow the rules or their designees, use of graduated sanctions that depend on the seriousness of misbehavior, easy access to conflict resolution mechanisms for those who participate in allocation decisions, and the ability for those who participate in allocation decisions to devise their own institutional structure (Ostrom, 1990).

■ CONCLUSION

While it is unrealistic to expect that health care delivery can be completely efficient, sufficient efforts to improve efficiency are warranted before rationing can be justly carried out. We recommend the use of benchmarks for efficiency for the definition of sufficient efforts and for evaluation purposes. Additional practice-oriented strategies need to be used for the selection of and adherence to such benchmarks. We describe the adherence to such benchmarks as a necessary (and often neglected) but clearly not sufficient requirement for just bedside rationing. Needless to say, further substantial and procedural principles should be acknowledged when making all-things-considered judgments about just or unjust cases of bedside rationing (Emanuel, 2000; Hurst & Danis, 2007; Daniels 2008).

■ ACKNOWLEDGMENT

This chapter has been published previously by the authors. See Strech, D., & Danis, M. How can bedside rationing be justified despite coexisting inefficiency? The need for 'benchmarks of efficiency.' *Journal of Medical Ethics,* 2012 Dec 20. [Epub ahead of print]

Note
1. We should clarify here that we are not saying that a clinician should avoid bedside rationing until he has improved efficiency. Rather, we are saying that bedside rationing merely remains less legitimate and less fair if it is done in the absence of efforts to reduce inefficiency.

REFERENCES

ABIM Foundation, ACP–ASIM Foundation and European Federation of Internal Medicine. (2002). Medical professionalism in the new millennium: a physicians' charter. *Lancet, 359*(9305), 520–522.

Bigos, S., Bowyer, O., Braen, G., Brown, k., Deyo, R., Haldeman, S., Hart, J. L., et al. (2011). Acute low back problems in adults: US Dept of Health and Human Services AHCPR Clinical Practice Guideline No. 14: AHCPR Publication No. 95–0642. Retrieved May 24, 2011, from http://d4c2.com/d4c2-000038.htm.

Brody, H. (2010). Medicine's ethical responsibility for health care reform—the Top Five list." *New England Journal of Medicine, 362*(4), 283–285.

Buyx, A. M., Friedrich, D. R., & Schone-Seifert, B. (2011). Ethics and effectiveness: rationing healthcare by thresholds of minimum effectiveness. *British Medical Journal, 342*, d54.

Cabana, M. D., Rand, C. S., Powe, N. R., Wu, A. W., Wilson, M. H., Abboud, P. A., & Rubin, H. R. (1999). Why don't physicians follow clinical practice guidelines? A framework for improvement. *Journal of the American Medical Association, 282*(15), 1458–1465.

CATT Research Group. (2011). Ranibizumab and Bevacizumab for neovascular age-related macular degeneration." *New England Journal of Medicine, 364*(20), 1897–1908.

Chisholm, D., & Evans, D. B. (2010). Improving health system efficiency as a means of moving towards universal coverage. World Health Report (2010) Background Paper, No 28. Retrieved May 21, 2014 from http://www.who.int/healthsystems/topics/financing/healthreport/28UCefficiency.pdf.

Daniels, N. (2008). *Just Health: Meeting Health Needs Fairly.* New York: Cambridge University Press.

Emanuel, E. J. (2000). Justice and managed care. Four principles for the just allocation of health care resources. *Hastings Center Report, 30*(3), 8–16.

Emanuel, E. J., & Fuchs, V. R. (2008). The perfect storm of overutilization. *Journal of the American Medical Association, 299*(23), 2789–2791.

Fojo, T., & Grady, C. (2009). How much is life worth: cetuximab, non-small cell lung cancer, and the $440 billion question. *Journal of the National Cancer Institute, 101*(15), 1044–1048.

Garber, A. M., & Skinner, J. (2008). Is American health care uniquely inefficient? *Journal of Economic Perspectives, 22*(4), 27–50.

Haas, J. S., Phillips, K. A., Gerstenberger, E. P., Seer, A. C. (2005). Potential savings from substituting generic drugs for brand-name drugs: medical expenditure panel survey, 1997–2000. *Annals of Internal Medicine, 142*(11), 891–897.

Holloway, R. G., Ringel, S. P., Bernat, J. L., Keran, C. M., Lawyer, B. L., et al. (2000). US neurologists: attitudes on rationing. *Neurology, 55*(10), 1492–1497.

Hughes, R. G. (2008). Tools and Strategies for Quality Improvement and Patient Safety. In Hughes, R. G., ed. *Patient Safety and Quality. An Evidence-Based Handbook for Nurses.* Rockville, MD: Agency for Healthcare Research and Quality.

Hurst, S. A., & Danis, M. (2007). A framework for rationing by clinical judgment. *Kennedy Institute of Ethics Journal, 17*(3), 247–266.

Hurst, S. A., Slowther, A. M., Forde, R., Pegoraro, R., Reiter-Theil, S., Perrier, A., Garret-Mayer, E., et al. (2006). Prevalence and determinants of physician bedside rationing: data from Europe." *Journal of General Internal Medicine, 21*(11), 1138–1143.

IOM [Institute of Medicine]. (2009). *Conflicts of Interest in Medical Research, Education, and Practice.* Washington, DC: National Academies Press, Institute of Medicine.

Kent, D. (2010). Just-as-good medicine. Less expensive, lower-quality innovations abound in every economic sector—except medicine. *American Scientist, 98*(2), 98–102.

Korenstein, D., Falk, R., Howell, E. A., Bishop, T., Keyhani, S. K. (2012). Overuse of health care services in the United States: an understudied problem. *Archives of Internal Medicine, 172*(2), 171–178.

Kramer, J. M. (2009). Balancing the benefits and risks of inhaled long-acting beta-agonists— the influence of values." *New England Journal of Medicine, 360*(16), 1592–1595.

Liu, X. (2003). Policy tools for allocative efficiency of health services. Geneva: World Health Organization.

NICE [National Institute for Health and Clinical Excellence]. (2007). NICE equality scheme and action plan: implementation plan. London: National Institute for Health and Clinical Excellence.

NICE. (2008). Social value judgements. Principles for the development of NICE guidance. 2nd edition. London: National Institute for Health and Clinical Excellence.

NICE. (2009). NICE annual equality report 2009. London: National Institute for Health and Clinical Excellence.

NICE. (2010). NICE revised equality scheme 2010–2013. London: National Institute for Health and Clinical Excellence.

O'Connor, A. M., Llewellyn-Thomas, H. A., & Flood, A. B. (2004). Modifying unwarranted variations in health care: shared decision making using patient decision aids. *Health Affairs (Millwood)* Supplemental Web Exclusives: VAR63–72.

Ostrom, E. (1990). *Governing the Commons: The Evolution of Institutions for Collective Action.* New York: Cambridge University Press.

Phillips, K. A., Shlipak, M. G., Coxson, P., Heidenreich, P. A., Hunink, M. G., Goldman, P. A., Williams, L. W., et al. (2000). Health and economic benefits of increased beta-blocker use following myocardial infarction. *Journal of the American Medical Association, 284*(21), 2748–2754.

Qaseem, A., P. Alguire, P. Dallas, Feinberg, L. E., Fitzgerald, F. T., Horwitch, C., Humphrey, L., et al. (2012). Appropriate use of screening and diagnostic tests to foster high-value, cost-conscious care. *Annals of Internal Medicine, 156*(2), 147–149.

Shrank, W. H., Joseph, G. J., Choudhry, N. K., Young, H. N., Ettner, S. L., Glassman, P., Asch, S. M., et al. (2006). Physicians' perceptions of relevant prescription drug costs: do costs to the individual patient or to the population matter most? *American Journal of Managed Care, 12*(9), 545–551.

Sima, C. S., Panageas, K. S., & Schrag, D. (2010). Cancer screening among patients with advanced cancer. *Journal of the American Medical Association, 304*(14), 1584–1591.

Storz, P., & Egger, B. (2010). [The debate about priority setting and rationing in the statuatory health insurance: Overdue or unnecessary überflüssig?]. *Gesundheits- und Sozialpolitik,* 1, 11–18.

Strech, D., Danis, M., Lob, M., & Markmann, D. (2009). "[Extent and impact of bedside rationing in German hospitals: results of a representative survey among physicians]." *Deutsche Medizinische Wochenschrift, 134*(24), 1261–1266.

Strech, D., Hurst, S., & Danis, M. (2010). The role of ethics committees and ethics consultation in allocation decisions: a 4-stage process. *Medical Care, 48*(9), 821–826.

Strech, D., Persad, G. & Marckmann, G. (2009). Are physicians willing to ration health care? Conflicting findings in a systematic review of survey research. *Health Policy, 90*(2–3), 113–124.

Strech, D., & Tilburt, J. (2008). Value judgments in the analysis and synthesis of evidence. *Journal of Clinical Epidemiology, 61*(6), 521–524.

The Good Stewardship Working Group. (2011). The "top 5" lists in primary care: meeting the responsibility of professionalism. *Archives of Internal Medicine, 171*(15), 1385–1390

Truog, R. D. (2009). Screening mammography and the "r" word. *New England Journal of Medicine, 361*(26), 2501–2503.

Ubel, P. A., & Goold, S. D. (1998). 'Rationing' health care. Not all definitions are created equal. *Archives of Internal Medicine, 158*(3), 209–214.

Ward, N. S., Teno, J. M., Curtis, J. R., Rubenfield, G. D., Levy, M. M. (2008). Perceptions of cost constraints, resource limitations, and rationing in United States intensive care units: results of a national survey. *Critical Care Medicine, 36*(2), 471–476.

WHO [World Health Organization]. (2010). *The world health report—Health systems financing: the path to universal coverage.* Geneva: World Health Organization.

13 The Collective Action Problem

■ ROBERT E. GOODIN

A classic collective action problem has the following structure. Each actor would be better off if everyone were to perform a certain action. But each actor would be even better off than that if everyone *except her* were to perform that action. Each one of them is thus tempted to let the others perform the action, while not doing so oneself. Yet each of the others, being identically situated, does the same. So no one ends up doing it at all.

That is the "tragedy of the commons" (Hardin, 1968). The tragedy lies in the fact that there is an outcome that would have been better for all concerned, if only they could have organized to act collectively in pursuit of it; but that outcome is virtually impossible to obtain through uncoordinated private action (Olson, 1965; Hardin, 1982; Ostrom, 1990).

For a familiar example, consider the case of fisheries. All fisherfolk would be better off if all of them restricted their catch to sustainable levels. Each of them, however, has a private motive to catch more than that. Yet if all of them do so, overfishing will lead to the exhaustion of the fishery. None of them wants that to happen: quite the opposite. But no one of them (and no small group of them) can, by desisting, prevent that from happening. So each acts on his private motive, and overfishing ensues.

Real-world collective problems are vastly more complicated than those examples might imply. Even regarding fisheries, restrictions might rightly concern not merely how many fish you can catch but what kinds, what sizes, and where. Likewise, restrictions on the use of a common pasture might have to stipulate a trade-off schedule among various different animals that might be put out to graze there or specify trade-offs between grazing and cultivating the common lands. In medical applications, the schedule for restricting allocation of resources according to conditions and prognoses will be even more complicated than that, by many orders of magnitude. Without meaning in the least to downplay the difficulty of coming up with a remotely defensible schedule, I merely observe that the structure of the problem is the same across all these cases.

In connection with bedside rationing, the common pool resource that is most commonly discussed is health care funding, be it in the form of a fixed national healthcare budget or some smaller pot of funds in the case of more decentralized systems.[1] As such the issue is labeled "cost containment." Of course, just how much importance should be assigned to containing costs of health care is contentious. Some would insist that "economic...consider-ations are not germane to ethical medical practice" at all (quoted in Aaron & Schwartz, 1984, p. 127). Indeed, Wyller has argued this point in chapter 15. Even those not disposed toward that extreme view must nonetheless acknowl-edge that pressure on the health budget could be reduced in at least two ways: one would be by reducing demand, through rationing; another would by increasing supply, through increased health care funding or making more effective use of available resources.

Cost containment looks like a classic common pool resource only if we regard the health budget as strictly fixed. That, many would say, is not some-thing we should easily concede. Perhaps in the long term we should not. Perhaps we should instead campaign for increased health care funding, or even an open-ended commitment to meeting health care needs regardless of cost. Perhaps we should campaign for improved effectiveness of the medical use of resources. Those are important long-term projects that may eventually bear fruit.[2]

In the short term, however, matters are typically otherwise. The supply of health care resources available at any given time is ordinarily strictly fixed and limited. Where that is so, the supply of those fixed resources would indeed be a common pool resource, and bedside rationing to maximize the health ben-efits derived from it would pose a collective action problem of the sort just described.

The bulk of this chapter will indeed discuss bedside rationing primarily in terms of cost containment. But it bears emphasizing that it is not purely a matter of cost containment alone. Collective action problems of a strictly analogous sort arise in other respects as well. Let me offer just two other health-related examples, to suggest the generality of the issues involved.

Consider, for one other example, the role of overprescribing in leading to the emergence of antibiotic resistant bacteria. All patients have a common interest in that not happening. Assuming there is any chance at all that the drug might be even minimally efficacious, each patient has an interest in being prescribed the drug by his own physician. Each patient hopes that all other physicians exercise restraint, while his own does not. Yet if each gets what he wishes for in his own case, no restraint will be exercised by any, and the effi-cacy of the antibiotics will be eroded for all.

For another example, consider a vaccination that carries some slight risk of adverse consequences. Any given patient might prefer to avoid that risk by not receiving the vaccination, trusting that enough of the others around him will have been vaccinated to provide "herd immunity" (Anderson & May, 1985). But of course if everyone does that then there will be no herd immunity. If each physician respects the wishes of her own patient in this regard then the common pool resource is extinguished.

Supposing the health budget to be strictly fixed, the same is true of bedside practices of prescribing treatments that are somewhat less efficacious but substantially less expensive, or refraining from the use of marginally effective treatments altogether. Each patient hopes his physician will provide him with the very best treatment available, whatever the cost, while hoping that physicians prescribe lower-cost treatments (or no treatments) to others to protect the health budget that is paying for his treatment. But again, if each gets what he wants in his own case then the overall health budget is seriously eroded.

Collective action problems lie at the heart of all of those cases. Much though each wishes she could be the sole exception, each would be better off if everyone's physician respected the general rule of treating everyone (herself included) as she ideally wishes her physician to treat everyone except her. The trick lies in how to secure that outcome in the absence of some external enforcement.

The problem is that, if left to her own devices, each physician is naturally tempted—some would say (wrongly, I shall go on to argue) "professionally obliged" (Levinsky, 1984)—to promote the best interests of her own patient. Doing that in the context of a collective action problem would, however, mean deviating, in each and every case, from the general rule that would be best for all.

■ PARTICULAR INTERESTS VERSUS THE COMMON GOOD

Collective action problems arise from the constellation of preferences of each of the actors involved and from the way in which those interact. Specifically, collective action problems arise from agents choosing to act on the basis of some "particular interest" rather than on the basis of the "common good" of all (Runciman & Sen, 1965).

In the case of the fisherfolk, that "particular interest" took the form of a self-regarding private motive: increasing their own catch and hence their own profits. In the case of the physicians as discussed above, that "particular interest" is presumed to take the form of an other-regarding motive: benefiting one of their own patients.[3] What is crucial in generating a collective action problem is not whether the agent acts from self-regarding or other-regarding motives. What is crucial is, instead, that the agent acts with a view to doing what is best not for all those who are affected by the action but rather for some subset of them.

That fact suggests one simple solution to collective action problems. If all agents act purely with a view to doing what is best for all agents, no collective action problem arises. With anything short of "all" and "purely," collective action problems can still arise, however.

For example, a collective action problem would persist, to some greater or lesser extent, even if physicians partially internalized the "common good" alongside the "particular interests" of their own patients. The more heavily they weigh the former as compared to the latter in their decision making, the more often the former will trump the latter for them in deciding what to do and the less severe the collective action problem will be in consequence. But collective action problems would be precluded altogether only if physicians give absolute priority to the "common good" over the "particular interests" of their own patients in cases of conflict.

Ignoring altogether the "particular interests" of one's own patients—even if only where those actually conflict with the "common good" of all patients taken together—simply does not come naturally to medical practitioners. It clashes with the conceptualization of the first duty of physicians as being to their patients (Levinsky, 1984; Snyder, 2012, p. 86 and passim).

■ THE PERMISSIBILITY OF PARTICULARISM

We might query whether that is the correct way to conceptualize the duty of the physician. Maybe physicians have no duty to (or maybe even a moral duty not to) help patients pursue every one of the "particular interests" that they might happen to have. That might include even some health-related interests.

I shall analyze that issue in two steps. First I shall address the question of whether it is morally permissible for any given patient to seek special treatment for her own health care needs over and above that devoted to everyone's similar health care needs. I shall then address the question of whether, even if it is morally permissible for any given patient to seek such special treatment, it is morally obligatory for physicians to give any patient such special treatment.

From the Patient's Perspective

Remember, patients are moral agents too. They are not merely bearers of interests, desires, and impulses; they are also the bearers of moral duties. The charge to a physician to attend assiduously to the particular interests of her patients is a moral charge. And one can be morally charged to assist others only in pursuing interests that are morally permissible for those other agents to pursue.

Thus, in asking what a physician ought to do in furtherance of her patients' interests, we have to ask what sorts of interest the patient might himself take in his own health. What will be of most concern to us in relation to collective action problems is the sort of interest a patient might take in his "relative health status"; that is, in his own health status and resources devoted to his own health care in comparison to that of others. What sorts of such interests are morally permissible for the patient to take?

Here are three sorts of attitudes one might take to the health of others, compared to one's own: (1) indifference, (2) comparative advantage, and (3) no comparative disadvantage.

Take first the case of someone who is indifferent to the health of others. He wants purely to maximize his own health, and he does not care one iota about anyone else's health. If all patients are of this sort, and each physician internalizes the interests of her own patients thus understood, that gives rise to a collective action problem of the sort discussed above. Such patients (and physicians acting pursuant to their interests thus specified) want to maximize their own absolute well-being without regard to the impact of doing so on others. If others exercise restraint, such a patient (and a physician acting on his behalf) would have no hesitation in taking advantage of that fact to further his own interests.[4]

Consider next the case of someone who is not indifferent to the health status of others but rather seeks comparative advantage over others in that respect.[5] He might seek to be healthier than others as an end itself. Or, he might seek it as a means to some other ends. Being more malnourished than your competitors for the same job puts you at a comparative disadvantage in the labor market (Dasgupta & Ray, 1986/1987). So too does being less healthy than your competitors. Insofar as health is a means to other ends that one harbors, one might seek comparative advantage over others in the realm of health in order to gain more of those other end-use goods (Sen, 1983).

Finally, consider the case of someone who is concerned merely not to be put at a comparative disadvantage from exercising restraint that others do not reciprocate.[6] Someone thus motivated simply does not want to be "played for a sucker." Experimental economists have shown that the impulse toward "strong reciprocity" is ubiquitous, not only among people in Europe and North America but also across a wide range of cultures (Bowles & Gintis, 2002).

Among those preference structures, which count as morally permissible? It would seem clearly impermissible to seek comparative advantage over others in the realm of health—certainly insofar as that is achieved by actually worsening the health status of others. Giving others some wasting disease or preventing them from being cured of one, just so one can get a job ahead of them, is morally unacceptable. Whatever interest a patient might have in doing that, it is not an interest that her physician can be morally obliged to help her pursue.

Displaying utter indifference to the health of others might be almost as bad. Giving complete weight to one's own health interests and absolutely none to those of others is morally obnoxious as a failing of human sympathy, most would probably agree. But giving somewhat more weight to one's own health than that of others might strike us as morally permissible. And remember, the collective action problem in view arises, to some greater or lesser extent, whenever patients (and physicians acting on behalf of them) give any extra weight whatsoever to their own particular interests.

Consider finally the third stance: merely not wanting to be played for a sucker. That may not be the most attractive stance that is morally conceivable. Morally, surely it is good to do good for others, whether or not they do good for you. But while that is certainly morally good, not all actions that are morally good are morally obligatory for you always to perform. Some are supererogatory, above and beyond the strict call of duty, the stuff of saints and heroes. In other cases the duty to perform a good action takes the form of an imperfect duty, one (like the duty of charity) that you should perform on some occasions but you need not perform on all occasions.

It is unclear precisely what description best fits the duty people (or physicians acting on their behalf) have to refrain from using health resources that would yield more health benefits if devoted to others. But, as I have already said, there seems to be no strict duty to do so. It seems morally permissible for people to weigh their own interests more heavily than those of other people, at least to some extent, at least sometimes or in certain sorts of circumstances. And if it is permissible for them to do so unconditionally, it is unclear why it should not be permissible for them to do so conditionally—specifically, conditional on reciprocity, if and only if others do likewise.

From the Physician's Perspective

The upshot of the previous discussion is that it is morally permissible—at least sometimes, to some extent—for a patient to display a preference for his health needs to be met instead of those of other people with similar health needs. But it does not automatically follow from that fact, necessarily, that it would be morally obligatory (or maybe even morally permissible) for that patient's physician to act on those preferences.[7]

I have spoken above in terms of the physician being the agent of her patients, acting on their behalf. From the principal's point of view, the whole point of hiring an agent is to get someone to do what you want them to do for you. It is in the nature of the relationship, however, that the agent always acts with some latitude in pursuit of the principal's objectives, and she may well end up doing other than exactly as the principal would wish. It is not simply that that might happen: it may, in the sense that it is proper that it should. A large part of the point of hiring an agent is that the agent should have discretion to exercise her independent judgment in ways to pursue the principal's objectives better than the principal would have done on his own.

Furthermore, there are some things that you morally may not instruct an agent to do for you. Obviously, this includes things that you are morally prohibited from doing altogether: morally, it is wrong to hire an agent to commit a murder for you for the same reason, morally, it is wrong to commit the murder yourself. But there may also be things that would be morally permissible for you to do yourself that it would not be permissible to instruct an agent to do for you. Morally, it may be permissible for you not to jump in and save every drowning child you see at a crowded beach yourself. But it would be morally impermissible for you, when hiring a lifeguard for that beach, to instruct her to do the same.[8]

The last two thoughts, taken together, suggest some considerable scope for conceptualizing the duties of the physician-cum-agent as being somewhat detached from the preferences and particular interests of her patient. The patient may have an understandable preference for his interests to be served ahead of others'. But that does not automatically translate into a duty on the part of his physician slavishly to do so, particularly not if the patient's own larger interests would be better served by the physician's doing otherwise in certain respects.

The latter is likely to be the case, in turn, because of the nature of the collective action problem in view. Everyone would be better off if everyone (or, rather, everyone's physician acting on his behalf) exercised restraint. Everyone is symmetrically situated; no one can have any reasonable, realistic expectations of being treated differently than anyone else. If it must be the case either that all exercise restraint or that none do, each patient is clearly better off in the former case than the latter.[9]

■ PROFESSIONAL NORMS ENCOMPASS ALL PARTICULAR INTERESTS

As I said at the outset, collective action problems arise from people pursuing particular interests rather than the common good of all. One very standard solution to the problem is to create a collective group agent responsible for serving the interests of all and to charge that collective group agent with the task of making decisions for the group as a whole. Representing as it does the group as a whole, that collective group agent has no particular interests apart from the common good of all. The collective action problem is thus straight-forwardly resolved.

That is the way Nordic countries traditionally avoided the counterproductive consequences of dispersed wage bargaining. Inflation arises from (among other things) wage competition. Trade unions strive to obtain competitive advantage for their own members in seeking higher wage rates than workers in other sectors of the economy. But if all independently pursued their particular interests in that respect, all workers would be worse off; the ensuing inflation would more than erode the purchasing power of all nominal wage gains. In Scandinavia, the solution historically took the form of a single umbrella organization (such as Sweden's LO, the *Landsorganisationen*) being charged with the task of negotiating wages for workers across the country as a whole. Encompassing the interests of all workers as a whole, the LO avoided the problem of counterproductive pursuit of sectoral advantage (Olson, 1982, pp. 89–92; cf. Hernes, 1991). The common good of all was secured in this way by entrusting its pursuit to some organization whose sole interest was in the good of all.

Professions can be like that. Even if particular physicians feel duty bound to internalize the interests of their own particular patients, the profession (and associations representing the profession as a whole) can internalize the interests of all the patients of all the physicians.

Where what is good for each will be undermined by independently pursuing what is good for each, a better outcome for each can be achieved by collectively pursuing the good of all. That is the general thought.

As applied to the case of health care rationing, the thought is simply this. Every patient will be better off than he would otherwise have been if (1) profession-wide norms of good practice in the effective use of medical resources were imposed rather than (2) rationing decisions were entrusted to the discretion of particular physicians at the bedside of particular patients one by one. In bowing to those norms, the physician is doing precisely what a good agent ought to do—pursuing her principal's (i.e., patient's) interests in ways different from but better than they would be if the principal- cum-patient's own particular preference in the matter were slavishly respected.

Far from breaching their professional duties of care toward their patients, then, physicians would actually be best discharging them by developing profession-wide standards of health care rationing that all those physicians then all implement. Bedside rationing systematically governed by such professional norms would be not only for the good of all. It would also be for the good of each, seen from a broader perspective. Each trying to get more than that would lead, ultimately, to each getting less than that.[10]

How is it to be enforced? Like any other professional norm of good practice: with esteem for good practice and scorn, culminating in sanctions (*in extremis* being struck off the medical register), for bad practice (Brennan & Pettit, 2004).

■ THE PHYSICIAN'S "FIRST DUTY"—NOT "ONLY DUTY"

To say that "the physician's first and primary duty is to the patient" (Snyder 2012, p. 86) is not to say that that is the physician's only duty. Nor is it to say that that "first and primary duty" cannot itself be overridden by other weighty considerations from time to time.

Wendler (2010) offers various examples of exceptions to the rule always to do what is in a patient's best interest. That occurs, for example, when an attending physician allows her intern to insert the central line rather than doing it herself, even though that poses somewhat more risk to the patient, on the grounds that learning-by-doing is the only way for new physicians to be properly trained.

More generally, the rule always to do what is in your patient's best interest is violated whenever you have multiple patients whose needs make competing demands on your time, attention, and resources (Mechanic, 1992, pp. 1731–2). This happens most clearly in emergency medicine, whenever one patient's treatment is postponed to allow treatment of another patient with more urgent needs. In order to do what is in the latter patient's best interest, the emergency physician has to do something that is not in the former patient's best interest (postpone treatment).

Indeed, the rule always to do what is in your patient's best interest, when you have multiple patients with competing claims, involves a notorious logical fallacy familiar from Bentham's initial sloppy statement of the fundamental rule of utilitarianism as "the greatest good to the greatest number" of people. The rule, as stated, demands the maximization of two separate parameters at once—such a double maximand is a nonsense. What does good for "the greatest number of people" might be one thing, what does the "greatest good" aggregating the good done to all people might be something else altogether. The rule always to do what is in your patient's best interest, when you have multiple patients whose interests are not necessarily perfectly aligned, involves an identical nonsense. It involves a maximization exercise that is logically impossible to perform.

The duty always to do what is in your patient's best interest is thus the physician's first but not only duty. Among other things, the physician has identical duties to her other patients. She has one duty qua "this patient's physician"; she has another duty qua "that patient's physician"; and insofar as their medical needs make conflicting claims on her, discharging those twin duties as best she is able will typically preclude the physician from doing literally what is in the very best interests of either of the two patients.

Let us now generalize one step further, from (1) "the duty of the physician, qua 'this patient's physician,' to this particular patient"; to (2) "the duty of the physician, qua 'these patients' physician,' to all of her patients"; to (3) "the duty of the physician, qua physician (to all patients)." The sorts of trade-offs involved in (2) (between the competing claims of all of the physician's own patients) provide a model for the sorts of trade-offs that are involved in (3) (between the competing claims of all patients of physicians in general) (Tavaglione & Hurst, 2012, p. 11). Those latter trade-offs lie at the heart of the duty of "stewardship of resources" enunciated in the Ethics Manual of the American College of Physicians.[11]

What is undeniably true is that the sorts of trade-offs involved in both (2) and (3) are best governed according to rules set down somewhere other than at the bedside (Snyder, 2012, p. 90). At the bedside, the physician's "primary role" is indeed "as a [particular] patient's trusted advocate." But in determining what she may or may not legitimately do to best further the interests of that particular patient, the bedside physician must reflect on a wider set of laws, rules, and professional norms crafted with the aim of best furthering the interests of all patients. The rule that the physician should not lie to insurance companies to maximize her patient's payout is one such rule, from a very different realm (Snyder, 2012, p. 89).[12] Another is the rule that the physician should "use all health-related resources in a technically appropriate and efficient manner" and "plan work-ups carefully and avoid unnecessary testing, medications, surgery and consultations" (Snyder, 2012, p. 90). Rules like that are best made by reflecting upon the duties of the physician to all of her patients (in 2) or upon the duties of physicians as a whole to all of their patients (in 3), and then imposed as constraints on the decision making of any particular physician at any particular patient's bedside.

Seen as a solution to a collective action problem, such profession-wide setting of rules and norms to govern bedside practice will have the effect of doing the best that realistically can be done for patients themselves. If every patient's physician tried to do better for her own patient than that, the upshot would be that everyone's patients (including, over the long term, that patient herself) would be worse off. Physicians binding themselves to a system of restraint in that way is what truly serves the best interests of their patients, individually as well as collectively, over the long haul.

■ OTHER SOLUTIONS

I have recommended a system of professional norms that could systematically guide bedside rationing, as my preferred mechanism for managing those trade-offs collectively. That is not the only conceivable way to solve the collective action problem surrounding health care resources, of course. Considering the limits of the alternatives, however, I think it the best.

One class of alternatives would involve the direct regulation of medical practice by state authorities. One solution, for example, would be simply to enact legislation that restricts undesirable practices and/or imposes better medical practices. We might be able to do that in rare cases. We might legislate to compel all school children to be vaccinated against certain specified diseases, for example. Or, in centralized health care systems such as the British National Health Service, authorities can simply "remove some services completely . . . off the list of services that they make available to patients in their regions" (Rogers & Braunack-Mayer, 2004, p. 84). But as a general strategy, that is politically unrealistic in most places. It is probably medically ill-advised as well. Politicians writing general rules cannot hope to capture the nuance of particular cases; the exercise of some physician discretion, operating under looser forms of professional norms, would lead to better health outcomes (Goodin, 1982, ch. 5; Braithwaite et al., 2007).

A weaker version of that might be to require physicians to get specific permission from some central authority for prescribing particularly expensive treatment, requiring the physician to justify that treatment in the particular case. The Australian Pharmaceutical Benefits Scheme operates that way with respect to a restricted list of particularly expensive medicines. Or maybe it might suffice just to impose a requirement for physicians to file a report to some central authority when opting for hyperexpensive treatments. Simply "knowing they're being watched" might encourage physicians to self-censor their overuse of expensive products and procedures. Such solutions might go some way toward ameliorating collective action problems, but they cannot be expected to eliminate them altogether.

A second class of alternatives works on the supply side to avoid overuse of especially expensive medical products or procedures. For capital-intensive branches of medicine, for example, you can simply not buy the machine. In that way you can guarantee that no one overuses a machine that is not available (Aaron & Schwartz, 1984, p. 128). But of course that guarantee comes at the cost of no one being able to use a machine that is unavailable, even if such a machine has been developed and marketed.

A third class of alternatives works on the demand side. Among a small and stable group of actors, collective action problems can often be reliably overcome through systems of reciprocal forbearance, enforced by breaches being punished by tit-for-tat retaliation in subsequent rounds of the game. I'll refrain from overfishing if you do; but if I see your catch exceeded your daily quota today, I'll do the same tomorrow (Axelrod, 1984; Ostrom, 1990). Sometimes that might work in a health care context. In a small community with only a handful of physicians, access to a local hospital might be successfully controlled in that way. I'll refrain from ordering expensive but almost certainly unnecessary tests for my patients if you do the same; but if I see you ordering them for yours, and my patients want the same, I'll order them too. But as a general strategy for a very large municipal (much less national) community of patients and physicians, that solution is simply not viable.

A fourth class of alternatives involves *partial* implementation of the scheme described above for solving collective action problems through the use of all-encompassing organizations. If you want an organization that is literally all encompassing—that is responsible for looking after the interests of literally all patients—then you will need to be thinking in terms of something like the profession as a whole.[13] But partial versions of that strategy are available and have sometimes been implemented with limited success.

An example of that is the GP Fundholder scheme introduced into the British National Health Service under the Tories in 1991 and its successor (the Primary Care Trusts) under the subsequent Labour Government. That scheme had the effect of making each medical practice internalize the interests of its portfolio of patients as a whole. Resources devoted to one of a practice's patients were resources that would not then be available to other patients of that same practice, toward whom physicians associated with that practice had just the same professional obligations.

Such schemes encourage physicians to think in terms of the common good of patients in their practice. But they still leave physicians pursuing the particular interests of the patients in their *own* practice at the expense of patients in *other* practices. That is a flaw that is endemic to any partially encompassing solution to a collective action problem.[14]

■ CONCLUSION

Physicians confront collective action problems all the time. Each vigorously pursuing the interests of each of their patients often leads to outcomes that are worse for all patients. Each physician's patients would typically be better off if all physicians exercised restraint in the use of health care resources. That might be accomplished, after a fashion, in any of many ways. But the best is almost certainly one that leaves room for the exercise of clinical judgment while subjecting that judgment to some collective discipline. The medical profession as a whole ought to develop norms to govern the appropriate use of scarce health care resources. Physicians engaged in bedside rationing can be guided by such norms, confident in the knowledge that in abiding by them they are indeed doing their best by their patients overall.[15]

■ ACKNOWLEDGMENTS

I am grateful to Marion Danis, Alan Wertheimer, and Dave Wendler for discussion of these issues and to Len Fleck and Annette Rid for comments on a previous draft of this chapter.

Notes
1. Asch and Ubel, 1997; Ubel and Goold, 1997. Just as there are more fish for everyone if fisherfolk practice sustainable fishing, so too is there more utility to be derived from a fixed number of health dollars if those are rationed rightly.

2. So too is improving health worldwide. But for purposes of this chapter I set aside issues of global justice and concentrate on issues of health care within one country.

3. In a fee-for-service system there might also be self-regarding motives for physicians. But I set that possibility aside for purposes of my discussion here.

4. In the terms of game theory, these represent Prisoner's Dilemma style preferences (Luce & Raiffa, 1957, pp. 95–102).

5. In terms of game theory, these represent Status Good preferences (Shubik, 1971).

6. In terms of game theory, these represent Assurance Game preferences (Sen, 1967).

7. There are various other situations, too, in which a physician might not be obliged to act on a patient's preferences, as when a patient requests an operation whose risks are excessive or amputation of a healthy limb in cases of body integrity disorder.

8. Permissions in general are not transferable. When I give you permission to enter my house, that does not give you any right to give permission to others to enter.

9. If it is the case that some need not exercise restraint so long as others do, the strategic structure of the game changes: it is then not a pure collective action (Prisoner's Dilemma) game, but rather an instance of a Chicken game nesting within a Prisoner's Dilemma (Taylor & Ward, 1982).

10. That is, over a substantial run of relevantly similar cases. Of course, the Keynesian aphorism, "In the long run, we're all dead," can apply with special force in some medical cases.

11. "Physicians have a responsibility to practice effective and efficient health care and to use health care resources responsibly. Parsimonious care that utilizes the most efficient means to effectively diagnose a condition and treat a patient respects the need to use resources wisely and to help ensure that resources are equitably available" (Snyder, 2012, p. 87; see similarly p. 90).

12. At least not unless the physician is operating in an "unjust restrictive environment" (Tavaglione & Hurst, 2012).

13. Or the state. The reason the state *can* resolve collective action problems is that it has coercive powers with which to enforce its edicts. The reason it *does*, when it does, is that it internalizes the interests of all those under its jurisdiction.

14. That is not the only flaw with such schemes, of course. Worse is the risk that practices will "cherry-pick" good patients who are cheap and easy to care for, while patients with costly or complex conditions prove unable to find care.

15. Some may be tempted to respond "there is no such thing as 'the medical profession as a whole, merely all sorts of competing subspecialties trying to maximize resources available to them.' " In response to them I would simply repeat the last two sentences of the text. Competition among subspecialties for scarce resources is simply another collective action problem, in which all would benefit if all exercised restraint; and that is best accomplished via coordination orchestrated by the most all-encompassing group ("the medical profession as a whole"). Where that group is not yet collectively organized, the first task, of morality and extended prudence alike, is to see to it that it gets effectively organized.

REFERENCES

Aaron, H. J., & Schwartz, W. B. (1984). *The Painful Prescription: Rationing Hospital Care.* Washington, DC: Brookings Institution.

Anderson, R. M., & May, R. M. (1985). Vaccination and herd immunity to infectious diseases. *Nature,* 318 (#6044), 323–329.

Asch, D. A., & Ubel, P. A. (1997). Rationing by any other name. *New England Journal of Medicine, 336*(23), 1668–1671.

Axelrod, R. (1984). *The Evolution of Cooperation.* New York: Basic Books.

Bowles, S., & Gintis, H. (2002). Homo reciprocans. *Nature, 15*(6868), 125–128.

Braithwaite, J., Makkai, T., & Braithwaite, V. (2007). *Regulatory Ritualism and the New Pyramid: Governance of Aged Care Across Three Decades in Three Nations.* Cheltenham: Elgar.

Brennan, G., & Pettit, P. (2004). *The Economy of Esteem.* Oxford: Oxford University Press.

Dasgupta, P., & Ray, D. (1986/1987). Inequality as a determinant of malnutrition and unemployment. *Economic Journal, 96,* 1011–1134 and 97, 177–188.

Goodin, R. E. (1982). *Political Theory and Public Policy.* Chicago: University of Chicago Press.

Hardin, G. (1968). The tragedy of the commons. *Science, 162,* 1243–1248.

Hardin, R. (1982). *Collective Action.* Baltimore, MD: Johns Hopkins University Press.

Hernes, G. (1991). The dilemmas of social democracies: the case of Norway and Sweden. *Acta Sociologica, 34* (4), 239–260.

Levinsky, N. G. (1984). The doctor's master. *New England Journal of Medicine, 311*(24), 1573–1575.

Luce, R. D., & Raiffa, H. (1957). *Games and Decisions.* New York: Wiley.

Mechanic, D. (1992). Professional judgment and the rationing of medical care. *University of Pennsylvania Law Review, 140*(5), 1713–1754.

Olson, M. Jr. (1965). *The Logic of Collective Action.* Cambridge, MA: Harvard University Press.

Olson, M. Jr. (1982). *The Rise and Decline of Nations.* New Haven, CT: Yale University Press.

Ostrom, E. (1990). *Governing the Commons: The Evolution of Institutions for Collective Action.* New York: Cambridge University Press.

Rogers, W. A., & Braunack-Mayer, A. J. (2004). *Practical Ethics for General Practice.* Oxford: Oxford University Press.

Runciman, W. G., & Sen, A. K. (1965). Games, justice and the general will. *Mind, 74,* 554–562.

Sen, A. (1967). Isolation, assurance and the social rate of discount. *Quarterly Journal of Economics, 81,* 112–124.

Sen, A. (1983). Poor, relatively speaking. *Oxford Economic Papers, 35,* 153–169.

Shubik, M. (1971). Games of status. *Behavioral Science, 16,* 117–129.

Snyder, L., for the Ethics, Professionalism and Human Rights Committee of the American College of Physicians. (2012). American College of Physicians Ethics Manual: sixth edition. *Annals of Internal Medicine, 156*(Jan 3, pt 2), 73–104.

Tavaglione, N., & Hurst, S. A. (2012). Why physicians ought to lie for their patients. *American Journal of Bioethics, 12*(3), 4–12.

Taylor, M., & Ward, H. (1982). Chickens, whales and lumpy public goods: alternative models of public-goods provision. *Political Studies, 30,* 350–370.

Ubel, P. A., & Goold, S. (1997). Recognizing bedside rationing: clear cases and tough calls. *Annals of Internal Medicine, 126*(1), 71–80.

Wendler, D. (2010). Are physicians obligated always to act in the patient's best interests? *Journal of Medical Ethics, 36*(2), 66–70.

14 Statistical versus Identified Lives

Why Not to Use the "R" Word

■ PAUL T. MENZEL

There are many plausible reasons for claiming that bedside rationing by clinicians is morally dubious. First, their primary, though not by any means only, loyalty ought to be to their patients. Second, if decisions allocating scarce resources have to be made, they should be made either out of some sort of agreement or contract between subscriber-patients and the entity which funds their care or through a public process in which their views and values are fairly considered along with those of others who have stakes in such decisions. Clinicians are thought not to be well situated to be proper decision makers on either of these grounds. Third, for clinicians, patients are identified individual persons. They represent "identifiable" not "statistical" lives. Identified patients call forth more strongly the moral responses of both compassion and respect for individual persons.

In this chapter I will focus largely on the third reason for moral skepticism about bedside rationing. I will argue that even if the distinction between so-called statistical and identified lives is morally relevant, its careful application to clinical settings has weaker implications than typically thought. Once this is well understood, not only is the sting of bedside rationing reduced but the choice to speak of "rationing" care cannot be justified in most clinical decision-making situations; "prioritizing" care is less misleading and more accurate. Avoiding the "R" word in these common situations is thus not cowardice, euphemism, or subterfuge, but perceptive and justified choice of language. Speaking of prioritizing rather than rationing is especially important when no global budgeting imposes immediate resource limits on a health care system or health plan, precisely the context where denial of care at the bedside is often viewed as particularly problematic morally. And even in fixed-budget contexts—either unitary national systems or "accountable care organizations" in a pluralistic system—care that is denied for essentially the same reasons it would be in non–limited-budget contexts should be spoken of as "prioritized" not "rationed."

■ STATISTICAL VERSUS IDENTIFIED LIVES

Views on whether the statistical versus identified lives distinction is morally relevant vary widely. From a utilitarian perspective, the distinction would seem to have little if any moral relevance. A life lost (or preserved) is still a life with all its same value, whether the individual who has that life is identified at the time of action or not. In Kantian moral views, the distinction is more likely to be relevant. Obligations grounded in respect for individual persons are presumably the most obvious when the people to whom they are owed are identifiable individuals. Moral philosophies that put an emphasis on virtue may also accord the distinction moral relevance. Compassion, for example, is a particularly strong and expected moral virtue when people stand in relation to each other as identified individuals.

The distinction is likely part of any explanation of the greater priority that treatment seems to have over prevention in people's minds and in much of health care practice (Menzel, 2012, pp. 199–201). The decision-making framework within which prevention typically saves lives is statistical. For example, only one out of every 1,900 women in their 40s who routinely receive an annual mammogram will actually have her life extended by such care.[1] In treatment, by contrast, the lives saved seem identifiable; we say that a person's bypass surgery, for example, saved his life.

This difference has implications for how we think about limiting the provision of treatments as compared to preventive services. The statistical perspective typical of prevention makes setting limits on—saying no to—particular preventive services easier to swallow than setting limits on treatment. By their respective yardsticks, both a preventive measure and a treatment may be effective,[2] but if a prospective recipient is denied the prevention, the threat to her welfare and the assault on her dignity seems slight by comparison. The life at stake is only "statistical"—we really have no idea whether *her* life is going to be saved by such measures, and thus we do not even see the life that is at stake as hers. In general, placing limits on services below a certain level of effectiveness or cost-effectiveness, when the probability that those services will benefit any individual patient is low, is likely to be received as more acceptable than placing limits on treatments that are seen as benefiting distinct individuals because their chance of success is much higher.

Despite this general pattern, it must be noted that people sometimes are as troubled about the exclusion of a preventive service as they are by limits on treatment. This is amply illustrated by some angry reactions to the 2009 report of the U.S. Preventive Services Task Force on breast cancer screening. The task force recommended against any *routine* annual use of mammography on women aged 40–49.[3] It cited comparative life-extension benefits: statistically, more than 1,900 women in their 40s have to receive mammograms annually for a decade to extend one life (extend it at all), noticeably more than the number of women in their 50s who have to be screened to extend one life (U.S. Preventative Services Task Force, 2009, p. 719). Adding to the case against routine annual mammography in women's 40s is the fact that the more than 19,000 screenings which have to be done over a decade (1,900 women x 10 annual screenings) to extend one life generate more than 1,000 false positives, all of which have to be followed up on extensively (Aronowitz, 2009).

Part of what lay behind the storm of controversy that followed the report[4] was that people who are aware of even a low risk of disease can imagine vividly what happens to the individual who turns out to be the unlucky *one* out of 1,900. The appropriate statistic in the case of women in their 40s who go without routine annual mammograms may actually be more like one unlucky person out of 6,000, not 1,900[5] but even then, people sufficiently attuned to the disease can still see *that one person* in their minds. When people become distinctly aware that the incidence of serious diseases to which they are vulnerable really can be reduced by prevention, they become capable of imagining vividly that they in particular might be a future victim. A policy decision to exclude a relatively inefficient preventive measure with low chance of benefit is then nearly as difficult for patients to accept as excluding elements of acute care with higher odds of benefit.

But notice what is going on here: in a situation of exposure to relatively low risk from forgoing a procedure, people still see the one person who will eventually suffer in *identified individual* terms—typically, perhaps, even themselves. The reaction to the task force's report may seem to be a case where statistical lives exert the same pull on people as identified ones, but arguably it is not an example of that at all. Instead it illustrates that when a statistical life is at stake, people in their perceptions can turn it into an identifiable one. The resistance to prioritizing in the mammography case does not indicate that people find it as difficult to accept limits on statistical lifesaving as limits on lifesaving treatments of identifiable patients. Instead, it shows that when people perceive a statistical lifesaving situation as if it were a matter of saving identifiable lives, they resist limit setting just as much as they do for treatments seen right from the start as saving identifiable lives.

My argument now comes into view. Just as people can turn the lives that are statistically at stake in prevention into virtually identifiable ones, the converse obtains, too, and in a more objective sense: the seemingly identifiable lives saved in many treatment situations are significantly statistical. Not only can they be seen that way; as we shall see upon more careful examination, they *are* that way. To discern this, we need to refine the statistical/identifiable distinction.[6]

■ REFINING THE DISTINCTION

In our preconception of the prevention/treatment comparison, we think of those whose well-being is at stake in treatment as identifiable individuals, whereas those who benefit from prevention remain statistical. Not only with but after the provision of preventive measures, we do not know specifically who the beneficiaries are.

Such a preconception of how the prevention/treatment difference and identifiable/statistical distinction intersect greatly oversimplifies reality. In any clearheaded application of the distinction to clinical situations we must distinguish *recipients* from *beneficiaries*. Recipients of a service might be identifiable individuals although its beneficiaries are not—not yet, at least. Four combinations of recipient/beneficiary and identifiable/statistical are possible.

(a) *Neither the recipients nor beneficiaries are identifiable; both are statistical.* This situation characterizes some public health measures, where even recipients are only a group of anonymous individuals. Meat inspection for bacterial contamination in meat packing plants, for example, may apply to all meat sold in a given area, but because we do not know which individuals buy meat, the "recipients" of this food safety measure remain unidentified. As for beneficiaries, the measure is thought to have many, but who exactly they are—just who are the persons who would have suffered from contaminated meat had the sanitation measures not been taken, and therefore who will actually have been helped—is not known at the time of action and may never be.

(b) *Recipients are identifiable but beneficiaries are not.* This situation is typical of clinical prevention—vaccinations, screening tests, and so forth. Known individuals receive the service, but the identity of beneficiaries remains unknown. For one thing, the risk diminished by these measures is usually already so low that it becomes very difficult to discern who benefits. People certainly do not know who benefits when the measure is administered, and seldom do they know even later. If a vaccinated person ends up not getting the flu, we still do not know she has benefited; she may well not have contracted the flu anyhow. And when a nonvaccinated person gets influenza, we cannot be sure he became a victim because of his lack of vaccination; he might have contracted the flu regardless (a strain different than the one targeted by the vaccine, for example).

(c) *Beneficiaries are identifiable but recipients are not.* This category is probably vacuous.

(d) *Beneficiaries as well as recipients are identifiable.* It is typically treatments that people locate in this category. And indeed, many times in treatment the beneficiaries as well as recipients are identifiable. In many cases of treatment, however, they are not. Just as in typical prevention,[7] the beneficiaries remain unknown. The *recipients* are identifiable at the time of treatment, but who will actually benefit is not—frequently not at the time of treatment and often not even after the treatment has had time to play out. Spinal surgery, for example, may be seen a year later as having led to a patient being relatively pain-free; both surgeon and patient will naturally tend to think of the patient as having benefited from that procedure. Perhaps, though, appropriate rest and good physical therapy, along with medication, exercise, and so on, would have yielded the same result. To use a more striking example, prostate surgery may leave its recipient alive for 20 years believing he has benefited, although actually, had he gone without surgery, the tumor would have grown so slowly as not to be fatal.

To be sure, the beneficiaries of some treatments are afterwards identifiable. A relatively advanced malignant tumor may be of a sort virtually certain to be fatal if not surgically removed or irradiated. If after treatment the patient survives for years, we justifiably see this individual as being a beneficiary. Sometimes even at the time of treatment, especially if the treatment has an extremely high likelihood of benefit, we discern identifiable beneficiaries. Certain kinds of emergency trauma surgery, for example, may have such a good track record and be so necessary to avoid otherwise certain death that we are justified in seeing the individual patient as a beneficiary already at the point of action. Even short of such relative certainty, however, we can legitimately identify patients as beneficiaries at the point of provision because a considerable enough reduction of risk is itself seen as a benefit. A given person's treatment might not work when it lowers a 90% risk of death to 40%, for example, but the proportion of reduction in risk in this high-risk situation is so great that most of us will see the risk reduction itself as a benefit to the patient. If it turns out that the patient does not survive, of course, it cannot be claimed, in the strict sense of medical benefit, that the treatment has benefited the patient—but it is still plausible to say that the patient "benefited" from the treatment. After all, she jumped from having very little chance of survival (10%) to having a better than 50–50 chance! Many patients living through such a scenario will experience a greatly increased chance as a real benefit, even if they do not in the end get its primary benefit, actual survival.

In many cases, of course, the situation is quite the opposite: a treatment has some chance of bringing about some net improvement compared to no treatment or to other alternatives, but not much chance; or it has a greater chance, but of only a very small net benefit. *These are the situations that are far and away most likely to obtain when treatment is not provided because it has been assigned very low priority*. By contrast, any treatments that reduce a sizable risk significantly, and where the eventual stake is itself substantial and not minor, is very likely *not* to be assigned low priority as a means to achieve potential cost control.

It is very important to note this fact about realistic prioritizing in the actual world of health care. A realistic case for prioritizing clinical medicine builds in steps.

(1) Focus first on what priority to assign to preventive services. Prioritizing these will be seen as relatively acceptable because of the low risk to which any given individual is exposed when a preventive service is forgone. Routine annual mammography in women's 40s or routine PSA testing in men without prior family history or other specific risk may be good examples of measures not provided. The point is not these examples in particular but that inevitably *some* preventive measures will not be pursued because their statistical return is seen as too low to justify either their side effects or their cost. People correctly see these as cases where no identifiable individual is deprived of benefits. The recipients of preventive care in clinical settings are identifiable, but we are willing to accept assignment of low priority and not view it as disrespectful of individual patients in part because the losing beneficiaries—those who would have benefited had they received the care—are not identifiable.

(2) In many clinical treatments, however, beneficiaries are also not identifiable. The recipients are, but recipients are identifiable in clinical prevention, too. Perhaps because treatment applies to individuals who are perceived to be already "in trouble," while prevention applies to those who are not in trouble (or at least do not see themselves as that),[8] we resist seeing the similarity in the two cases. The similarity is still objectively there, however: in neither can the *beneficiaries* be identified. When we come to recognize this similarity, we are less likely to criticize the assignment of low priority to low-chance-of-benefit treatment. We do not see the decision not to offer treatments because of their low priority as greatly different from the same decision regarding clinical prevention.

(3) In both cases, the effect of not seeing identifiable persons as the would-be beneficiaries of the care is to enable us to see the situation in its societal whole. In our lives generally, we struggle with resource shortages of all sorts and do not shrink from making allocation choices, even though we know that real people (often ourselves) will end up bearing the consequences. Maturity involves confronting and taking risks. We do not turn every decision that involves risk into an assault on individuals. One ramification of the unpredictable way that risk will

end up affecting each of us, or what I will call the *veil of risk*, is to enable us to see ourselves as members of a larger pool of people, and it is the pool that will be affected. Risk buffers us from the prospect of being the individual who loses. We do not know who that individual is.[9]

One aspect of European physicians' responses in the Values at the Bedside study likely reflects something close to this role of risk. In all four countries, Italy, Norway, Switzerland, and the United Kingdom, physicians registered their highest positive agreement with rationing in responding to the proposition, "Physicians should adhere to clinical guidelines that discourage the use of interventions that have a small proven advantage over standard treatment but cost much more" (Hurst et al., 2009, p. 6). Interventions with "a small proven advantage over standard treatment" certainly include procedures with low chance of benefit because they either accomplish only a very small reduction in risk, or the risk they reduce is one of only small loss.

▪ LANGUAGE: THE "R" WORD

Building this kind of case for prioritizing clinical care requires that prioritizing be focused on procedures with relatively low chance of benefit. I will argue that these are precisely the situations where "prioritizing," not "rationing," is the right language. If procedures with low chance of benefit are what this process will in fact end up denying to patients, speaking of that denial as rationing rather than prioritizing is downright misleading. Calling it rationing is likely to be terribly counterproductive as well.

There are contexts where people readily accept rationing referred to as such. One is battlefield triage. Another is natural disasters and epidemics of emergency proportions, where a range of items such as personnel, equipment (ventilators, e.g.), or facilities (ICU beds) may suddenly be in ineradicably short supply. The context with which people in developed countries are most familiar is organ transplantation, because stubbornly short supply has characterized the situation for decades. In these contexts rationing is marked by the fact that we have no choice but to do it. Care cannot be provided for all who need it, because a sufficient supply of one or more of its critical elements is simply not available to treat everyone. Even when a shortage is arguably correctable by adequate foresight and planning, as in some temporary shortages of important drugs, ineradicable shortage is still the stubborn present reality within which decisions have to be made. People have no choice but to ration.

Whenever an obviously scarce resource thus has to be allocated the need for rationing, spoken of as such, is not disputed. How to ration may continue to be a matter of debate, even fierce debate, but in no sense does "rationing" become "the R word." Moreover, it is accepted even though those who lose may be as identifiable individually as potential beneficiaries of care ever are. The individuals with organ failure who are listed on the transplant waiting list and who have an excellent prognosis if they become organ recipients in all likelihood will lose their lives if they do not receive organs, and those who do have successful transplantation have very likely gained life they otherwise would not have had. The losers as well as the winners are identifiable.

The context in the cases where this is readily accepted is a relatively absolute shortage that cannot be relieved within the time frame in which the immediate item in short supply is needed. This does not characterize all allocation situations. In cases where "we"—somebody—set(s) a limit, things may be seen very differently. People might, of course, think there is a need to announce that resources are in short supply: when health care costs are thought simply to be getting too high and need to be controlled, for example. Limits that then get set—a "global" budget for health care in the society, established, for example, by national commission or legislature—are endorsed by the "society" including those who are denied selected care. The shortage is voluntarily created, but those who created it are not blamed; having limits is viewed as justified. This apparent social equilibrium, however, is prone to instability. *Are* the costs that are going up getting "simply too high," so that limits must be set? *When identifiable lives are going to be lost*, what amount of resources spent really *is* excessive, and therefore what limits really *are* justified? Such questions know no easy answers, for it is not clear what limit is a socially acceptable price for an identifiable individual life. Asking what such a price would be may itself meet resistance, manifesting a conviction—at least suspicion—that identifiable individual life has *no* acceptable price. The limits on resources that should be spent to save lives lose their anchor in any willingness, explicit or implicit, to discern a monetary value for life and therefore a limit to what we should be willing to do to save it.

A lot of this changes when we see lives behind a veil of risk. With high risk, of course, people still see the situation as one in which their individual life is at stake.[10] In low-risk situations, however, or ones in which only a very small reduction in a rather high risk can be accomplished, they much more easily see themselves as members of a statistical pool, only some of whom (an *unidentifiable some*) will eventually be identifiable winners and losers. When this is the applicable context, people can much more readily accept limits on resources as proper and appropriate. In decisions to set global limits, a larger social context of macro-allocation frames decisions. Similarly, at the clinical level, when it is low risks that can be lowered further or only very small reductions in not terribly high risks that can be accomplished, even individual patients end up having to view decisions from a perspective that is, in effect, larger and societal. In the world of their own perceived reality they become members of a statistical pool.

For this sort of situation we need a different language. We already have a language for situations of stubborn scarcity of health care resources where not everyone can be saved and where typically the beneficiaries (losers and winners) are known individuals: we "ration." For this other kind of situation my suggestion is that what we do is "prioritize."[11]

If we do not use different language for these two situations, we are only asking for trouble. In the United States the merest mention of limiting Medicare or other insurance reimbursement for procedures of little or no known benefit, or even of *known* no benefit, elicits charges of "rationing!" The more the proponents of controlling costs by setting priorities that discipline reimbursement for care of low or unknown benefit refer to what they support as "rationing," the more they give the game away to their opponents, who can then portray them as willing to deny care to known beneficiaries who become known individual victims. Surely people who support setting priorities so that we do not throw more money at health care than is worth its benefits do not have in mind priorities that deny people lifesaving ventilators and ICU beds in an emergency epidemic, where there are fully identifiable individual winners and losers. If that is not what any remotely fair criticism of setting priorities should be allowed to allude to, then *supporters of controlling costs by setting priorities must stop handing the argument to their critics on a silver platter by using misleading language that plays into their hands.*[12]

The linguistic practice should be this. Confine "rationing" to two situations: (1) Resources are unalterably scarce (e.g., organ transplantation). (2) Scarcity has been created deliberately by human beings, and the rationing that is subsequently necessary creates identifiable individual losers and winners at the point of clinical decision. A third sort of situation is different: (3) Individual beneficiaries—winners and losers—are not identifiable at the point of clinical decision and will not be with any certainty, even well after the time of clinical decision. For this third sort of situation we should speak of "prioritizing care" or "setting priorities," not "rationing."

Such a linguistic practice is not deceptive or manipulative. It is a matter of fact that people under the veil of relatively low risk can and often do see themselves differently than they do when risk is high and they naturally see themselves as identifiable individual beneficiaries. To refer to prioritizing and denial of low-chance-of-benefit care in the former case as "rationing" is an invitation to misinterpret prioritizing as denial of care to identifiable losers of life and health, which have such great value. If setting priorities to avoid spending large amounts of money on extremely low-benefit care is justified, it is because, from the societal perspective of being members of a larger pool of citizens or subscribers, people do not want to spend more on health care than the benefits are worth. The benefits of health and life that know virtually no limit in monetary value when they accrue to identifiable individuals become amenable to more limited investments when veil of risk is one's perspective. We need language that enables us to draw meaningful distinctions when those distinctions matter for our action. The difference between rationing and prioritizing is one of those.

■ THE RANGE OF LEGITIMATE PRIORITIZING IN CLINICAL SETTINGS

Insurance distorts patient and provider decisions about the value of interventions: any prospective positive net benefit, no matter how small, gets pursued regardless of cost. Assume that people understand that *in such a context of insurance*, in order to prevent resources from being drained to the point where the investment seems much greater than what is justified by results, practice guidelines will need to be formulated at a level prior to clinical practice. The formation of such guidelines will involve, among other things, some truly substantive prioritizing. Not everything with positive statistical net benefit will be appropriate care. I have argued that in the third situation described earlier, where beneficiaries are not identifiable at the time of treatment, the denial of care that flows from setting guidelines and carrying them out in clinical practice should be referred to as "prioritizing" care, not "rationing" it. Although the scarcity of resources is deliberately created by human agents and is not natural or altogether stubborn, the lives jeopardized by such prioritizing do not rise to the same extremely high level of value claimed for identifiable individuals. Because the losers and winners are not identifiable, such prioritizing can be seen as morally acceptable as long as the procedures for determining scarcity and setting guidelines have social legitimacy. Any special moral burden of justification then falls not on clinicians who follow such guidelines and say no to selected treatments but on those who would fail to follow them and overprescribe.

This is hardly the end of the matter, however. Two situations in clinical practice remain problematic. One occurs because of an ambiguity about identifiability: here, initially, though the benefit of treatment is only a small to modest risk reduction and beneficiaries cannot be identified at time of treatment, later, after results have played out, individual beneficiaries can be identified. In at least a relative if not strict sense, the identity of winners and losers is eventually known. Imagine, for example, that the likelihood of a person surviving for several years without a given treatment is very low. The treatment, which is known to have a small chance of reducing mortality, is provided, and the person survives that long. Her recovery is very likely due to the treatment, not to some natural recovery or other intervening factor. Normal people reacting to circumstances like this—carefully thinking people, not merely wishfully thinking ones—will see a specific, identifiable person as having benefited from the treatment. Beforehand, moreover, it can be seen that generally, for the treatment–condition pair in question, the beneficiaries will eventually become identifiable.

Now suppose further that for this kind of situation, when cost and size of achieved reduction in risk are considered, a treatment is given low priority and is not covered by insurance. Is this better termed "rationing" or "prioritizing"? Because there are no identifiable beneficiaries in view at the time of clinical action, I would argue that it is more logical to call this prioritizing than rationing, with its identifiable losers and winners at the time of clinical decision. Regardless of that decision about language, however, it is undoubtedly more difficult for patients and clinicians to follow a no-saying guideline here than in cases where no identifiable beneficiaries can be discerned even after the results of treatment have played out. I suspect that it takes some considerable experience with prioritizing in a variety of situations before people will know what they want to say about the acceptability of this kind of situation.

A second problematic situation, long viewed as such, is classic "bedside rationing." Clinicians deny or forego care not by applying an already existing guideline, but by using their own substantive discretion in deciding what care is worth the investment of resources. Because it is much more difficult to expose such decisions to critical discussion within a socially transparent process, they are more problematic than clinical decisions to apply already formulated guidelines that have independent legitimacy. I will not wade into the full debate about such discretionary bedside rationing, but others in this volume and elsewhere address this.[13] The previous discussion, however, throws light on the matter.

The case for substantive physician discretion to prioritize care in this kind of case begins with the claim that not all wise decisions in the art of medicine can be represented by practice guidelines; there are simply too many variables in real situations for guidelines to account for. Therefore, the argument goes, we are likely to achieve greater effectiveness and value for money not by relying solely on prior guidelines for setting priorities in clinical practice but by using less guideline-setting and making up the difference with clinicians' own substantive discretion. Then the key point: denial of care that emerges from such discretion will be most acceptable to patients and insurance subscribers when the identity of beneficiaries is hidden by risk and probability, especially at the time of treatment. If this is a key element in the acceptability of setting substantive priorities through practice guidelines and in making policy, why would it not also play a constructive role in justifying a similar segment of discretionary bedside prioritizing?

This point adds to the role of the statistical/identifiable beneficiary distinction in justifying substantive prioritization of care. The distinction, refined to be attentive to beneficiaries and not only to recipients, helps justify the setting of priorities that deny statistically beneficial care to some, and it does that both at the level of guidelines and policymaking and at the level of individual clinician discretion. Both will gain in legitimacy if they do not reach as far as denying treatments that have identifiable beneficiaries. Both can then proceed without apology as prioritizing, not rationing.[14]

To be sure, discretion to prioritize at the bedside will always have to be contained, morally speaking. It is not just in setting practice guidelines that policymakers should be accountable for reasonableness; providers at the bedside need to see themselves similarly accountable. Even when a patient—a potential recipient of care—who is denied care could not likely be an identifiable beneficiary, the reasons for assigning low priority and not giving him the care must be ones that fair-minded people can agree are relevant.[15] Even when patients are not identifiable beneficiaries, it would be egregiously wrong to deny them care, for example, because they were less "likeable" than other patients in the provider's eyes. Physicians carry a burden of trust as societal decision makers, behaving responsibly in a context where guidelines made by others would be too crude, and preserving the "art" of medicine through their discretion is deemed beneficial. Just because many of the patients in question will not end up as identifiable, "real" beneficiaries, clinicians cannot escape the burden of making their decisions for reasons that fair-minded persons would find relevant. None of that precaution, however, weakens my primary argument that it is more accurate to speak of prioritizing than rationing in situations where the factual ingredients that could at least approximate identifiability for the beneficiaries are missing.

Notes

1. Screening tests are among the measures referred to as "secondary prevention." Although the patient may already have the disease at issue, secondary prevention increases the likelihood of catching the disease at an early enough stage to be treated more effectively.

2. And equal in their cost-effectiveness. A $200,000 treatment with a 1:10 chance of extending a life 10 years, for example, is as cost effective ($200,000/year of life extended) as a $200 screening test done 10 times on each of 2,000 women that extends one of their lives 10 years.

3. They did not recommend *against* mammography for women 40–49 and certainly did not deem it to be of no value; they just recommended against *routine annual* use of mammography in that age group.

4. This was only part of what explains the controversy, to be sure. Another part was a significant misunderstanding of what the task force had recommended previously, in 2002. At that time it had made only a *weak*, not a strong, recommendation for routinely screening women 40–49 (Kolata, 2009). Having been adopted as pervasive practice in the meantime, however, the fact that the previous recommendation was weak was lost on the public by 2009.

5. One gets the 6,000 number rather than 1,900 by focusing on a crucial factual dimension not addressed by the task force, probably because it was too elusive to be specified with precision: the *marginal* benefit of routine over discretionary screening for women 40–49. Nonroutine mammography screening at the discretion of a woman and her physician, which the task force *did* still recommend, catches a considerable proportion of the one in every 1,900 whose life is extended by routine screening. The marginal "catch" ratio for routine screening, then, is probably more like one in every 6,000. Such an estimate is plausible if, as would seem likely, discretionary screening would still be done on the highest-risk women. It catches, say, two-thirds of the cancers in women 40–49 that would be caught by routine screening. In this case the *marginal* benefit of routine screening in that age group is to extend life not in one out of every 1,900 but one of every 5,700 women screened annually for 10 years. Simplified, this is 1:6000.

6. The first seven paragraphs of the following section are a revised segment from Menzel, 2012, pp. 199–203.

7. To be sure, in a few instances—secondary prevention, most likely—prevention, too, can have identifiable beneficiaries. Suppose that an early-stage cancer is found with an exploratory procedure or screening test and that the cancer can then be cured. If it is a very aggressive form that is highly likely to have been fatal had it not been caught early, the patient has almost certainly benefited from the screening. We have good reason to think that without it, *she* would have died. Some primary prevention may also fall into this category: virtually all the recipients of chlorinated water in an extremely highly cholera-infested area are beneficiaries, for example.

8. If treatment does not correlate well with the identifiable half of the statistical/identifiable distinction, what does? At least three other distinctions track the prevention/treatment difference better than statistical/identifiable does. One of them—"in trouble" versus "not (yet) in trouble"—tracks it best. The other two are low versus high baseline risk, where baseline risk is typically low for prevention and higher (sometimes very high) for treatment, and small versus large magnitude of the reduction in one's risk that is accomplished, where the reduction treatment accomplishes is usually greater in magnitude than what effective prevention accomplishes. See Menzel, 2012, pp. 201–202.

9. None of this is to say that we do not or should not take risk seriously. We are, however, able to approach many risk assessment situations without seeing them as cases where *we* are going to be the victim.

10. This is captured by the insightful comment of one of the economists early involved in monetary-value-of-life studies, Ezra Mishan (1985, pp. 159–160). Mishan quipped that he had yet to meet a colleague "who would honestly agree to accept any sum of money to enter a gamble in which, if at the first toss of a coin it came down heads, he would be summarily executed." That is, looked at in a high-risk context, life has no price. In lower-risk gambles, of course, people frequently do trade life for money. They are unwilling to pay more than so many dollars to reduce a certain risk of death, for example, or they will accept higher than normal occupational risks for an adequate wage premium. In portraying the trades that empirically ground the so-called monetary price of life, it should not be claimed that people are willing to trade life directly for money; it is only that they are unwilling to spend more than so much to reduce a relatively low risk. For further clarification of so-called "willingness to pay" approaches to the value of life, see Menzel (1990), pp. 37–39, 45–53.

11. In many health care economies this is linguistic practice. The most prominent organization that meets annually to discuss allocation of scarce health care resources is

the International Society on *Priorities* in Health Care (my emphasis), not rationing health care. See the ISPHC website org.uib.no/healthcarepriorities/. My occasional experience in Australia and Scandinavia has been that the American habit of speaking of "rationing" is met with something ranging from mild perplexity to frank correction (to "prioritizing").

12. A consistent, eloquent critic of the continued talk of "rationing" by some policymakers and many bioethicists has been H. R. Moody in his newsletter as Director of Academic Affairs for the American Association of Retired Persons (AARP), "The Soul of Bioethics." In the September 15, 2011 issue he comments on the fact that an article entitled "Rationing Just Medical Care" had been recently published in a prominent journal: "Do bioethicists not read the newspapers? Yes, we need serious public debate about setting priorities and cutting costs in our health care system. But we will never have that debate as long as bioethicists insist on using the 'R' word in their discourse. Please: let's just stop talking about rationing."

13. Ubel, 2000, at pp. 99–110 and 137–152, provides a fair treatment and vigorous defense of such discretionary bedside rationing. Another valuable analysis is presented by Hurst and Danis, 2007, reproduced here in Chapter 17.

14. I stop short of making the strong claim that the distinction between the lives of identifiable and statistical beneficiaries is actually morally justified, not just of relevance in articulating how prioritizing care can gain acceptability and public legitimacy. For some of the further refinement needed to determine how much ultimate moral justification can be marshaled for the distinction, see Menzel, 2012 at pp. 203–211.

15. Daniels and Sabin (2008, pp. 45–58) include four conditions needed to achieve what they term "accountability for reasonableness": publicity, relevance, mechanisms for revision and appeal, and regulatory oversight—some public or voluntary private process to ensure that the previous three conditions are met. The "fair-minded" reason language I use here is part of Daniels' and Sabin's articulation of the relevance condition. I leave open the matter of whether the other three conditions in their accountability for reasonableness framework—publicity, revision and appeal, and regulatory oversight—ought also to be seen as constraining bedside provider discretion.

REFERENCES

Aronowitz, R. (2009). "Addicted to Mammograms." *New York Times*, 20 October, p. A35.

Daniels, N., & Sabin, J. (2008). *Setting Limits Fairly: Learning to Share Resources for Health*, 2nd ed. New York: Oxford University Press.

Hurst, S., & Danis, M. (2007). A framework for rationing by clinical judgment. *Kennedy Institute of Ethics Journal*, 17(3), 247–266.

Hurst, S., Pegoraro, R., Slowther, A-M., Perrier, A., Forde, R., Reiter-Theil, S., & Danis, M. (2009). "The Values at the Bedside Study: Physicians' Attitudes Towards Clinical Rationing in Four European Health Systems." Material for symposium on Rationing Health Care Fairly, Brocher Foundation, July 8–10, 2009. Based on the publication by Hurst, Forde, Reiter-Theil, Slowther, Perrier, Pegoraro, and Danis. (2007). Physicians' views on resource availability and equity in four European health care systems. *BMC Health Services Research*, 7, 137–147.

Kolata, G. (2009). "Mammogram Debate Took Group by Surprise." *New York Times*, 20 November, p. A16, reproduced here in Chapter 17.

Menzel, P. T. (1990). *Strong Medicine: The Ethical Rationing of Health Care.* New York: Oxford University Press.

Menzel, P. T. (2012). The Variable Value of Life and Fairness to the Already Ill: Two Promising but Tenuous Arguments for Treatment's Priority. In Faust, H. S., & Menzel, P. T., eds. *Prevention vs. Treatment: What's the Right Balance?* pp. 194–218. New York: Oxford University Press.

Mishan, E. J. (1985). Consistency in the valuation of life: A wild goose chase? In E. Paul, E., F. Miller, F., & J. Paul, J., eds. *Ethics and Economics,* pp. 152–167. Oxford: Basil Blackwell.

U.S. Preventive Services Task Force (USPSTF). (2009). Screening for breast cancer: U.S. Preventive Services Task Force recommendation statement. *Annals of Internal Medicine, 151*(10), 716–727.

Ubel, P. A. (2000). *Pricing Life: Why It's Time for Health Care Rationing.* Cambridge, MA: MIT Press.

15 Give to the Doctor What Is Due to the Doctor!

Why "Fair Rationing at the Bedside" Is Impossible

■ VEGARD BRUUN WYLLER

This book concerns how health care professionals can contribute to fair rationing and distribution of scarce medical resources at the bedside. The present
essay, however, provides a critical appraisal. I shall elaborate on the immoral
and contradictory implications of such a practice from a political, clinical, and
moral perspective, thus defending a radical proposition: "Fair rationing at the
bedside" is impossible. Furthermore, I argue that a return of the physician
to the classical role of the Good Samaritan dissolves the dilemmas. In short,
I maintain that the doctor should be given what is due to the doctor.

Some definitions seem pertinent: I take attention to *fairness* as equivalent
to distributive justice, as is common in contemporary debate on the topic
(Ubel, 2002; Schneiderman, 2011; Churchill, 2011). For *rationing* I adopt the
definition provided by Ubel (2002): "[. . .] rationing occurs whenever [patients
receive] less than the most beneficial healthcare service." "Bedside" implies
that rationing is included in the practice of clinical medicine and occurs at the
discretion of the physician who is at the same time in charge of clinical care. To
put it succinctly: "Fair rationing at the bedside" means that a physician decides
to give a patient suboptimal treatment because he finds it morally more acceptable to prioritize someone (or something) else.

■ THE POLITICAL PERSPECTIVE

Principally speaking, distributive justice concerns the allocation of some
goods, including any goods that may have economic value, within a society.
Thus, distributive justice is primarily related to *politics*. As pointed out by
Rawls: "The central ideas and aims of this conception [i.e., justice as fairness]
I see as those of a philosophical conception for a constitutional democracy"
(Rawls, 1999, p. xi). Thus, working toward distributive justice should be a
primary concern for political institutions, as is evidently demonstrated in the
development of the Norwegian welfare state (Østerud & Selle, 2006). There
will, however, be disagreement about the practical application of distributive
justice. People disagree about what is fair, and they may even possess different

conceptions of fairness. While this may be an overly simplistic statement, it points to the importance of *political processes,* which could be regarded as institutionalized procedures to handle such disagreement. Thus politics is a normative practice, not a scientific one: the traditional task of the politician is to *choose* a certain distribution of goods, not to perform a calculation that tells with certainty what the fairest distribution would be.

This has important implications for my initial proposition. First, the total amount of resources allocated to health care is not a fixed quantity—it is the product of a political choice. Politicians are free to move goods to and from the health care system, thus *deciding to what extent rationing is needed* (Loughlin, 2002, p. 174). In Norway this is particularly evident: the combination of a wealthy state and a public health service could almost dissolve the question of health care rationing at the macro level, given—say—a doubling of the central health budget. I realize of course that most other nations do not have the same fiscal opportunities. Still, the principle remains valid: *how much* we need to ration depends upon politics.

Second, given that we have to ration, the distribution of goods to different parts of the health care system is also a normative challenge deeply rooted in politics. As stated above, people disagree about what is fair and what fairness is; within a pluralistic democracy, however, these different opinions have *equal weight.* Based upon "one man, one vote," we elect those representatives that serve our interests and our conceptions of fairness. Thus, it could be argued, a democratic constitution acknowledges and grants every citizen the power to participate in decisions about distribution of goods within the health care system. Indeed, people seem to regard such participation as a fundamental constitutional right (Katz, 2010).

These two aspects seem to be more or less neglected in contemporary discussions on rationing (Schneiderman, 2011; Churchill, 2011; Tauber, 2003; Williams, 2005). For instance, Tauber states that "the reality of scarce medical resources demands prioritization" without admitting that the degree of scarcity as well as the scarcity-driven prioritization depend upon normative political choices.

The underlying explanation for this neglect might be the close link between distributive justice and *efficiency*—fairness in health care seems to demand knowledge of who will benefit most from a certain allocation of resources. Often, the health budget is taken as a matter of fact where health economics reigns—in particular through the use of cost-benefit analyses—to make practical rationing decisions. This, however, appears to be a *categorical fallacy* in which normative issues are substituted with science, thus violating the distinction between *is* and *ought* and seriously obscuring the political essence of the matter.

The concept of QALY (quality adjusted life years), which is a commonly applied tool in rationing, constitutes a pertinent example (Dineen, 2011; Katz,

2010). As Katz observes, QALY seems to presuppose that "human life has a defined value that is capable of entering into mathematical calculation" and that "some years of human life are more valuable than other years of human life" (Katz, 2010). Laughlin, being even more critical, questions the very meaning of "quality," accusing its proponents of "persuasive definitions" (Loughlin, 2002, p. 73). I would argue that the concept of a QALY is incompatible with the traditional ethos of health care professionals. I shall return to this later, but for now it suffices to emphasize that QALY is *also* incompatible with the foundations of a constitutional democracy, as it creates the illusion that "fair" decisions depend solely upon advanced arithmetic and therefore could be left to health economists.

However, this observation does not imply that health economists and bio-ethicists neglect *their own* political influence. Rather, they seem to actively *seek* such influence, apparently based on the assumption that they possess the "right" answer to the rationing issue at stake (Tauber, 2003; Stark, 2011). Some even propose a refinement of language, for instance substituting "rationing" with "stewardship" in order to make rationing decisions more "palatable" for politicians and society in general (Fine, 2011).

Summing up, within the field of health care there is a *transfer of political power* from traditional political institutions to experts and bureaucrats, in particular health economists and bioethicists. This is part of a more general tendency: in most areas of public welfare, an analogous power transfer has been thoroughly documented in empirical research (Østerud, 2006; Katz, 2010). In other words, the concern for distributive justice has become an administrative and bureaucratic challenge instead of a political one. Bringing this concern all the way to the bedside, as the title of this book implies, seems to me to be an extreme variant of power transfer.

From a political perspective the consequences of such power transfer are threefold: first, traditional politics becomes devoid of *meaning*. Elections are purposeless if politicians are not accountable for normative decisions that are of vital importance for the life of individuals, such as access to health resources. Rational public discourse is reduced to empty rhetoric when normative challenges are obscured as scientific. Second, health economists and bioethicists— and eventually physicians—become too *mighty*. Their normative influence is controlled neither by the parliamentary processes of funding and legislation nor by the legal system of appellate processes for individuals who are denied access to a particular health service on the basis of rationing (Katz, 2010). Third, a certain ideology, often entitled "New Public Management" (NPM), is thereby tacitly promoted (Laughlin, 2002, p. 98 ff). The observed transfer of power from a political to a bureaucratic level is neither coincidental nor neutral. It relates to a much larger trend in society, characterized by neoliberalistic ideas and "the language of business" gaining increasing influence in public affairs (Østerud & Selle, 2006). In NPM, health care is transformed into "production," the patient becomes a "consumer," and medical treatment turns into a "commodity." The fundamental contrasts to the traditional ethos of the physician will be elaborated below. From a political perspective, however, it should be noted that the ideology of NPM—being highly controversial—should be subjected to democratic processes such as the rationing dilemmas themselves, rather than being implemented more or less unconsciously.

To put it succinctly: "Rationing at the bedside" means that the physician becomes a powerful politician, the politician becomes a powerless celebrity, and the hospital becomes an enterprise. I do not see that this serves any good purpose; rather, from a political perspective, bedside rationing should be *avoided* as much as possible. While many might agree with this ideal, they nevertheless maintain that *some* extent of bedside rationing is inevitable given the scarcity of resources in most circumstances. My approach to this challenge is outlined at the end of this essay; first, however, a discussion of the clinical perspective is pertinent.

■ THE CLINICAL PERSPECTIVE

"Rationing at the bedside" has profound implications for the clinical encounter. Given this concept of rationing, a *third party*—be it the next patient in the corridor or some anonymous person or undertaking in society—is included in the doctor–patient relationship. The argument that Levinsky pursued 30 years ago that the classical ideal of the medical profession—being the patient's advocate—is equally justified nowadays: "[...] physicians are required to do everything that they believe may benefit each patient without regard to costs or other social considerations" (Levinsky, 1984). In contemporary debate this stance is frequently labeled as "utopian" and rejected without further arguments (Paris, 2011). I maintain, however, that it deserves serious consideration.

First, bringing a third party to the clinical encounter might influence patients' fiduciary negatively (Weiner & Rice, 2001; Schafer, 2001). Commitment is a prerequisite of basic trust; even a suspicion of being abandoned by your physician for the benefit of someone or something else might seriously jeopardize the doctor–patient relationship. Of note, this relationship is not some secondary or "external" good; it should be regarded as an intrinsic part of medical practice, being directly related to the quality and outcome of the health service (Skirbekk & Nortvedt, 2011). However, the "cost" of fiduciary loss cannot be easily quantified, which may explain why this perspective tends to be absent from most analyses of health economics. While patients' fiduciary loss is recognized as a main challenge by most debaters, some proponents of bedside rationing, such as Ubel, frankly claim that: "[...] we need to make sure that physicians ration in ways that do not greatly reduce patient trust. I think this is achievable" (Ubel, 2002). He does not provide any further argument, but as long as his statement is contrary to reason, intuition, and established beliefs, I do believe that he—not I—should be obliged to provide evidence.

Second, health care providers experience a conflict between two responsibilities: toward the patient and toward the society (Levinsky, 1984; Maxwell, 2009). The physician feels compelled to find some sort of compromise between two divergent moral claims: individual beneficence and collective distributive justice. As the ideology of NPM expands to include the clinical encounter and "confronts" the traditional ethos of medical care, the physician is expected to combine cost-benefit analyses and compassionate care (Maxwell, 2009). The physician is expected to be both a Samaritan and a gatekeeper. Evidence suggests that the experience of this conflict is increasingly widespread, problematic, and morally distressing in parallel with the gradual transfer of rationing responsibilities to the bedside. It threatens professional flourishing and eventually causes burn-out or cynicism (Austin et al., 2003; Førde & Aasland, 2008; Maxwell, 2009; Simpson et al., 2005).

Thus, the physician is in a crossfire. The clinical perspective suggests that the dilemmas of rationing might be interpreted as a consequence of *competing moral philosophies*. To this issue I now turn.

■ THE MORAL PERSPECTIVE

In *After Virtue*, MacIntyre outlines how moral reflection in contemporary Western society is greatly influenced by the development of moral philosophy from the Enlightenment to the nineteenth century (MacIntyre, 1984). In other words, our moral conceptions and beliefs—whether they are classified as utilitarian, deontological, or emotivist—are all a product of *modernity*. Indeed, Rawls in his highly influential *Theory of Justice* acknowledges his debt to the Enlightenment philosophers (Rawls, 1999). It seems superfluous to point out in detail how this influence extends to the various branches of bioethics, health economics, and rationing discussions.

A central claim in *After Virtue*, however, is that our inclination to a modernistic stance towards morality is not based upon a philosophical superiority or vindication of the underlying moral theories. On the contrary, the hegemony of modernity is a product of a cultural context; it continues despite serious criticism of its foundation in recent philosophical literature and the presence of competing moral theories. For my present topic, two of these competing theories are of particular importance.

First, an *ethics of proximity* has been developed within the field of phenomenology, in particular by the contemporary Lithuanian-French philosopher Emmanuel Levinas. The focal point of this ethics is the unique relationship between two persons, between an "I" and a "Thou"; *responsibility for the Other* is the fundamental source of morality (Vetlesen, 1997; Bauman, 1993). This responsibility is rooted in our very existence as human beings—or, even more radically, it constitutes us as humans. Thus, an ethics of proximity acknowledges the relevance of emotions (such as compassion) and intuition for moral action and opposes the modernistic reliance on pure, context-independent reason. The relevance of this philosophy for health care workers seems obvious; indeed, it is sometimes labeled "ethics of care" (Nortvedt, 2003; Clifton-Soderstrøm, 2003; Nortvedt & Nordhaug, 2008; Nordhaug & Nordtvedt, 2011).

Second, the ancient ethics of Aristotle and its medieval revisions, in which morality is related to vices and virtues (i.e., traits of character), represents a tradition that is still alive (MacIntyre, 1984). For Aristotle the faculty of reason is vital for performing moral judgments, but reason cannot be separated from an established mode of life; thus, this tradition also opposes the abstraction and context-independence of moral judgments that characterize modernity (Vetlesen, 1997). When applied to a certain practice, such as medicine, the Aristotelian tradition emphasizes the particular end or *telos* for which this practice exists (Pellegrino, 2001; Armstrong, 2006; Maxwell, 2009; Laughlin, 2002). Thus a physician ought to act in a way that improves patients' health; the more he cultivates his virtues (such as justice), the more he will flourish in practical wisdom and the better he will serve this particular *telos* of his practice.

A general discussion of these moral theories is beyond the scope of this essay. What is more important here is their relevance for the problem of "fair rationing at the bedside." As noted previously, "fair rationing" belongs to the vocabulary of distributive justice and thus to the moral apprehensions of modernity. Distributive justice is regarded as a universal principle and as such encompasses all human beings in the present and future generations. Limiting its scope to a certain group of individuals, for instance the citizens of a nation, seems to violate the very principle. While this might constitute an ideal for global policymakers, it does seem totally infeasible when it comes to medical practice "at the bedside." It would demand that each and every physician weigh the effect of a certain health "commodity" against all other possible applications of the same amount of resources. Even a more restricted application of the principle will confront the physician with an immense—and indeed impossible—task, and may turn out to be quite arbitrary and inefficient (Schafer, 2001; Lauridsen, 2009).

As opposed to "fair rationing," a focus on the "bedside" implies a focus on individualized clinical care. As outlined above, both the Aristotelian and Levinasian ethics seem to be more congruent with the traditional stance toward the moral foundations of medical practice (Clifton-Soderstrøm, 2003; Pellegrino, 2001). Indeed, evidence suggests that even nowadays, despite the hegemony of modernity, nurses and physicians possess tacit concepts of professional moral obligation that are more in line with these alternative traditions (Skirbekk & Nordtvedt, 2011). Furthermore, these traditions articulate a draconian criticism of the modernistic conception of ethics; in particular the formalistic, impersonal, and universalistic aspirations of modernity (Vetlesen, 1997; MacIntyre, 1984; Bauman, 1993). For instance, some proponents of the ethics of proximity radically maintain that the moral responsibility towards the Other constitutes a protection toward the possible brutal consequences of pure distributive fairness and the related ideology of NPM:

> In the spirit of Levinas one may argue that the distributive maximization of health care jeopardizes the essence of this care itself. The other is reduced to a number, and ethics becomes economy. Not the vulnerable sensitivity for the other, but the clever rationality of justice then justifies the moral order. [...] This does not merely open up for brutality, *it is brutality* (Nortvedt, 2003).

Similarly, from an Aristotelian-inspired point of view, Laughlin accuses the radical proponents of distributive justice of cynicism, stating that

> ... [they] do not view it as morally outrageous that some people who could in principle be relieved will instead suffer and die. The pain, terror, and despair of the 'de-prioritised' are of course 'regrettable' but it is not the moral problem ... [it is] ... the unsystematic way in which such pain, terror and despair are currently distributed (Laughlin, 2002, p. 157).

Thus "fair rationing at the bedside" seems to possess an inherent *conflict* between competing moral theories. "Fair rationing" belongs to modernity and concerns universal justice at a political level. "At the bedside" belongs to an Aristotelian or Levinasian tradition and concerns particular care at the individual level. In short: the two parts of the phrase are at home in different spheres. An attempt to fuse them, as has indeed been advocated by some theorists (Nordtvedt, 2003), might have several unwanted consequences for both society and the individual patients, as outlined previously in this essay. Furthermore, considering the inner characterizations of the underlying moral theories, such a fusion seems insuperable—"fair rationing at the bedside" is simply impossible. So why even try?

▪ GIVE TO THE DOCTOR WHAT IS DUE TO THE DOCTOR!

I maintain that we should not try. Indeed—we *do not have to try*. While I acknowledge that a universal moral theory is a legitimate aim for philosophy, medical ethics might have a much more modest ambition: to furnish the *role as caregiver* with a moral framework. In other words: we do not need to worry about distributive justice and fair rationing; this problem could (and in my opinion should) be left to the politicians, while we give the doctor what is due to the doctor, namely the right to remain faithful to his traditional ethos.

From antiquity, the role of the caregiver is the role of the Good Samaritan:

> But a Samaritan who was travelling came to where the injured man was, and when he saw him, he felt compassion for him. He went up to him and bandaged his wounds, pouring oil and wine on them. Then he put him on his own animal, brought him to an inn, and took care of him (The Bible, Luke 10, 33–34).

The Samaritan did not consider whether a part of his limited resources should be reserved for another individual or spread among all the poor in Palestine. His moral obligation was awakened by the particular individual in need. Remark, however, that the parable is the answer to a most provocative challenge: "Who is my neighbor?" Thus, the particularity of the story infers a universal vocation as has always been emphasized in the teaching of the Church: every human being who incidentally comes in my way deserves my compassionate care.

In an analogous manner, both the Aristotelian and the Levinasian tradition recognize a universal moral obligation, despite having a particularistic foundation and starting point. For instance, a Levinasian will infer our sense of justice for mankind from our care for the Other, whereas an Aristotelian will maintain that a man excelling in the virtue of justice will promote a just society. Indeed, some will argue that a universalistic ideal is actually *better* protected within these traditions. As Bauman observes: "The humankind-wide moral unit is thinkable [...] as the [...] emancipation of the autonomous moral self and vindication of its moral responsibility" (Bauman, 1993, p. 13).

In other words, returning to the ideal of the Good Samaritan and adopting a Levinasian or Aristotelian foundation for medical practice is *not* a naïve position; it is not a kind of "moral nearsightedness," which is a commonly uttered criticism (Tauber, 2003). In particular, it does provide a framework for moral actions in situations characterized by acute discrepancy between means and needs. As mentioned previously, health care workers may to some extent be confronted with such situations; indeed, this is an everyday experience in underdeveloped parts of the world. However, it is not at all obvious, although it is often taken for granted, that the modernistic interpretation of justice as fairness should be applied. An alternative moral theory might result in an equal (or even more) just outcome, and might also be more in line with our intuitive apprehension of morality (MacIntyre, 1984, p. 244 ff). The terrorist massacre on a Labor party youth camp (Utøya) in Norway is a pertinent example: immediately after the attack, a few lay people provided immense support to the victims in a situation of severe resource constraints. However, the rescuers did not act according to a rational plan of maximizing some particular gain; their intuitive practice was not founded on a calculus of distribution and efficiency. Rather, their actions seem to be directly related to their virtuous character (following Aristotle) and their compassionate care (following Levinas). And for this, they were unanimously celebrated as heroes afterwards; no one claimed that that the outcome was unjust because it was not a product of distributive justice and pure, context-independent reason.

Summing up, the traditional ethos of the Good Samaritan and the moral theories of Levinas and Aristotle provide a *sound foundation for the social role of the caregiver*. I believe this is of vital importance for the caring professions. And I think that society as a whole will benefit from it. Quoting Levinsky once more: "When practicing medicine, doctors cannot serve two masters. It is to the advantage both of our society and of the individuals it comprises that physicians retain their historic single-mindedness. The doctor's master must be the patient" (Levinsky, 1984).

■ ACKNOWLEDGMENTS

I thank Reidun Førde, Arne Johan Vetlesen, Hanne Kraugerud, Torgeir Bruun Wyller, Liv Holtan-Hartwig, Kari Bruun Wyller, and Thomas Chr. Wyller for thoughtful discussions and comments on drafts of the manuscript.

REFERENCES

Armstrong, A. E. (2006). Towards a strong virtue ethics for nursing practice. *Nursing Philosophy, 7*, 110–124.

Austin, W., Bergum, V., & Goldberg, L. (2003). Unable to answer the call of our patients: mental health nurses' experience of moral stress. *Nursing Inquiry, 10*, 177–183.

Bauman, Z. (1993). *Postmodern Ethics*. Oxford: Blackwell.

Churchill, L. (2011). Rationing, rightness and distinctively human goods. *American Journal of Bioethics, 11*, 15–16.

Clifton-Soderstrøm, M. (2003). Levinas and the patient as the other: the ethical foundation of medicine. *Journal of Medicine and Philosophy, 28*, 447–460.

Dineen, C. (2011). Finding the right way to ration. *American Journal of Bioethics, 11*, 26–28.

Fine, R. (2011). Rationing or stewardship in pursuit of just medical reform. *American Journal of Bioethics, 11*, 22–23.

Førde, R., & Aasland, O. G. (2008). Moral distress among Norwegian doctors. *Journal of Medical Ethics, 34*, 521–525.

Katz, M. (2010). Towards a new moral paradigm in health care delivery: accounting for individuals. *American Journal of Law & Medicine, 36*, 78–135.

Lauridsen, S. (2009). Administrative gatekeeping—a third way between unrestricted patient advocacy and bedside rationing. *Bioethics, 23*, 311–320.

Levinsky, N. G. (1984). The doctor's master. *New England Journal of Medicine, 311*, 1573–1575.

Loughlin, M. (2002). *Ethics, Management and Mythology. Rational decision making for health service professionals*. Oxon: Radcliffe Medical Press.

MacIntyre, A. (1984). *After Virtue*. Indiana: University of Notre Dame Press.

Maxwell, B. (2009). Just compassion: implications for the ethics of the scarcity paradigm in clinical healthcare provision. *Journal of Medical Ethics*, 35, 219–223.

Nordhaug, M., & Nortvedt, P. (2011). Justice and proximity: problems for an ethics of care. *Health Care Analysis*, 19, 3–14.

Nortvedt, P., & Nordhaug, M. (2008). The principle and problem of proximity in ethics. *Journal of Medical Ethics*, 34, 156–161.

Nortvedt, P. (2003). Levinas, justice and health care. *Medicine, Health Care and Philosophy*, 6, 25–34.

Østerud, Ø, & Selle, P. (2006). Power and democracy in Norway: The transformation of Norwegian politics. *Scandinavian Political Studies*, 29, 25–46.

Paris, J. J. (2011). Rationing: "A decent minimum" or "consumer driven" health care system? *American Journal of Bioethics*, 11, 16–18.

Pellegrino, E. D. (2001). The internal morality of clinical medicine: A paradigm for the ethics of the helping and healing professions. *Journal of Medicine and Philosophy*, 26, 559–579.

Rawls, J. (1999). *A Theory of Justice*. Oxford: Oxford University Press.

Schafer, A. (2001). Bedside rationing by physicians: The case against. *Healthcare Papers*, 2, 45–52.

Simpson, C. S., Hoffmaster, B., & Dorian, P. (2005). Downward delegation of implantable cardioverter defibrillator decision-making in a restricted-resource environment: the pitfalls of bedside rationing. *Canadian Journal of Cardiology*, 21, 595–599.

Skirbekk, H., & Nordtvedt, P. (2011). Making a difference: a qualitative study on care and priority setting in health care. *Health Care Analysis*, 19, 77–88.

Schneiderman, L. J. (2011). Rationing just medical care. *American Journal of Bioethics*, 11, 7–14.

Stark, M. (2011). Shifting the focus of rationing discussions. *American Journal of Bioethics*, 11, 20–22.

Tauber, A. I. (2003). A philosophical approach to rationing. *Medical Journal of Australia*, 178, 454–456.

The NET Bible, The Biblical Studies Foundation. See http://bible.org/netbible. Accessed October 24, 2011.

Ubel, P. (2002). Physicians, thou shalt ration: The necessary role of bedside rationing in controlling healthcare costs. *Healthcare Papers*, 2, 10–21.

Vetlesen, A. J. (1997). Introducing an ethics of proximity. In Vetlesen, A. J., & Jodalen, H. *Closeness. An ethics.* pp. 1–19. Oslo: Scandinavian University Press.

Weiner, S. K., & Rice, C. L. (2001). Cutting healthcare cost without rationing at the bedside: preserving the doctor–patient fiduciary relationship. *Healthcare Papers*, 2, 38–44.

Williams, A. (2005). Thinking about equity in health care. *Journal of Nursing Management*, 13, 397–402.

PART FOUR

Strategies for Promoting Fair Bedside Rationing

16 Priority Setting in Hospital Care

Implementing National Legislation and Guidelines in a Hospital Trust

■ ODD SØREIDE, STENER KVINNSLAND, AND TORHILD HEGGESTAD

In this chapter we will outline how national legislation and regulations relevant to priority setting in health care were incorporated into clinical work and in management in a hospital trust (which also included a large university hospital) in Norway.

■ THE CONTEXT: THE NATIONAL HEALTH SERVICE IN NORWAY

The health care system in Norway has been outlined by Førde in Chapter 5. In brief, the majority of health care services in Norway are publicly owned. The Norwegian health care system—serving a population of 5 million—is organized on three levels: national, regional, and local. Overall responsibility for the health care sector lies at the national level with the Ministry of Health and Care Services[1] (Johnsen, 2006).

Specialist health care is the responsibility of Regional Health Authorities and is in principle free at the point of delivery and need. The Norwegian health care system is primarily funded through taxes. Some user charges that are set by the government apply for ambulatory and day care treatment and for ambulatory radiology services. Health care spending is well described by the Organisation for Economic Co-operation and Development (OECD, 2010). In terms of health spending per capita, Norway ranked second highest among OECD countries in 2008 (after the United States), spending US $5,003 (adjusted for purchasing power parity), well above the OECD average of $3,060 (OECD, 2010).

National reforms of the health care system have focused on three broad areas: responsibility for providing health care services, priorities and patients' rights, and cost containment.

▪ PRIORITY SETTING IN NORWEGIAN HEALTH CARE

Priority setting in the health services in Norway is closely linked to the development of legislation for stronger patients' rights and to the concept of the right to necessary health care. Patients' rights were strengthened with the passing of the Patients' Rights Act in 1999 (Patients' Rights Act, 1999). Its main purpose was to ensure equality of access to good-quality health care. A description of the guiding principles of health legislation in Norway and of patients' rights has recently been published by Molven and Ferkis (2011).

Under the Patient- and User's Rights Act, patients are given broad rights: the right to a medical evaluation, the right to a second opinion, the right to choice of hospital, the right to participation and information, the right to consent to health care, the right of access to medical records, special rights for children, and access to the patient ombudsman system.

The right to necessary health care contained in section 2-1 of the Patient- and User's Rights Act[2] is a key provision with respect to priority setting.

> *The patient is entitled to receive necessary health care from the specialist health care services.*
>
> *This right only applies if the patient can be expected to benefit from the health care and if the costs are reasonable in proportion to the effect of the measure.*
>
> *The specialist health services shall set a time limit within which it is medically appropriate for a patient entitled to such a right to receive necessary health care.*

On the basis of section 2-1 of the Patient- and User's Rights Act, the Ministry has formulated regulations called the Regulations on Priority Setting (FOR 2000-12-01 no. 1205).

Section 2 of the Regulations ("right to necessary health care from the specialist health services")[3] states the basic criteria that must apply for the conferral of rights and for understanding the notion of the right to necessary health care.

> *The patient has the right to receive necessary health care from the specialist health care services pursuant to section 2-1, second paragraph of the Patient- and User's Rights Act when:*
>
> 1. *The patient will have an impaired prognosis in terms of length of life or not insignificantly impaired quality of life if the health care is delayed, and*
> 2. *The patient, with the exception given in section 3, second paragraph, can be expected to benefit from the health care, and*
> 3. *The anticipated costs are reasonable in proportion to the effect of the measure.*

> *"Not insignificantly impaired quality of life" means that the patient's quality of life without treatment will be noticeably impaired as a result of pain or suffering, problems relating to vital life functions such as intake of food, or reduced physical or psychological functional level.*

"Expected to benefit from the health care" means that it is well documented that active medical or multidisciplinary specialist treatment may improve the length or quality of the patient's life for a certain length of time, that the condition may deteriorate without treatment or that possibilities for treatment may be lost by delaying the treatment.

There are two other guarantees added in the legislation for patients with need for necessary health care (i.e., prioritized patients). One empowers patients by giving them the right to receive immediate care at an alternative hospital once their individual maximum time limit (see Patient- and User's Rights Act, section 2-1) is exceeded. The second imposes penalties on hospitals which fail to provide treatment within the set time limit, as they have to pay for alternative treatment elsewhere (in the private sector or abroad).

The Patient- and User's Rights Act and the subsequent Regulations on Priority Setting show that Norwegian legislators specify that:

- Priorities shall be set for specialist health care services.
- The legislators have defined the criteria on which priorities must be based.
- Time limits must be set for providing prioritized health care.
- Priority setting, including the setting of time limits, must be professionally appropriate.

The term "professionally appropriate" in this context is of particular interest. In Norway, the concept of appropriateness is a legal norm regarding the health services that will be provided. From a medical perspective and for hospital managements with responsibility for complying with the Regulations on Priority Setting, "appropriateness" could be paraphrased as "good quality health care." In other words, a specialist health service is founded on a commonly agreed upon, professional (health and medical) standard.

The background for and development of the Patient- and User's Rights Act and the Regulations on Priority Setting can be seen in the draft legislation for the Patient- and User's Rights Act (Ot. prp. nr. 12, 1998–1999) and in the Recommendation of the Social Committee on the Patient- and User's Rights Act (Inst O. nr. 91, 1998–1999). A legal description of the development of patient rights to necessary treatment from the health services has been published by Kjønstad (2011).

We argue that development and use of the prioritization criteria in the Norwegian specialist health services, the legal basis for which is provided in the Regulations on Priority Setting, is founded on three cornerstones:

- A political ambition to ensure treatment for the sickest patients within a reasonable length of time and a goal to ensure patients a more or less equitable provision of treatment, regardless of where they live and to which regional hospital district they belong. In addition, a general goal is to create effective use of health service resources so that more patients can be treated.

- A political ambition to introduce a waiting-time guarantee and thereby a system of priority setting in the specialist health care services whereby, for example, the sickest patients would receive treatment within a given time limit. This work was first entrenched in legislation in 1990 by means of the regulations concerning waiting-list registers and the prioritization of patients.

- The significance of a legitimizing public debate over priority setting as expressed in two Norwegian Official Reports (NOU 1987:23 and NOU 1997:18).The basic criteria on which laws and regulations for priority setting are based draw on the thinking in these two official reports and on NOU 1997:18 in particular.

Norwegian health legislation confers patients with rights. Due to the way in which Norwegian legislation is formulated, a patient population can be divided into three categories (*Figure 16.1*): patients who require emergency care, and elective patients who are either given priority under the law (the right to necessary health care) or who seek specialist health care but are given lower priority. This categorization will be used in the following descriptions of priority-setting practice.

The Patient- and User's Rights Act and the Regulations on Priority Setting have two areas of application: determining *access to* the specialist health care services for individual patients (waiting list management) and *allocation of* specific health care services (examination, treatment, rehabilitation) in the specific patient situation. The specific application of laws and regulations in practical clinical work in hospitals is the subject of this chapter.

■ FROM LEGAL FRAMEWORK AND LAW TO IMPLEMENTATION: PRIORITIZING AND OPTIMIZING THE DISTRIBUTION OF CARE

Despite the introduction of the Regulations on Priority Setting in 2000, it is fair to say that its provisions generated little discussion or attention in the health services sector. The introduction of a waiting-time guarantee for priority patients in 2004, with time limits for when the health care should be provided, significantly changed this situation both politically and in terms of management attention.

However, the focus was for the most part limited to issues relating to waiting times and queues in the specialist health care services.

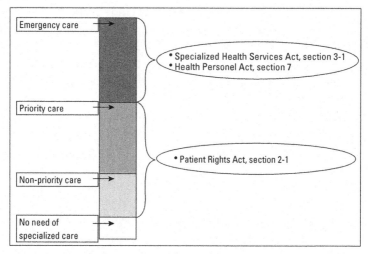

Figure 16.1 Theoretical distribution of hospital patients in priority groups with corresponding legal framework determining whether they receive specialized care or primary care instead.

Access to Services: Waiting Times and Waiting List Management

In 2004–2005 Bergen Hospital Trust was charged by its owner (Western Norway Regional Health Authority) with the task of creating guidelines and a regional system that ensured compliance with the provisions of the Regulations on Priority Setting in the practical, clinical work of the hospitals. The authors of this chapter were given responsibility for performing this task.

This coincided with a period in which the hospital faced major challenges in achieving cost control without reducing allocative efficiency.

The authors—responsible for developing a priority-setting instrument at a time of turbulence caused by what clinicians and other health professionals perceived as dramatic cuts in hospital spending—established three guiding principles:

A. Establishing operational criteria for clinical priority setting
B. Development of practical tools for documentation and transparent monitoring
C. Leadership—using information in hospital management decisions.

A. Establishing Operational Criteria for Clinical Priority Setting

Each clinical department was given the task of formulating diagnosis-based or symptom-based clinical guidelines—based on the criteria given in the

Regulations on Priority Setting—which should guide priority setting (including time limits for treatments). The process was professionally led and driven by consensus. No attempt was made to harmonize priority-setting criteria across medical specialities. The process was supported and supervised by a leading academic with a proven track record in medical ethics and priority setting in health care.

This pragmatic, simple, time-efficient process led to practical priority-setting guidelines for more than 20 medical specialties, including psychiatry, that were adopted by the Trust and, in 2005, by the Western Norway Regional Health Authority.

As an extension of this work and in order to operationalize different levels of priority for planned elective treatment, each department was asked to place each patient referral into one of the three categories specified in the national legislation for priority to access necessary health care. The guiding principle for the practical work was the simple question of how the prognosis of the patient would be affected if care were to be delayed:

P1: *reduced life expectancy*
P2: *other potential prognostic loss (defined as potential organ failure)*
P3: *substantial reduction in quality of life*

B. Development of Practical Tools for Documentation and Transparent Monitoring

The second principle of the strategy was to formulate indicators related to priority setting using routinely registered patient administrative data (hospital episode statistics). Registration of any necessary new data to document the categorization of patients as specified above was integrated into the patient administration system as an obligatory element.

This information was made available in electronic format to ensure transparency across departments and was actively used to monitor the development of the hospital's clinical activities and distribution of priority groups. Online presentations of the chosen indicators was developed using online reports updated and made available on the hospital's intranet.

Importantly, the information system enabled clinicians and heads of departments to follow their priority-setting practices on a daily basis, including tools to identify patients with long waiting times and those with waiting times exceeding those specified in the Regulations on Priority Setting.

An example of the reports used, particularly at the hospital level, was the categorization of hospital activity in different priority groups (*Figure 16.2*, emergency care included) broken down by clinical departments. The distribution

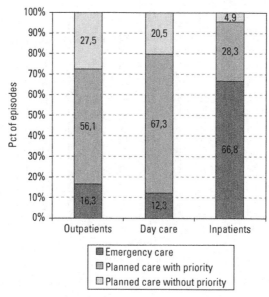

Figure 16.2 Distribution of hospital episodes by priority group (2009).

of priority groups differs greatly by type of department or medical specialty (*Figure 16.3*).

A high proportion of inpatient care for most departments consists of emergency admissions. The group with the highest priority (right to necessary health care) accounted for approximately 30% of the total patient volume and represented roughly 80% of all elective (planned) inpatient admissions (*Figures 16.2* and *16.3*).

Categorization of priority patients (i.e., right to necessary health care) into the priority subgroups outlined above according to the national legislation, as well as their corresponding waiting times, are given in *Figure 16.4*.

The volume of the group with the highest severity (Priority Group 1 in *Figure 16.4*, left-hand panel) is smaller than the other two priority subcategories. Furthermore, this subcategory showed a high degree of variation between different departments or medical specialties. By far the largest category was that of patients admitted for treatment facing the risk of significant reduction in quality of life (Priority Group 3 in *Figure 16.4*).

An essential analytical dimension was to include patient-perspective relevant information (i.e., access) and not only episodes of hospital activity. In a resource allocation discussion, such information is helpful to separate between activities that primarily increase services to patients already in the system versus those which increase accessibility.

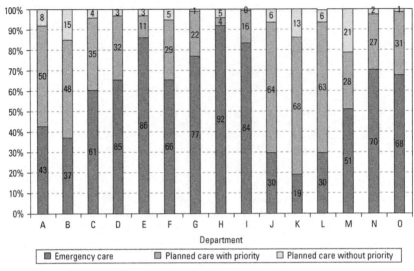

Figure 16.3 Distribution of episodes (in %) of inpatient care by priority group and department (2009).

When monitoring results, observation of waiting times was essential in addition to the relative distribution of the groups. Importantly, there are differences—as we would anticipate—in waiting times for patients within the categories specified in national legislation; patients with more severe prognoses experienced the shortest waiting times (*Figure 16.4*, right-hand panel).

An information system based on the same principles as outlined above was later implemented for the Regional Health Authority, providing information

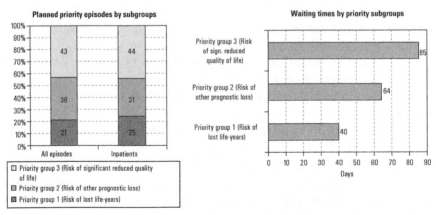

Figure 16.4 Distribution of high-priority subgroups defined in Norwegian law as measured by hospital episodes, and their corresponding mean waiting times (2009).

about 280,000 new elective (planned) referrals per year in addition to 140,000 emergency admissions.

C. Leadership: Using Information in Hospital Management Decisions

The information outlined above and accrued longitudinally was actively and openly used in the resource-allocation processes, which are an integrated and important part of hospital management as we discuss further below.

Documenting the effects and development over time was an essential part of the follow-up. The monitoring system was actively used in management over time. In our opinion this had a pedagogical effect that raised the whole organization's awareness on this subject.

We also consider it essential that the principles of priority were widely used as basic guidance in different kinds of management discussions and decisions, constituting a basis for logical argumentation and communication. Such a set of fundamental principles may be important in cases of counterveiling incentives, for instance in relation to the activity-based financing system.

Without elaborating extensively on this issue, we found it easy to communicate and discuss such information with clinicians and clinic managers. An important prerequisite is full and open information sharing and transparency in the informational elements used by hospital management.

Based on data for actual priority setting in clinical practice, we conclude that we achieved the objective of implementing a system of priority setting throughout the hospital where the waiting times for different groups were in accordance with their listed priority. Significant variations in priority between different groups of patients and medical disciplines are easily identified, which also makes this system a potentially potent tool to execute the very difficult horizontal priority setting and resource allocation.

■ LATER NATIONAL INITIATIVES

Following the changes in the Regulations on Priority Setting implemented in 2004, and with increasing political attention to waiting lists and waiting times, it soon became obvious that the hospitals varied in their interpretation of the regulations. The proportion of patients with the highest priority (right to necessary health care services) varied significantly between health regions, hospitals, between internal medicine and surgical specialties, and between subspecialties such as orthopedics and rheumatology. Waiting times for the priority patients (those with a right to necessary health care) varied, and many patients did not receive treatment within the established time limits. This

274 PROMOTING FAIR BEDSIDE RATIONING

challenged the principle of equality that is so pivotal in Norwegian health care services.

In 2007 the Norwegian Directorate of Health and the regional health authorities were therefore charged by the Ministry of Health and Care Services with the task of formulating national guidelines to serve as a tool for assigning the right to necessary health care to patients in 30 areas of medicine and to give recommended time limits based on medical professional judgement (National Guidelines for Priority Setting in Specialist Health Care, 2011).

The guidelines, used for 30 medical specialties, consist of two parts. The first part is an introduction to the law and regulations with emphasis on definitions and interpretations of legal terms for clinicians intended to be uniform for all specialties. The second part contains disease or symptom-based information for recommended priority status (right to necessary treatment or lower priority), diagnostic investigations or treatments, suggested grading according to criteria set in the Regulations on Priority Setting, group-level maximum waiting times, and individual factors that should be considered and might influence waiting times.

The national guidelines, having a normative status, replaced the local and regional priority-setting tools.

The Regulations on Priority Setting not only govern access to services but are also applicable for the treatment of individual patients. Whereas access and waiting times can be monitored as described above, it is more difficult, indeed impossible, to document that the myriad of clinical decisions that occurs in day-to-day clinical practice follows the criteria set in the Regulations on Priority Setting to the letter.

We would argue that application of the priority criteria in the Regulations will, in essence, be synonymous with the concept of evidence-based medicine. We acknowledge that some clinical decision making leads to inappropriate treatment—that is, treatment that falls outside scientifically indicated care (McGlynn et al., 2003)—but we believe that the Regulations on Priority Setting represent a strong incentive and reminder to the clinical staff in the execution of their day-to-day activities.

To support evidence-based practice, the Western Norway Regional Health Authority (the owner of the hospital trust) has facilitated the development of tools for use by clinicians to support decision making. In particular, a database for new technologies based on the concept of early warning or scanning of the horizon (drawing heavily on international experience) was developed and introduced regionally and nationally (http://mednytt.no). The Health Authority also developed a tool for mini–HTA (Health Technology Assessment) to aid decision support when new medical technologies are considered.

■ APPLICATION OF THE REGULATIONS ON PRIORITY SETTING IN END-OF-LIFE DECISIONS

Three abbreviated patient case histories illustrate that the Regulations on Priority Setting have been used in extremely difficult and sensitive end-of-life situations and highlight issues relevant for the discussion here.

Patient number 1. A 4-year-old child was admitted and underwent intensive care for trauma including a severe head injury. After intensive care treatment on a ventilator for 4 weeks and after repeated examinations, it was concluded that the child had irreversible brain damage but did not fulfill universal and national criteria for brain death. It was advised to terminate medical treatment. This professional conclusion was challenged by one of the parents and was debated extensively in the public domain.

What is relevant here is that the Norwegian Board of Health Supervision, a national public institution organized under the Ministry of Health and Care Services, supported the hospital's opinion that the patient did not fulfill the criteria specified in the Patient- and User's Rights Act and in the Regulations on Priority Setting regarding the right to necessary health care. Active treatment was suspended after 20 weeks.

Patient number 2. A family with one healthy child was expecting a second child. A routine ultrasound examination of the fetus revealed a cerebral cyst in the embryo. The results of an amniocentesis were found at 31 weeks to reveal the chromosomal disorder, trisomy 18. Uncomplicated, induced delivery occurred 18 days past due date.

The physical features of the baby were consistent with the diagnosed chromosomal disorder. The infant was weak and passive but had otherwise normal organ status. The chromosomal disorder was confirmed by further blood tests. The baby's condition gradually deteriorated, with prolonged eating difficulties, arrested development, and increasing and more prolonged breathing difficulties. The child died after 3 months.

The medical advice was not to put the patient on a respirator but instead to provide relief in the form of breathing support when breathing difficulties occurred. The parents did not agree with this, and the case was referred to the Norwegian Board of Health Supervision and brought before a court. The Norwegian Board of Health Supervision did not agree that this was a case of a right to priority health care, nor did the court uphold the parents' claim, commenting that, by virtue of the nature of the case, it had no place in the legal system.

Patient number 3. A 10-year old girl received treatment for acute leukemia. Her treatment was completed in 6 months, after which she showed no signs of illness.

A relapse in the patient's leukemia was detected one year later. She received several rounds of treatment but consequently suffered from prolonged side effects on normal bone marrow cells and a fungal infection in the lungs. She received all the treatments available but presented increasing changes in the lungs despite specific treatment.

This time the patient responded badly to the treatment for leukemia. Experimental support treatment was given. There was a brief period of clinical improvement, but the effect was temporary and accompanied by pronounced side effects and increasing lung disease. The girl died after an illness trajectory of 26 months.

The parents disagreed with the decision to stop medical treatment and the experimental support treatment. International experts many places in the world were consulted; all of them endorsed the medical evaluations made by the hospital. The case was referred to the Norwegian Board of Health Supervision, which agreed with the medical decision not to continue the treatment. The conditions for the right to priority health care were not met.

▨ REFLECTIONS AND CHALLENGES

The Norwegian system for priority setting in specialist health care with its base in Norwegian law is not necessarily easy for stakeholders such as politicians, the public, administrators, and professionals to understand.

In essence, there are four basic elements in this system:

a. Clear principles and criteria formulated in national legislation
b. Clear case-processing routines (diagnostic and therapeutic time limits for priority patients).
c. Treatment time limits are set in accordance with medical appropriateness (as a legal term).
d. A "punitive" system with payment obligations if the rights for the sickest patients are not met

We are not aware of any similar system for priority setting in health care elsewhere. There is a clear distinction between the role of the politicians and lawmakers as they establish the basic principles and criteria for priority setting rooted in Norwegian legislation and the role of health care providers who are responsible for clinical application and execution of these principles.

Our main argument for endorsing the principles and criteria for priority setting is that they are the best tools we have seen so far that support the *equity* or *fairness principle*, particularly in regulating and governing access to services. In our view, an explicitly formulated priority-setting mechanism and a system for monitoring priority-setting practice, despite their limitations and

TABLE 16.1. *Priority-Setting System Requirements (based on Daniels & Sabin, 2002) and the Norwegian Basis for Priority Setting as we view it*

Priority-Setting System Requirements	Norwegian Basis
• The basis for priority-setting decisions must be public (*"publicity condition"*).	Norwegian Official Reports (1987 and 1997). Patient- and User's Rights Act legislative history and the Recommendation of the Social Committee on the Patient- and User's Rights Act (8).
• The basis (evidence, principles) must be considered relevant to the priority-setting decisions (*"relevance condition"*) by people who possess a sense of justice (*"fair-minded people"*)	
• There must be mechanisms in place for reevaluating decisions and for reviewing them in the light of new evidence and arguments ("appeals condition")	Second opinion according to law
• There must be a voluntary or public regulator of decision-making processes to ensure that conditions 1 to 3 are met ("enforcement condition")	National guidelines (Norwegian Directorate of Health)

weaknesses, are preferable to clinical decision-making processes in which priorities are made on the basis of inexplicit criteria, medical specialty interests, and individual professional preferences.

We also argue that the Norwegian normative grounds for priority setting and the principles on which they are based go a long way toward satisfying the requirements of an open, fair, and good priority-setting system posited by Norman Daniels and James Sabin (2002) (TABLE 16.1).

The Norwegian System for Priority Setting: The Clinical Perspective

The main criteria given in Norwegian law—impaired prognosis (i.e., disease severity), effect of intervention, and cost effectiveness—should be at the core of good clinical practice. Knowledge about the potential loss of a health care benefit if treatment is not given must be fundamental in all clinical decision making. Similarly, the effect-of-treatment criterion points directly to a clinical practice based on sound scientific evidence and the principle of evidence-based medicine.

A problematic criterion is the cost-effectiveness or cost utility principle. This criterion is difficult to understand and accept for many health care professionals and patients, policymakers, and the public at large, particularly because many feel that health care should be given irrespective of cost. Similarly, the concepts of cost effectiveness and cost utility do not have the same evidence base as that of treatment benefits, are more difficult to understand for the practicing clinician, and are perceived by the public, politicians, and clinicians to be a theoretical exercise.

There are, in principle, two main reasons for seeking health care: patients with symptoms or signs who are referred to hospitals for establishing a specific diagnosis and subsequently receiving treatment, and patients with a need for treatment of a specific illness. Categorization of referred patients into priority groups on the basis of symptoms and/or signs may represent a challenge, particularly in terms of how to define "commencement of treatment" and thus determining that waiting time has ended. The national guidelines (National Guidelines for Priority Setting in Specialist Health Care, 2011) have discussed this issue extensively.

Despite obvious challenges in practicing the Regulations on Priority Setting, it is our opinion that the system nonetheless works. Normal clinical judgment suggests that electively hospitalized patients are more severely ill than patients receiving day care, and that these patients are in turn more severely ill than patients who are undergoing outpatient clinic evaluation and care. *Figure 16.4* shows that the actual clinical priority setting practiced in hospitals reflects this situation.

The Norwegian System for Priority Setting: The Administrative Perspective

In our experience, systematic priority setting in hospitals requires a hospital administration or management team with the interest, insight, and will to use the regulations and its criteria actively. We also find that one must adhere to and place importance on priority setting over time, including in processes where priority setting in clinical enterprises is not traditionally emphasized such as in budgeting and activity management.

Traditionally, hospital budgets have been structured on the basis of historical precedent. Projections have rarely resulted in large redistributions. New measures have often been given priority, particularly if they have been put forward by prominent specialists. But otherwise the expectation has been that new measures should be implemented with the use of additional resources. For many years the Haukeland University Hospital Health Trust has worked on medical priority setting as a tool for adapting to the given financial framework. Within an overall framework it ought to be that needs are budgeted according to medical importance, and all patients with the same prognosis should have the same access to resources. This would mean that all patients with a need for specialist health care services (from cancer to drug dependence) would be included in an evaluation.

Consequently, the concept of prognosis gains considerable significance. A simple and practical understanding of the concept of prognosis is that a prognosis takes into account severity and effect of treatment. Prognosis cannot be disconnected from effect of treatment if it is to serve as a useful tool for allocating resources.

In this context, the Regulations on Priority Setting have been widely used. All referred elective patients are evaluated and assigned a priority. One can then produce departmental profiles (*Figure 16.3*). These are ascribed considerable weight when allocating resources as part of the budgetary process. Other factors that are used include productivity indicators (such as wage expense per DRG points and total cost per bed day), teaching load, night/day/outpatient clinic relationships, proportion of emergency admissions, proportion of outpatient surgery in total surgery, and so on. During the past 3 years, priority setting based on prognosis has increasingly been assigned the most weight.

There is no doubt that these principles have considerably eased the budgetary process. The use of professional priority setting as a common fundamental principle in the institution has gained considerable and growing support from the specialist communities, which are more willing to look at the use of resources outside their respective areas of specialization.

■ LIMITATIONS, PROBLEMS, AND VARIATION

While public debate shows that the specialist communities understand and accept priority setting as an integrated and necessary part of medical practice, many clinicians perceive the Regulations on Priority Setting and the political attention to waiting times and breaches of time limits as bureaucratic rules that hold little relevance for clinical activities. In our opinion, this dualistic view—acceptance of the necessity for priority setting on the one hand and skepticism about open and transparent criteria for priority setting on the other—does not safeguard the rights and interests of patients and leaves room for random variation and inequality in patient care.

One particular problem is that other legal considerations may also influence priority setting; in this case, which patients and how many patients are accorded the right to necessary health care. This became evident in connection with the preparatory work on the national guidelines; for example, the UN Convention on the Rights of the Child had a bearing on the medical criteria for ascribing the right to necessary health care within the specialty of Child and Adolescent Psychiatry. For those who must adhere to and practice the Regulations on Priority Setting with emphasis on its main criteria, such "external" considerations could lead to impaired professional legitimacy of the priority-setting system.

There are also unexplained differences between the regional health authorities, and even within a region where one would expect the patient populations to be relatively homogeneous (TABLE 16.2). In addition, there are different profiles for different medical specialties. There may be different interpretations of such variations. Standardization and reduction of practice variation are declared goals, and as a consequence reduced variation will be expected. So far, large geographical variations within identical medical specialties

TABLE 16.2. *Variation in Priority given to Patients Referred to Planned Hospital Care during the First Third of 2010*

	Variation in percentage of patients with high priority—mean and range given
SOMATIC HEALTH CARE	
Norwegian regions (4 health authorities)	60 (47–77)
Within Western Norway Health Authority	65 (54–75)
Between medical specialties (selected)	39 (18–76)
• General surgery	75 (65–81)
• Orthopedics	58 (36–89)
• Gastroenterology (medical)	88 (69–95)
• Urology	80 (72–87)
• Pediatrics	
PSYCHIATRY—ADULTS (> 18 YRS)	
Norwegian regions (4 health authorities)	87 (66–91)
Within Western Norway Health Authority	78 (61–87)
CHILD PSYCHIATRY	
Norwegian regions (4 health authorities)	73 (70–91)
Within Western Norway Health Authority	92 (86–98)

Data obtained from national statistics (Ventetider og pasientrettigheter, 2010) and administrative data from Western Norway Regional Health Authority.

remain, which may be interpreted as a failure to achieve the goal of equity at the national level. But over time, there appears to be regression toward a common mean, probably due to the standardization efforts.

In addition to and in spite of the national guidelines, there is ample room for variation in practice. The recommendations in the guidelines are based on knowledge of patient group levels, allowing opportunities for individual judgment. Such individuality is stressed in the legal framework, allowing for adjustments from patients and physicians. Professional judgments are, of course, also influenced by more subjective criteria and, as is known, the status of medical specialties vary (Norredam & Album, 2007; Album & Westin, 2008).

Variation between specialties is, however, to be expected, and it is difficult to judge which rate is right in each case. Furthermore, the national guidelines were drawn up separately by the different medical specialties. No attempt was made to standardize the judgment of priorities for patients belonging to different specialties.

In measuring the distribution of priorities by relative portions as in TABLE 16.2, the question of systematic differences in the denominator is disregarded. The point is that the threshold for treatment or "inclusion criteria" may differ by region. As a consequence there may be case-mix differences even at the regional level. In addition, there are other ways of adjusting the practice, as was found by comparing two university hospitals: the situation at a hospital with the higher proportion of priority patients was adjusted by allocating them much longer waiting times.

Such data raise the question of which level is the right one; in other words, what is the Norwegian "standard"? We would argue that it is impossible to define which level is the right one—the "right" proportion of patients entitled to necessary health care. But in reality, with a health care system that in principle is available to everyone and where differences in degree of sickness in the Norwegian population is not that great, there ought to be less variation. Large and inexplicable differences threaten the principle of equality in the Norwegian health care system and consequently challenges national policy.

The "right" practice of the Regulations on Priority Setting could lead to marginalization of low-priority patients; among other consequences, estimated severity and potential life prolongation through treatment would be accorded greater weight than quality of life, ability to function, and the subjective perception that needs are being met. If we end up in a situation where it is predominantly the patients with the right to necessary health care who are offered treatment, this would clearly run counter to any expectations and legitimate demands that patients and society—represented here by the media, politics and the professions—may have. And if all patients who are referred are given the status of patients entitled to necessary health care, the Regulations on Priority Setting will lose its effect.

■ FINAL COMMENTS

We suggest that the mechanism for priority setting outlined here is an effective tool in clinical practice and in the management of hospitals. We feel that we have moved from a situation where priority setting in planned treatment was nontransparent and varied considerably between medical specialties—even for the sickest patients, as illustrated in the left-hand panel of *Figure 16.5*—to a situation where priority setting is better harmonized across specialties for patients with high priority (i.e., need for necessary health care; right-hand panel in *Figure 16.5*).

In a situation with priority-setting mechanisms based on national law and a fixed health budget, we may anticipate that the question of defining groups that should be denied access to publicly financed specialized care will be raised (illustrated by the broken circle in the right-hand panel of *Figure 16.5*). This is a contentious issue. A pragmatic solution to the problem is probably not to deny access but to increase the waiting times for those falling into the low-priority group.

We also have to admit that the public and political legitimacy of the law and regulations is weak. A parliamentary debate and a public discussion in the media in the spring and summer of 2010 illustrate this. Leading spokespersons from most of the political parties essentially demonstrated that all parties have health care areas or disease groups they prioritize without being

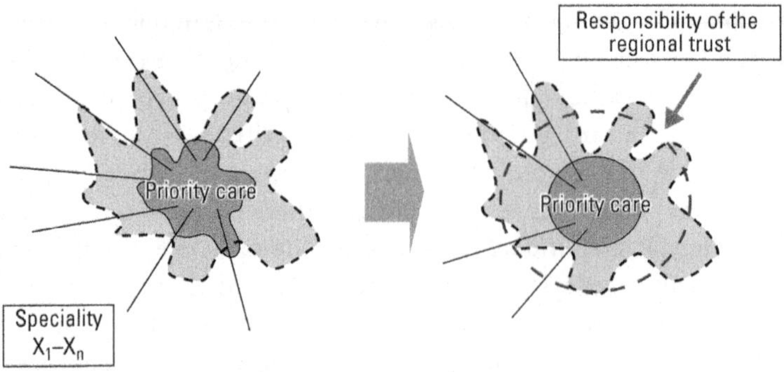

Figure 16.5 A schematic description of priority setting before and after the Regulations on Priority Setting came into force.

specific about the inherent consequences of such statements. No reference was made to the relationship or contrast between public political rhetoric and national legislation on priority setting determined by political decisions. The political dimension of priority setting in health care is further demonstrated by the appointment of a new national commission which, for the third time in 25 years, will formulate a Norwegian Official Report on priority setting in Norwegian health care.

Notes

1. Information given in this part is taken from "Health Systems in Transition: Norway" published by European Observatory on Health Systems and Policies, 2006 (Johnsen, 2006). Reproduced with permission granted from the World Health Organization (October 24, 2011).

2. Unofficial translations of law and regulation are shown in italics.

3. Amended by Regulations of 7 July 2004 no. 1121 (entered into force 1 September 2004), 27 June 2008 no. 740, and 25 July 2008 no. 833.

REFERENCES

Album, D., & Westin, S. (2008). Do diseases have a prestige hierarchy? *Social Science & Medicine, 66*(1),182–188.

Daniels, N., & Sabin, J. E. (2002). *Setting Limits Fairly: Can we learn to share medical resources?* Oxford: Oxford University Press.

FOR 2000-12-01 nr 1208: *Forskrift om prioritering av helsetjenester, rett til helsehjelp fra spesialisthelsetjenesten, rett til behandling utlandet og om klagenemnd (prioriteringsfor-skriften).* Regulation on priorities of healthcare services, the right to health care from specialist health services, the right to healthcare abroad and about the appeals board (priority regulations) (Available at: http://www.lovdata.no/cgi-wift/ldles?doc=/sf/sf/sf-20001201-1208.html.

Innst. O. nr. 91. *Innstilling fra sosialkomiteen om lov om pasientrettigheter (pasientrettighet-sloven)*. Ot. prp. nr. 12 (1998-99). Proposal from the social committee on "Act relating to patients' rights [Patient- and User's' Rights Act].

Johnsen, J. R. (2006). *Health Systems in Transition: Norway*. Copenhagen: World Health Organization Regional Office for Europe on behalf of the European Observatory on Health Systems and Policies. Available at: (http://www.euro.who.int/__data/assets/pdf_file/0005/95144/E88821.pdf.

Kjønstad, A. The right to specialized healthcare. In Molven, O., & Ferkis, J., eds. *Healthcare, Welfare and Law. Health legislation as a mirror of the Norwegian welfare state*. pp. 71–92. Oslo: Gyldendal Akademisk.

Lov 1999-07-02 nr 63: *Lov om pasient- og brukerrettigheter (pasient- og brukerrettighet-sloven)*. Available at: (http://www.lovdata.no/all/hl-19990702-063eng.pdf. Also available in English on http://www.ub.uio.no/cgi-bin/ujur/ulov/sok.cgi?type=LOV; Patients' and Users' Rights Act. Act of 02.07.1999.

McGlynn, E. A., Asch, S. M., Adams, J., Keesey, J., Hicks, J., DeChristofaro, A., & Kerr, E. A. (2003). The quality of health care delivered to adults in the United States. New England Journal of Medicine, 348(26), 2635–2645.

Molven, O., & Ferkis, J., eds. (2011). *Healthcare, Welfare and Law. Health legislation as a mirror of the Norwegian welfare state*. Oslo: Gyldendal Akademisk.

National Guidelines for Priority Setting in Specialist Health Care (in Norwegian) http://www.helsedirektoratet.no/vp/multimedia/archive/00043/Generell_veileder-_P_43849a.pdf (generell del; 27.04.2011) og http://www.helsebiblioteket.no/Retningslinjer/Prioriteringsveiledere (for medisinske fagområder; 27.04.2011).

Norges Offentlige Utredninger. *Retningslinjer for prioriteringer innen norsk helsetjen-este*. NOU 1987:23 [Norwegian Official Report. Guidelines for priority setting in Norwegian health care].

Norges Offentlige Utredninger. *Prioritering på ny. Gjennomgang av retningslinjer for prior-iteringer innen norsk helsetjeneste*. NOU 1997:18. [Norwegian Official Report].

Norredam, M., & Album, D. (2007). Prestige and its significance for medical specialities and diseases. *Scandinavian Journal of Public Health, 35*(6), 655–661.

OECD [Organisation for Economic Co-operation and Development]. Health data 2010. How does Norway compare. Available at: http://www.oecd.org/dataoecd/43/23/40905066.pdf.

Ot.prp. nr. 12 (1998-99) Lov om pasientrettigheter (pasientrettighetsloven). Available at: http://www.regjeringen.no/nb/dep/hod/dok/regpubl/otprp/19981999/otprp-nr-12-1998-99-.html?id=159415.

Ventetider og pasientrettigheter 2010. Norsk Pasientregister Rapport IS-1895. Oslo Norwegian Directorate of Health 2011.

17 Rationing by Clinical Judgment

■ SAMIA A. HURST AND MARION DANIS

Increasing pressure to control costs is leading to a greater awareness of resource scarcity in health care. At the same time, there is considerable controversy regarding the acceptability of bedside rationing by physicians (Hiatt, 1975; Loewy, 1980; Levinsky, 1983; Morreim, 1991; Sulmasy, 1992; Pellegrino, 1994; Ubel, 2001). The obligation to advocate for patients (Hiatt, 1975; Loewy, 1980; Levinsky, 1983; Sulmasy, 1992; Pellegrino, 1997; Weinstein, 2001; Askin, 2002) and a lack of trust that physicians will make the right kind of rationing decisions (Veatch, 1997) have prompted reservations about physician involvement in health care rationing. However, physician involvement has also been defended on the grounds that physicians are entrusted with the stewardship of scarce resources (Morreim, 1991), could make cost control compatible with patient advocacy (Pearson, 2000; Hardee et al., 2005), and indeed may be in the best position to ration care in an appropriate and justifiable manner (Daniels, 1981; Pearson, 2000; Ubel, 2001).

Debates regarding whether or not rationing of health care is acceptable rarely truly dispute setting *some* limits on care. Usually some threshold, such as the current standard of care, or patients' wishes, is taken for granted, and discussion focuses on whether or not setting a more restrictive threshold would be justifiable. Rationing, defined as "any implicit or explicit mechanisms that allow people to go without beneficial services"(Ubel, 2001), must take place because the use of every single intervention that holds the smallest possibility of minute benefit seems financially untenable. Any clinical decision to place or accept a limit on benefits for a patient constitutes rationing. Examples include such mundane decisions as early discharge to follow-up when there is a very small remaining risk of complication, such as postoperative deep venous thrombosis under appropriate prophylaxis. As this example shows, some instances of clinical rationing are routinely accepted and would be difficult to describe as immoral. While some may criticize forgoing benefits in the abstract, few dispute that forgoing very marginal benefits may be reasonable.

Involvement of physicians in these decisions is and will remain a part of clinical practice. Physicians make decisions regarding whether or not a small benefit is worthwhile. They face requests for expensive interventions with little prospect of benefit to their patients (Hurst et al., 2005). Thus, physicians contribute to setting the threshold above which an intervention is "unreasonable." Such limit setting is a "mechanism that allows people to go without beneficial services" (Ubel, 2001). Furthermore, clinical judgment ought to contribute to these decisions: there will always be a degree of indeterminacy involved here that cannot, and perhaps should not, be addressed beforehand by rules.

The question, then, is not whether physician bedside rationing is ever acceptable, but which thresholds and which processes are acceptable. The way in which bedside rationing is applied is the key question when considering its acceptability. Despite some study of public and physicians' attitudes towards theoretical rationing situations, however (Ubel, DeKay, et al., 1996; Ubel, Loewenstien, et al., 1996; Ubel et al., 2000), little has been said about how bedside rationing ought to be practiced. Clinicians make rationing decisions (Hurst et al., 2006) but cannot currently refer to a generally applicable rule or to a widely accepted social understanding. The difficulty of such a controversial topic may play a part in this, but the very danger that bedside rationing could be done in an unacceptable way makes its examination all the more important. Explicit public understanding is needed to lend legitimacy to rationing decisions.

Our purpose in this paper is twofold. First, we wish to describe the kinds of activities that constitute bedside rationing. We also propose a framework and reasoning strategy to begin refining the processes of bedside rationing. Both aim to further the debate regarding the most justifiable way to practice bedside rationing.

▪ TYPES OF RATIONING BY CLINICAL JUDGMENT

Setting limits at the bedside can occur in a variety of ways. As Truog and colleagues have outlined, (Truog et al., 2005) clinicians ration generally by three mechanisms: in accord with external constraints, by rules of medical practice, or by exercising clinical judgment where the first two mechanisms do not apply. In this paper we examine the third of these mechanisms.

Rationing by clinical judgment itself also comes in three forms. First, it can occur as an instance of triage, where locally available resources are in obvious and immediate short supply and must be allocated between identified patients who are in competition with each other. Examples are decisions regarding the last available ICU bed, or organ transplantation (TABLE 17.1).

Second, rationing by clinical judgment can occur in a situation where resources are strained or subject to fixed limits. While there is no immediate competition between identified patients, candidates for an intervention are nevertheless compared to other patients who may potentially need the same resource: residents of a community served by a hospital, or population covered by a health plan (TABLE 17.2; Lee, 2004).

Third, rationing by clinical judgment can be based on an opinion that using a specific intervention in a specific case will bring an incremental gain in benefit that is not worth the additional human or financial effort that this intervention will cost. Here, the clinician judges that the contemplated intervention, as reported in the literature for a population of like patients, shows a benefit, but that this benefit is, in the light of the expected cost, too small to put the intervention over a certain threshold that is deemed reasonable (TABLE 17.3). This is different from rationing by rules of clinical practice, because it involves an individual case assessment, in contrast to a general cost-effectiveness analysis (CEA) on a population. For example, a clinician could judge that although a single drug was shown to be effective in his patient's condition, the incremental cost effectiveness of adding this drug to the many others already prescribed is low (Tinetti et al., 2004).

In these three circumstances, the clinician is situating the patient at hand in the context of increasingly wider circles of competing patients and deciding about the use of constrained resource pools with regard to these populations (*Figure 17.1*).

Importantly, many difficult end-of-life choices regarding when to initiate or continue "cure-oriented" treatments are not rationing decisions in this sense.

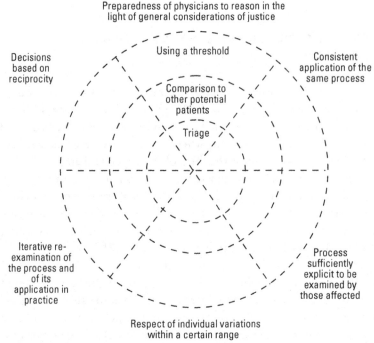

Figure 17.1 A framework for rationing by clinical judgment.

Clinical judgment that an intervention will cause the patient more harm than good is a different consideration. However, when an intervention contemplated in end-of-life care is indeed expected to bring more good than harm, but too little good to be indicated or reasonable, then forgoing it constitutes rationing by clinical judgment under this framework.

■ CONDITIONS FOR FAIRNESS AND LEGITIMACY IN RATIONING BY CLINICAL JUDGMENT

One of the fears regarding rationing by clinical judgment is that it may be susceptible to subjectivity and bias. It has been noted that concerns about justice infrequently come into physicians rationales for decision in the facing scarcity (Hurst et al., 2005). This is concerning, as it does suggest that links between general concerns for fairness and the clinical practice of bedside rationing may be weak.

Models have been proposed to increase consistency, openness, and participation by those affected in limit-setting decisions (Daniels et al., 1997; Pearson, 2000). Outlining an approach that respects general conditions for fairness in rationing by clinical judgment faces several difficulties. First, it must be consistent, and attentive to justice. In addition, it must be sensitive to relevant individual variations. These first two conditions can conflict with one another. In addition, any consistently applied framework must be revisable in the light of new theoretical and practical insights (Daniels et al., 1997), some of which will arise in the application of the process itself. All these features will be necessary for it to be a trustworthy process, able to lend moral legitimacy to rationing decisions by individual clinicians. The final difficulty is that a framework for rationing by clinical judgment must in practice be applicable in the three different kinds of cases outlined above, each of which poses certain specific difficulties.

■ ELEMENTS OF A FRAMEWORK FOR RATIONING BY CLINICAL JUDGMENT

A general framework must recognize that a legitimate diversity of values will be at play in rationing by clinical judgment. In this sense, Daniel and Sabin's *Accountability for Reasonableness* is convincing and influential (Daniels et al., 1997). However, applying it to rationing by clinical judgment is not straightforward. First, the substantial content of a reasonable rationale is too vague for use in clinical practice. Additionally, the reasoning strategy that could be used to apply it in this setting is unspecified. Based on Daniels and Sabin's four conditions of publicity, relevance, revisions and appeals, and enforcement, a justifiable model seems to us to require the consistent presence of six minimal elements (*Figure 17.1*).

Physician Reasoning Based on General Considerations of Justice

Physicians should be prepared to reason about rationing in the light of general considerations of justice. It is essential that clinicians appreciate the concept and importance of fairness and apply considerations of justice to rationing decisions. This requires them to be aware of the various traditional theories of justice. They should understand the basic elements of utilitarian, egalitarian, and prioritarian theories, and be aware that different theories of justice will lead to different outcomes. The requirement that physicians become knowledgeable regarding theories of justice may seem demanding. However, it is no more so than for other conceptual tools that medical practice now requires, such as the use of decision analysis in diagnostic approaches, or evidence-based medicine. Furthermore, physicians are already expected to have some understanding of medical ethics in general. They are quite familiar with issues of patient autonomy, beneficence and nonmaleficence. They are also taught some nonprinciplist approaches to bioethics such as virtue ethics and casuistry. However theories of justice are insufficiently taught. As it is necessary to address the competing duties to different patients in an evenhanded way, an important clinical outcome, this educational requirement appears justified.

Respect for Individual Variations

Respect for individual variations within a certain range can be in tension with general considerations of justice, as it seems to contradict the demand for consistency. On the other hand, the degree of indeterminacy involved in these situations seems to require this flexibility. In addition, it seems that the assurance that individual circumstances have been taken into account would be important to most of us in accepting limit-setting decisions if we were affected. Indeed, much of the value of physician involvement in rationing lies in their ability to do just this: to balance respect for individual variation and consistency. No other locus seems better for achieving this balance.

Decisions Based on Reciprocity

Rationing by clinical judgment should only take place where reciprocity prevails. The process thereby becomes defensible to all affected by being applicable not merely to the patient who forgoes a potential benefit for the sake of others, but also, and similarly, to others for the benefit of this patient. Reciprocal sacrifice is a basic benchmark if we are to justify sacrifices made for the benefit of others. It is a justified requirement because health care resources are shared resources, making them a common good to which rules of cooperative fairness will need to apply (Rawls, 2001). This requires that the decision take place in a closed system in which it would be possible for the patient to benefit from a reciprocally offered sacrifice.

Consistent Application of the Same Process

The same process should be applied in every case to introduce a minimal procedural equity into rationing by clinical judgment (Daniels et al., 1997). This is also necessary if the process is to be justified by reciprocity. Consistency is a limiting condition for the application of a process that could otherwise be applied in several different ways.

Explicit Process

The process should be sufficiently explicit to be examined by patients, physicians, and those who fund care (Daniels et al., 1997). In other words, the process must be outlined in a way that is understandable and accessible for examination by all those affected.

Iterative Reexamination of the Process and Its Application

There should be an iterative reexamination of the process, so that new theoretical and practical insights can be included as they are brought to light (Daniels et al., 1997). There should also be an iterative reexamination of practices, so that they can (1) be evaluated for application of the process and (2) be a source of insight for new input into the process.

■ APPLYING THIS FRAMEWORK

A framework for rationing by clinical judgment must be applicable in practice. For this purpose knowledge is important (Rest et al., 1994; Eastman et al., 2001), but insufficient. Bringing considerations of justice, respect for variation, reciprocity, consistency, explicitness, and revisability to bear on actual decisions requires the use of specific reasoning strategies, akin to a reasoning strategy for ethical thoughtfulness. This is similar to other reasoning strategies learned by physicians, such as decision analysis or evidence-based medicine

(EBM). Difficulties identified in getting physicians to use the reasoning strategies of EBM in clinical decision making include a persistent gap between theory and practice (Slawson et al., 2005). A similar gap exists between theory and practice in resource allocation (Hurst et al., 2005). Thus, we outline proposals for the application of the elements outlined above to rationing by clinical judgment.

The application of general considerations of justice raises several questions. Must all clinicians, or at least any given physician, always apply the same theory? One might argue that consistency in applying theory will lead to greater fairness. Physicians might consider which patients would benefit the most from resource use or who would face the least risk from having a resource withheld, using utilitarian logic. They might give priority to the patient who is the worst off. They might take an egalitarian approach and attempt to limit care on as even handed strategy as possible.

However, there will not necessarily be a uniquely applicable or justifiable theory of justice for every case. Indeed, the existence of these different views of distributive justice, all of which can be defended to some degree by reasonable people, makes this unlikely. The essential guide here should be that application of theories of fairness by individual clinicians should function in such a way as to reduce arbitrariness. Always applying the same theory might be one way, but individual patients treated by different clinicians may still be treated very differently. Alternatively, clinicians might agree that they will vary the theory they each apply according to the situation, but do this in a predetermined and consistent manner. One approach could be to always take all these views into account. The likely benefit from resource use, the degree of risk faced from having a resource withheld, and how badly off different patients are, will each vary from case to case. This means that, in some cases at least, the degree of unfairness linked to setting aside one kind of consideration of justice will vary, and some theoretical approaches will thus weigh more heavily than others in a given case. For example, one could be considering the two following patients in a triage situation: one stands to gain slightly more from the intervention, but the second is much worst off. In this case, setting aside the prioritarian consideration to favor the worst off would result in a much higher degree of injustice on this view, than giving up a slightly higher overall benefit would constitute on the utilitarian view. Thus, priority should be given to the worst off patient in this case. For this to be a consistent process, it is necessary to be prepared to reach the opposite conclusion in opposite circumstances, namely, if one patient was only slightly worst off, but the other stood to benefit much more. This is different from proportional satisfaction of moral reasons (Broome, 1991), because these are situations where the resource cannot be meaningfully split. It is also different from choosing the best consequences, which would lead to the opposite conclusion in our example. What this amounts to is choosing the smallest available wrong.

This also illustrates one of the ways in which the requirement for consistency will constrain the process. It will limit how reasoning in terms of justice can be applied to real cases. For example, it could dictate that the same theory of justice should be applied to all situations or that the strategy of weighing different theories of justice should be applied to all situations. In addition, there is a degree of tension between consistent application of the same process and respect for individual variations. Consistency will also dictate that the same kinds of individual characteristics of patients, such as preference, likelihood of benefit, degree of need, be considered in all circumstances.

In applying reciprocity, it should be understood that any organizational entity may support reciprocally offered sacrifices. In the United States, this could mean that any insured patient could be considered as part of one pool where reciprocal sacrifices will be accepted. On the face of it, a universal health care system appears to be a better environment for reciprocal rationing. However, it is not a necessary condition. A set of patients could be reciprocally sharing health care resources even in its absence. It could mean that all beneficiaries of hospital services in a given area form such a group. Applying rationing to them could take place in a closed system and be fair. This sort of system, however, could not be viewed as closed as regarded any person not within this circle. Rationing from someone who was not covered would thus not take place within a closed system; although it could sometimes be described as necessary, on our framework it would not be fair. Importantly, a universal health care system is not a sufficient condition for reciprocal rationing either. It only represents a more favorable set of initial circumstances. It does not, for example, preclude systematic discrimination against a specific group by a majority of health care providers.

Explicitness would require that physicians document these decisions, at least retrospectively. For example, intensive care units must regularly refuse patients who do not meet their criteria for inclusion, or who are in competition with other patients whose needs are, for example, greater. Some ICUs keep logs of refused referrals with documentation of the reasons. This can serve as a basis for review and critique later on. Such a system could be applied by surgical services to delays for elective procedures, or by hospital pharmacies for nonformulary requests. Decisions for rationing by clinical judgment could also be documented in patients' charts.

Clearly, all decisions could not be documented in this way all the time. If we wish to open these decisions to examination, however, we must start somewhere. Additionally, even if only some interventions are logged in such a way, or consigned to patients' charts, physicians will become better accustomed to thinking and justifying their decision in those terms in applying this process, and will be better able to compare their decisions with those of others. This is likely to improve rationing practice even in non monitored interventions. Documentation and examination would constitute a kind of quality control for the process. One could also, as a quality improvement effort, select certain routine decisions for review, such as hospital or ICU admission, or dialysis. The process should also be publicly available in some form, and thus accessible to critique by those affected.

Iterative reexamination could be done as a self-evaluation by a group of physicians of their rationing practices, with a result disclosed to individual physicians only along with a comparison to the typical practices of colleagues in similar situations. It should be explicit that this typical practice is not a norm in the moral sense. It may very well be that physicians could legitimately depart from typical practices. This evaluation should not serve to enforce a return to the mean, but to foster regular thoughtful reevaluation of rationing practices.

Like other reasoning strategies, such as those incorporated in evidence-based medicine, this framework could serve as a checklist for intuitive conclusions, or used to move forward in difficult situations. This would require that physicians take pause and at least briefly question each point when making rationing decisions. It could also serve to guide physicians' general reflections on how to ration by clinical judgment. Time could be set aside every now and then to share experience, as it is for other difficult decision-making skills such as diagnosis. Indeed, if rationing by clinical judgment is part of physicians' role such time should be set aside. This practice should be examined in the same kind of circumstances as other interventions are: continuing education time should be allocated to it.

■ SPECIFIC DIFFICULTIES FOR DIFFERENT TYPES OF RATIONING BY CLINICAL JUDGMENT

Unique issues will arise during rationing by triage, comparison to other potential patients, and using a threshold.

Triage of Identified Patients

During circumstances when triage is necessary the notion of reciprocity is not straight forward. When immediate demand exceeds fixed resources the circumstances do not permit immediate reciprocity and may not permit reciprocity in the future particularly in life-threatening circumstances. Thus the demand for reciprocity cannot dictate that reciprocity should be literally feasible at the given moment a rationing decision must be made. It would not be possible to adequately give in return at the moment that a critically ill patient must forgo some share of a potentially beneficial intervention such as a doctor or nurses' time. It should however be the case that if the patient who is about to forgo this resource were in the opposite situation, in the situation of the patient who will benefit from the sacrifice, the clinician would, upon reflection, be willing to parse out the necessary resource to her.

In such cases, reasoning based on general considerations of justice must take place in very limited time. This may imply using a simplified algorithm in certain cases. While this is clearly a less than optimal way to use general considerations of justice, any improvement in the systematic application of such considerations to triage is certainly desirable (Repine et al., 2005).

Comparison to Other Potential Patients

In situations where rationing by clinical judgment occurs by comparison to other potential patients who could benefit from the resources involved, the urgency of the rationing decision is not as obvious. The competition for resources is not as frenzied, which makes the notion of reciprocity more imaginable. Again, the clinicians should consider whether it is the case that if the patient who is about to forgo this resource were in the opposite situation, in the situation of the others who will benefit from the sacrifice, the clinician would, upon reflection, be willing to parse out the necessary resource to her.

An added feature of this level is the risk that the "potential patients" used in this hypothetical comparison could be defined very differently. Consistent application of the same process would seem to require that the type of patient physicians use in these comparisons be explicitly examined. It is not realistic to expect these hypothetical patients to be identical for all physicians. However, they should not be allowed to vary on points that could lead to discrimination. One simple example is that, were physicians to systematically compare their patients to people who were the same age as themselves, marginal benefits would be more likely to be denied to patients by those physicians not in their age range. They should also avoid comparison on the basis of characteristics considered morally non relevant (race or gender, for example).

Using a Threshold

In this circumstance, clinicians may judge that using a specific intervention in a specific case will bring an incremental gain in benefit that is not worth the additional human or financial effort that this intervention will cost. While the reasoning that the clinician will use under these circumstances uses the logic of cost effectiveness, the available literature does not suffice to answer the question of whether or not to intervene because the patient does not exactly match the patient population reported in the CEA literature.

The difficulty here is to maintain respect for individual variation when making a decision using analysis based on population data. An added difficulty is that there are in practice two thresholds. The first is the amount of expected benefit required to consider that an intervention is indicated, the second is the cost-effectiveness ratio required to judge that implementing an intervention is "reasonable." Each threshold can be examined at the level of rule setting, or at the level of clinical judgment. The specificity of the threshold problem at the level of clinical judgment is that the tension between data gathered from groups and the care of individual patients is more palpable at this level (Saarni et al., 2004).

Clinical Judgment of Expected Benefit

Clearly, the benefit expected of a specific intervention will contribute to determining whether or not it is indicated. Thus, it is important to know what prospective benefit can be expected for this particular patient. Comparisons must be made between the individual patient and the study group. This is a standard necessity, and a standard difficulty, in the application of evidence-based medicine (Slawson et al., 2005).

The result of this is an assessment of the amount of benefit expected from an intervention. Knowing if this benefit is sufficient for the intervention to be indicated will further require that there be an agreement on the level of expected benefit sufficient to warrant treatment. This is a value judgment that will vary individually. When costs are not considered, the main stakeholder is clearly the patient. The setting of clinical discussion can thus be legitimate and sufficient to set this first threshold on a case by case basis.

Clinical Judgment Regarding Expected Cost Effectiveness for a Patient

In making a clinical judgment regarding cost effectiveness and the reasonableness of paying for an intervention, a layer of complexity is added. The first question here is the prospective cost effectiveness level in this particular case. Here too, the best available evidence must be examined in the light of relevant patient characteristics. This is more complex than examining the question of benefit, because there are several parts to a cost-effectiveness ratio: the prospective benefit in terms of years of life gained, the prospective benefit in terms of quality of life, and the cost of the intervention. The standard unit of CEA is the cost per quality adjusted life year (QALY). The QALY is the number of years gained on average through the intervention, multiplied by the assessed value for the quality of life of the patient (V). This is a number between 0 and

1 where 0 is death, 1 is perfect health, and anything in between is life in less than perfect health.

The number of years gained from an intervention is based on data gathered from a study population. Thus, it is important to assess whether this patient differs from the study group. This is similar to the kind of clinical judgment required when applying any evidence based practice guideline to individuals who do not quite fit the study populations. Here, the legitimacy of considering individual cases in the light of clinical judgment is relatively straightforward.

The assessed cost of the intervention or of the alternative it is being compared to can also differ from the costs in the study group. As with the evaluation of differences between an individual patient and a study population on the question of a prospective health benefit, cost may not apply precisely to details in a particular clinical situation. Thus, there are circumstances where the literature on cost effectiveness suggests that a treatment is not cost effective and yet the cost of the intervention may be less than that indicated in the literature, placing this treatment above the threshold deemed reasonable. The opposite could happen in situations where the cost is greater than in the study population. For example, the indication of many preventive interventions, such as screening, is based on cost-effectiveness ratios. A physician who is deciding whether to schedule colonoscopies or mammographies will be basing her assessment on population-based data. If either the prevalence of the disease or the cost of the intervention in her area differs from that of the study population, the cost-effectiveness ratio may need to be tempered by this information. Currently, however, many cost-effectiveness analyses give clinicians insufficient elements to make this judgment. A clinician will typically be told the age range of the study group, whether they were male, female, or both, some information regarding prevalence of the studied disease, comorbidity and similar information. The same type of general information about costs in the study should also be made available to clinicians if they are to apply CEA with the same kind of thoughtfulness as evidence-based medicine.

The assessed value for the quality of life of the patient, V, could also be different for an individual patient if she differs sufficiently from the kind of patient used in reaching this evaluation. Here, however, a problem arises. In clinical practice it is considered important to leave the assessment of quality of life to the patient herself. In placing the value of V for CEA, however, this assessment is not left to the patient alone. Indeed, there is substantial controversy regarding what the best viewpoint for this assessment would be (Ubel, 1997; Menzel et al., 1999; Nord et al., 1999; Ubel, 1999; Ubel, Baron, et al., 2000; Ubel, Nord, et al., 2000; Ubel et al., 2001, 2003) In adapting the value of V to an individual patient who does not quite fit the study population, the difficulty regarding the best viewpoint from which to assess V is imported into clinical practice. If patient input is legitimate, then the clinical setting is the appropriate locale in which to allow this.

Importantly, then, there are elements of cost-effectiveness assessment that are compatible with respect for individual variations: the number of years gained, and the added cost of the intervention. Using input from clinical judgment in rationing through cost-effectiveness thresholds is thus already possible, and would be important. If a consensus could be reached regarding what constitutes a legitimate input by the individual patient on the assessment of V, this element may be adaptable as well.

Knowing how to adapt cost-effectiveness assessment to individual patients, however, goes only part of the way to deciding whether or not it is "reasonable" to implement an intervention in a specific case. Knowing if this level of cost effectiveness is sufficient for the intervention to be "reasonable" will further require that there be an agreement on the level of cost effectiveness sufficient to for this to be so. This is a value judgment that will vary individually. At this point, however, the patient is no longer the only stakeholder. Whether or not she remains the *main* stakeholder is controversial. If any limit whatsoever is placed on potentially beneficial interventions, even where the chance of benefit is small and remote, then the clinician will be considering the cost born by third parties: all enrollees into whichever program pays in a third party system; enrollees in a plan, or tax-payers in a state system. Considering that *some* threshold will be used, the question is how to legitimately decide where it should be. Whether the clinician's judgment carries legitimate authority that is sufficient to answer this question is contingent on the presence of the six elements we have outlined at the outset of our discussion.

■ CONCLUSION

The framework we have outlined here contains minimal requirements for fair rationing by clinical judgment. It is intended to begin attempts to refine the practice of rationing by clinical judgment. It needs to be judged realistic by other clinicians, as well as theoretically robust. By adopting minimal requisite conditions for rationing by clinical judgment, clinicians could practice bedside rationing more fairly. They would not cease using their personal values, or intuitions, but would be able to complement them and subject them to more systematic examination. They may also be able to advocate more effectively for their patients in situations where pressure could be exerted on them to ration without meeting these requirements. In addition, this framework could serve as the basis for clinical tools for bedside rationing. To the extent that rationing

TABLE 17.1. *Examples of Triage Situations in the ICU*

Limited time	The ICU team goes on rounds for 90 minutes each morning and has 10 beds in the ICU. Inevitably many of the patients require more than 9 minutes of the team's attention to fully evaluate their status, consider the options, and decide on a plan of care and communicate this to the ICU staff. The patients in the first beds often get more time on rounds and the last ones barely get adequate attention. The staff wonders about how to best ration their rounding time. Should they move from bed to bed every nine minutes? Give more time to the patients who are more unstable? Give most time to the patients who are likely to benefit the most from their care? Should they simply reverse the rounding order so they start at the back end of the ICU on alternate mornings?
Limited beds	The ICU team often receives patients admitted from the emergency department during the night. When these patients need ICU care the unit is often full and the question therefore arises as to whether there are any patients who could be transferred out of the ICU earlier than would otherwise occur. The team must review the ICU census and consider who is least likely to suffer adverse consequences if transferred. Should the patient with the poorest prognosis be moved? Or the patient who is most stable? Or the patient who is receiving the least monitoring?
Limited staff	The ICU has 5 nurses staffing each shift. This provides an average of one nurse for every two patients in the 10-bed unit. During one shift a patient in respiratory failure is so difficult to ventilate that the team judges that it is necessary to paralyze the patient and put him on volume control ventilation with a high I:E ratio. This will require that the patient have 1:1 nursing. The charge nurse must decide how to reassign the nurse in the ICU. Three patients will need to be assigned to one nurse to accommodate the nursing care needs of the patient in severe respiratory failure. Should a patient who is terminally ill and getting palliative care be one of them? Should a patient who is an acute asthmatic be one of them?

TABLE 17.2. *Examples of Comparison to Other Potential Patients*

Limited blood supply	A patient is utilizing a great deal of the supply of a particular blood product for treatment of a severe bleeding diathesis; use by this patient is expected to limit the blood supply in a certain region. There is no immediate call for competing use of this blood product, but use of it for this patient could cause a shortage that could pose a potential threat to the remaining population.
Influenza vaccination	A 40-year-old patient in good health consults for influenza vaccination. A vaccine shortage has been announced for this year, and vaccination campaigns for the elderly are still underway. Will the benefit of avoiding absenteeism from work and unpleasant symptoms in this patient warrant risking a lack of vaccine for someone in an age group at risk of mortality from the complications of influenza?

TABLE 17.3. *Examples of Using a Threshold in Rationing by Clinical Judgment*

Assessment of individual benefit	A patient suffers both from hormone-sensitive metastatic breast cancer and from ischemic heart disease. Guidelines for the secondary prevention of coronary heart disease include treatment of hypercholesterolemia with statins. Will the benefit to this patient be sufficient to warrant prescribing a statin in her case?
Assessment of individual cost	A patient presents with uncomplicated myocardial infarction. It has been shown that a length of stay of over 3 days is not cost effective,[1] but inpatient care is much cheaper in this area. How should this result be applied?

[1] Newby, L. K., et al. (2000). Cost effectiveness of early discharge after uncomplicated acute myocardial infarction. *New England Journal of Medicine, 342*(11), 749–755.

is unavoidable, and that making it more explicit and equitable is desirable, such a tool would be valuable. Finally, in including iterative reexamination of the process and its application, this framework could serve as an assessment tool for clinical rationing. This evaluation should help to foster regular moments of thoughtful reevaluation of rationing practices.

▪ ACKNOWLEDGMENTS

This chapter is a republication of the following manuscript: Hurst, S., & Danis, M. (2007). A framework for rationing by clinical judgment. *Kennedy Institute of Ethics Journal, 17,* 247–266.

The authors wish to thank John Rapoport and Robert Truog for reading and commenting on the manuscript.

SAH was funded by the Bioethics Institute at the University of Geneva, by the Centre Lémanique d'Ethique, and by the Swiss National Science Foundation. MD was funded by the Department of Clinical Bioethics at the National Institutes of Health. This work was written on behalf of the VERICC task force, which is funded by an unrestricted educational grant from Eli Lilly. The VERICC task force funded travel for one of the authors to a congress where a preliminary version of this work was presented.

The funding sources were not involved in the study design, the collection, analysis, or interpretation of data, in the writing of the report, or in the decision to submit the paper for publication.

The views expressed here are the authors' own and do not reflect the position of the National Institutes of Health, of the Public Health Service, of the Department of Health and Human Services, of the University of Geneva, of the Centre Lémanique d'Ethique, of the Swiss National Science Foundation, or of Eli Lilly.

REFERENCES

Askin, W. J. (2002). Bedside rationing. *Canadian Medical Association Journal, 166*(6), 711.
Broome, J. (1991). *Weighing Goods.* Oxford: Blackwell Publishers.
Daniels, N. (1981). What is the obligation of the medical profession in the distribution of health care? *Social Science & Medicine, 15F*(4), 129–133.
Daniels, N., & Sabin, J. (1997). Limits to health care: fair procedures, democratic deliberation, and the legitimacy problem for insurers. *Philosophy & Public Affairs, 26*(4), 303–350.
Eastman, J. K., Eastman, K. L., & Tolson, M. A. (2001). The relationship between ethical ideology and ethical behavior intentions: an exploratory look at physicians' responses to managed care dilemmas. *Journal of Business Ethics, 31*(3), 209–224.
Hardee, J. T., Platt, F. W., & Kasper, I. K. (2005). Discussing health care costs with patients. *Journal of General Internal Medicine, 20*(7), 666–669.

Hiatt, H. H. (1975). Protecting the medical commons: who is responsible? *New England Journal of Medicine, 293*(5), 235–241.

Hurst, S., Slowther, A., Forde, R., et al. (2006). Prevalence and determinants of physician bedside rationing in four European countries. *Journal of General Internal Medicine, 21*(11): 1138–1143.

Hurst, S. A., Hull, S. C., DuVal, G., & Danis, M. (2005). Physicians' responses to resource constraints. *Archives of Internal Medicine, 165*(6), 639–644.

Lee, T. H. (2004). Rationing influenza vaccine. *New England Journal of Medicine, 351*(23), 2365–2366.

Levinsky, N. (1983). The doctor's master. *New England Journal of Medicine, 311*(24), 1573–1575.

Loewy, E. H. (1980). Cost should not be a factor in medical care. *New England Journal of Medicine, 302*(12), 697.

Menzel, P., Gold, M. R., Nord, E., Pinto-Prades J. L., Richardson J., & Ubel, P. (1999). Toward a broader view of values in cost-effectiveness analysis of health. *Hastings Center Report, 29*(3), 7–15.

Morreim, E. (1991). *Balancing Act: The New Medical Ethics of Medicine's New Economics.* Dordrecht, Boston, London: Kluwer Academic Publishers.

Nord, E., Pinto, J. L., Richardson, J., Menzel P., & Ubel, P. (1999). Incorporating societal concerns for fairness in numerical valuations of health programmes. *Health Economics, 8*(1), 25–39.

Pearson, S. D. (2000). Caring and cost: the challenge for physician advocacy. *Annals of Internal Medicine, 133*(2), 148–153.

Pellegrino, E. D. (1994). Allocation of resources at the bedside: the intersections of economics, law, and ethics. *Kennedy Institute of Ethics Journal, 4*(4), 309–317.

Pellegrino, E. D. (1997). Managed care at the bedside: how do we look in the moral mirror? *Kennedy Institute of Ethics Journal, 7*(4), 321–330.

Rawls, J. (2001). *Justice as Fairness; A Restatement.* Cambridge, MA: The Belknap Press of Harvard University Press.

Repine, T. B., Lisagor, P., & Cohen, D. J. (2005). The dynamics and ethics of triage: rationing care in hard times. *Military Medicine, 170*(6), 505–509.

Rest, J. R., & Narvaez, D. (1994). *Moral Development in the Professions.* Hillsdale, NJ: Lawrence Erlbaum Associates.

Saarni, S. I., & Gylling, H. A. (2004). Evidence based medicine guidelines: a solution to rationing or politics disguised as science? *Journal of Medical Ethics 30*(2), 171–175.

Slawson, D. C., & Shaughnessy. A. F. (2005). Teaching evidence-based medicine: should we be teaching information management instead? *Academic Medicine, 80*(7), 685–689.

Sulmasy, D. P. (1992). Physicians, cost control, and ethics. *Annals of Internal Medicine, 116*(11), 920–926.

Tinetti, M. E., Bogardus, S. T. Jr., & Agostini, J. V. (2004). Potential pitfalls of disease-specific guidelines for patients with multiple conditions. *New England Journal of Medicine, 351*(27), 2870–2874.

Truog, R. D., Brock, D. W., Cook, D. J., Danis, M., Luce, J. M., Rubenfeld, G. D., et al. (2005). Rationing in the ICU. *Critical Care Medicine, 34*(4): 958–63.

Ubel, P. (2001). *Pricing Life: Why It's Time for Health Care Rationing.* Cambridge, MA: MIT Press.

Ubel, P. A. (1997). The role of community values in setting healthcare priorities. Ethically and financially viable, or merely a "modest proposal?" *MLO: Medical Laboratory Observer, 29*(7), 90, 92–93.

Ubel, P. A. (1999). The challenge of measuring community values in ways appropriate for setting health care priorities. *Kennedy Institute of Ethics Journal, 9*(3), 263–284.

Ubel, P. A., Baron, J., Nash, B., & Asch, D. A. (2000). Are preferences for equity over efficiency in health care allocation "all or nothing"? *Medical Care, 38*(4), 366–373.

Ubel, P. A., DeKay, M. L., Baron J., & Asch D. A. (1996). Cost-effectiveness analysis in a setting of budget constraints—is it equitable? *New England Journal of Medicine, 334*(18), 1174–1177.

Ubel, P. A., Loewenstein, G., Hershey, J., et al. (2001). Do nonpatients underestimate the quality of life associated with chronic health conditions because of a focusing illusion? *Medical Decision Making, 21*(3), 190–199.

Ubel, P. A., Loewenstein, G., & Jepson, C. (2003). Whose quality of life? A commentary exploring discrepancies between health state evaluations of patients and the general public. *Quality of Life Research, 12*(6), 599–607.

Ubel, P. A., Loewenstein, G., Scanlon, D., & Kamlet, M. (1996). Individual utilities are inconsistent with rationing choices: A partial explanation of why Oregon's cost-effectiveness list failed. *Medical Decision Making, 16*(2): 108–116.

Ubel, P. A., Nord, E., Gold, M., Menzel, P., Prades J. L., & Richardson, J. (2000). Improving value measurement in cost-effectiveness analysis. *Medical Care, 38*(9): 892–901.

Ubel, P. A., Richardson, J., & Menzel, P. (2000). Societal value, the person trade-off, and the dilemma of whose values to measure for cost-effectiveness analysis. *Health Economics, 9*(2): 127–136.

Veatch, R. M. (1997). Who should manage care? The case for patients. *Kennedy Institute of Ethics Journal 7*(4), 391–401.

Weinstein, M. C. (2001). Should physicians be gatekeepers of medical resources? *Journal of Medical Ethics 27*(4), 268–274.

18 Fairness and Transparency in Bedside Micro-allocation

Improving the Ethical Competence of Clinical Staff

■ JAN SCHÜRMANN, BARBARA
MEYER-ZEHNDER, MARCEL MERTZ,
HEIDI ALBISSER SCHLEGER,
MATHIAS SCHLÖGL, RETO
W. KRESSIG, HANS PARGGER,
AND STELLA REITER-THEIL

In this chapter we describe an approach that integrates various ways of help-ing clinicians to practice fair and transparent bedside allocation. A key com-ponent of this help is to improve the competence of clinicians in identifying ethical concerns and making ethically appropriate decisions in this challeng-ing area. The approach has been developed from the project, *Modular, Ethical, Treatment decisions, Allocation of resources at the micro-level, Process* (METAP), which began in 2009 with the aim of providing several forms of clinical eth-ics support including consultation (Albisser Schleger et al., 2012; Reiter-Theil et al., 2011a).[1] We first introduce briefly the problem of bedside resource allo-cation decisions and present background information about the METAP clinical ethics support project, its context, settings, and processes. Then we outline a concept of—ethical—competence as a theoretical foundation of the METAP approach. Two cases, one from acute geriatric care and another one from operative intensive care, are presented to illustrate how METAP is work-ing in clinical practice. This is followed by a critical appraisal of the compe-tences shown by the clinicians in the cases.

■ CLINICAL ETHICS SUPPORT AND BEDSIDE RESOURCE ALLOCATION DECISIONS

After a long period of neglect, fairness-sensitive difficulties at the bedside are now attracting considerable interest. These difficulties affect patient care every day and are ethical in nature but are often not identified as ethical by physi-cians, who more commonly describe ethical difficulties in relation to clinical decision-making challenges such as end-of-life care, patient's decisional capac-ity, and conflict between decision makers. It seems that clinicians do not easily recognize or "diagnose" problems of fairness in terms of ethics, or their lack of the relevant ethical vocabulary may contribute to an underestimation of the importance of "allocation ethics." The Values at the Bedside study helped to identify the dimensions and articulate the problem: it showed that physicians are aware of making distributive decisions, but also that they witness discrimination of certain patient groups (Hurst et al., 2006).

The study showed that European physicians do encounter scarcity-related ethical difficulties, and they are dissatisfied with the resolution of many of these cases (Hurst et al., 2007). However, they rarely seek ethics support for resolving such difficulties even when such support exists in their institutions. Physicians in the study thought ethics consultants could assist physicians in these decisions in a range of ways including making the process less difficult, helping to make decisions more ethically justifiable, and bringing considerations of justice to bear on real cases (Hurst et al., 2008). One important aspect of resource-allocation decisions at the bedside is the consideration of futility and knowing when to withdraw futile treatment. At least one study has shown that clinical ethics support can be effective in limiting futile treatment in an intensive care setting (Schneiderman et al., 2003). Thus there appears to be an unmet need for support for clinicians on ethical decision making related to bedside allocation decisions and some limited evidence that such support can be effective. However, standard clinical ethics support services based on individual ethics consultation may only impact on a few cases, reaching a minority of those needing help (Hurst et al., 2007). Even if the access to and the acceptability of these services will increase, proper clinical ethics consultation cannot be seen as an everyday component of clinical routine. In the vast majority of cases, clinical decision making relies on the competence of the responsible health care professionals. Therefore, any support program needs to include mechanisms for improving the day-to-day competency of clinicians to make these difficult decisions. The METAP project was specifically conceived to develop this broader range of ethics support in the specific context of clinician resource-allocation decisions.

■ CONTEXT, SETTINGS, AND PROCEDURES OF THE METAP PROJECT

METAP is a clinical ethics support project. It aims at improving the ethical quality of clinical decisions and relies on enhancing the ethical competence of the clinical staff involved in making these decisions by providing knowledge through material, procedures, and instruments, as well as education and advice (ethics support). The project has been developed for and with the Unit of Operative Intensive Care as well as with the Acute Geriatric Clinic in the University Hospital Basel—the two units where our illustrative cases come from. After a period of pilot implementation and step-wise improvements,

METAP is now working in various clinical settings in seven institutions in Switzerland including surgical and internal intensive care, acute and long-term geriatrics, surgery, and (forthcoming) hematology.

Its central idea is that the way in which the solution for a problem is sought should reflect the nature of the problem: some difficulties may just require a brief clarification by sharing relevant information; others will need a substantial discussion. Thus the approach constitutes four different levels of an "escalation model" (see TABLE 18.1) with procedures for problem solving to be chosen by the clinical staff whenever someone feels that a fairness-sensitive issue is arising in the care of a patient who may be at risk of being treated in an unfair way. A further characteristic of METAP is the use of specific knowledge provided in a comprehensive manual, in a short version and through complementary educational training prior to and during the implementation on the wards. The manual describes and summarizes empirical data from studies examining risk factors for undertreatment as well as overtreatment and provides ethical, medical, and psychological basic information and suggestions. It makes available to the clinicians the basic knowledge that is needed to deal with ethical problems and describes in detail the procedure of ethical case discussions in the clinical team (level 3 in the escalating model) and clinical ethics consultations (level 4). The short version, available as a pocket guide called "Leporello" (a small accordion-folded booklet), summarizes the information from the manual and offers procedures as well as checklists and tables for organizing these case discussions.

The preparatory phase of the implementation of the METAP approach in any setting includes the provision of specific training by members of the METAP manual authors, particularly for small groups of care team members nominated to become *facilitators*. In seminars (three 4-hour sessions) they familiarize themselves with the manual, the use of the short version, and particularly the instruments such as guidance for problem identification and checklists for preparing an ethical case discussion (ECD). An important part

TABLE 18.1. *The Escalating Model*

Level 1 of the escalating model means that a *staff member* who has an ethical concern will consult the short version for the core knowledge that is provided, for example on patient rights.

In **level 2**, the person will call upon the help of a trained *peer facilitator*—a member of the clinical team—either after level 1 failed to solve the problem, or directly if the problem appears too difficult for solving on one's own.

For problems of a higher complexity, **level 3** foresees an internal ethical case discussion (ECD) among the *care team* on the ward, to be chaired by a facilitator following an explicit guideline described in the manual/short version.

Level 4 is a clinical ethics consultation (CEC) on demand that includes an experienced *clinical ethicist* invited to discuss the problem with the care team. This option can be requested in cases where a previous ECD has failed or where the individual or team (immediately) feel that the problem is particularly complex and requires more experienced or independent support than is available from the peer group.

of the training is the instruction and practice of the ECDs using examples. The aim is to ensure that the facilitator is responsive to ethical requirements such as respecting patient wishes and is able to identify risks for unfair care, for example undercare due to discrimination. These trained facilitators share their knowledge with the other team members and motivate them to use the instruments. However, enhancing the competence of clinical staff in this way does not imply demanding from them the same degree of ethics knowledge that a trained clinical ethics consultant would have, who also needs to practice special skills (Reiter-Theil et al., 2011a).

The METAP manual is based on both research and consensus building, and it undergoes systematic evaluation and modification. Clinical partners have been actively involved in the developmental process from the beginning and contributed to the practical applicability and acceptance of the manual by discussing their needs regarding the whole tool kit. This partnership and the participatory approach have helped METAP to gain a foothold in the clinic (Reiter-Theil et al., 2011b). Implementation of such procedures calls for some sort of cultural change: personal involvement of the senior leaders, education of the team, and identification of implementation barriers are key factors for this process to succeed.

■ A CONCEPT OF ETHICAL COMPETENCE FOR CLINICAL PRACTICE

Competence is a central component of the theoretical framework underlying clinical ethics support in the METAP project (Reiter-Theil et al., 2011a; see also Mertz et al., 2014). In the following section we refer to and develop further our understanding of what ethical competence is and how it should be used in the clinical context, especially with regard to handling fairness-sensitive issues appropriately.

Clinical, Moral, and Ethical Competence—All Different and Yet the Same?

As a first approximation to the concept of *ethical competence*, we propose an understanding of ethical competence as the ability to articulate, analyze, and justify moral judgments in a reasoned manner and to promote actions accordingly. We distinguish it from the concepts of *moral competence* and *clinical competence* that are also important in patient care. *Moral competence* is the ability to act consistently according to the normative aspects of a personal, professional, or social ethos. This ability encompasses different skills and attitudes: sensitivity for the morally salient features of a situation, the power to formulate consistent moral judgments, and the strength of character to prioritize and act according to moral reasons (Jormsri et al., 2005; Narvaez et al., 2003; Rest, 1994). Excellence here is based on moral virtues such as attentiveness, sincerity, or integrity. For health care practitioners, the professional ethos of medicine and health care is of paramount importance. It contains substantial beliefs, virtues, and practices encompassing the various aspects of what it means to be a morally good physician, nurse, or therapist, and thereby provides a value basis or a "normative framework" for their conduct (Marcum, 2012; Pellegrino, 2002). *Clinical competence* can be defined as the ability to use clinical reasoning, technical skills, and communication in a professional manner for the benefit of the individual and community served in daily clinical practice (adapted from Epstein & Hundert, 2002; see also Batalden et al., 2002).

The interpretation of these three prima facie distinguishable competences and their functions in clinical ethics support are still open to discussion. Pragmatist or hermeneutical approaches tend to be skeptical about the possibility of justifying normatively binding decisions through ethical competence; they rather emphasize the facilitating roles of the clinical ethicist to strengthen the moral competence of the care team (Fins et al., 1997; Molewijk, Abma, et al. 2008; Widdershoven & Abma, 2007). Others emphasize the normative force of the ethical reflection presupposing a specific ethical competence (Gesang, 2010; Weinstein, 1994) or try to mediate between moral and ethical competence (Eriksson et al., 2007; Steinkamp et al., 2008). In order to clarify these functions, it should first be acknowledged that there are significant relationships between these abilities. Good clinical practice itself exhibits certain *moral* features, as its goal is to help vulnerable human beings in poor health conditions. Medicine is a genuine moral enterprise (Miller & Brody, 2001; Pellegrino, 2001). Thus, substantive values that morally competent practitioners can integrate rightfully into clinical decision making are drawn from the professional ethos of their medical profession. However, there are other sources of moral values such as personal convictions and character, social sensibility, or the acknowledgement of the vulnerability and dignity of human beings. Consequently, even highly specialized clinical experts participate at least in the moral idea of promoting health, even if they may not be able to deal with every moral situation competently. What of the relationship between moral and ethical competence? They seem to be mutually dependent: on the one hand, in everyday clinical practice, practitioners have to rely on their moral sensitivity and integrity to make ethically sound judgments that fit the given situation. On the other hand, in view of the morally demanding challenges of modern medicine typical for pluralistic societies, moral intuitions and beliefs often come into conflict with each other and lose their action-guiding force. Also clinical, as any, decision making is susceptible to reasoning errors (Albisser Schleger et al., 2011) and, as Agledahl, Forde and Wifstad (2010) argue, tends systematically to simplify the moral aspects of a situation. Therefore these beliefs are in need of critical examination, and this requires the reflective power of *ethical* competence.

This first, rather rough analysis suggests that these competences are different though not totally distinct: they exist and are exercised to some extent at the same time. This fact contributes to the complexity of the concept of an ethically justified clinical judgment that has not yet been discussed sufficiently in the literature (for a first step see Baeroe & Norheim, 2011). We suppose that the three competences are complementary in the process of developing an ethically justified clinical judgment, namely in deciding what is the reasonable and appropriate thing to do for this patient in this situation. In a nutshell, clinical competence provides the relevant alternative *procedures* and appropriate *means*; moral competence provides the substantive *moral goals* and proper *attitudes* (including intentions); and ethical competence allows for a *critical and principled reflection* of the unity of these elements, viz. ends, means, consequences and attitudes. Ethical competence alone is thus not sufficient to answer moral questions in the clinic, as it has to rely on a proper assessment of the clinical situation and a common moral foundation. Craftsmanship, mores, and reason contribute to the normative dimension of ethical decision making. It is a distinctive feature of the METAP approach, however, that the distribution of these competences among the participants is not straightforward. We cannot attribute them simply according to professional roles, for example; when it comes to morality, everyone has to act in accordance with his or her own conscience—that is the reason why moral responsibility cannot be delegated. The demand of an overall proficiency for all practitioners obviously fails to recognize the practical requirements in a clinical setting. Thus we prefer to speak of different *competence profiles* that can be developed by each participant of the clinical practice in varying degrees.

The Peculiar Nature of Ethical Competence

Before we elaborate further on our concept of competence profiles, we have to deal briefly with some objections that may question the legitimacy of such a concept altogether. Rasmussen (2011) summarizes different kinds of objections to the concept of ethical competence. The "epistemological objection" is the most forceful one: How is it possible for anyone to know about the good at all, and how could some know it better than others? The answer to these questions obviously depends on what kind of knowledge is involved in clinical ethics support. In our approach, we consider at least three different forms of knowledge to be necessary for making good treatment decisions: "knowing that," which encompasses empirical and theoretical knowledge on medical, psychological, and social aspects of a case; "knowing why," which is normative knowledge of moral values and ethical reasoning; and "knowing how," which is knowledge about how to realize good ethical conduct under the given circumstances. Each of these should be based on the best available evidence (Reiter-Theil et al., 2011a). "Knowing why," most often addressed by this objection, entails a substantial and a formal aspect. Moral claims are *substantially* sound if they cohere with the lived morals and values of a human community, for example the claim that a healthy life is valuable. Clearly we know a lot of these things in an ordinary way, because they determine what it means to be a member of such a community. The *formal* validity of such claims is assessed by formal principles such as (practical) consistency, transparency, justifiability, or generality. Knowledge of these principles is reflective, in other words it requires ethical reflection on the form of our moral judgments to make these explicit—what trained ethicists are more able to do.

But can't we avoid using the complex expression of "ethical competence" by formulating ethical guidelines for clinical practice instead? Such guidelines can provide a useful framework for institutionalizing procedures or defining a foundation of democratically and legally legitimized moral values (Bartels et al., 2007). However, the prescriptive content of a clinical-ethical guideline can never do complete justice to the individual case. Moreover, a difficulty of legitimization arises due to the fact that this kind of external knowledge is not necessarily accompanied by individual insight (Eriksson et al., 2007). To bridge this gap between prescriptive guidelines and moral practice, we have to conceptualize ethical competence as an ability that is reflective, dialectical, practical, communicative, and can be learned by reflective practice. Let us briefly consider these features:

1. *Reflexivity:* Ethical competence has to be understood as *reflective* since it is an ability to share and evaluate reasons for moral judgments in different, potentially new and complex situations. This activity is self-conscious, as it critically reflects the attitudes, responsibilities, and motivations of the judging subject. Narvaez (2010) calls this "moral metacognitions." This does not imply that the whole process of moral decision making is purely cognitive and conscious. The development of a moral perspective on specific situations relies heavily on moral intuitions, tacit knowledge, and emotional attitudes. Clinical ethical decision making is based on a complex interplay of intuitive, associative, and largely automatic processes and reasoning that is conscious, self-conscious, and conscious of other selves (Clark, 2000; Mercier, 2011; Musschenga, 2008, 2009; Narvaez, 2010; Paxton et al., 2010).

2. *Dialectical structure:* This reasoning process has to be oriented toward a *dialectical* model that takes into consideration all structural elements of possible actions under the given circumstances—ends, means, consequences, attitudes—and correlate these progressively with the

formal and substantive norms and principles of ethics. In this way, a step-wise approach can be conducted that takes into account both the normative requirements of ethics as well as the specific characteristics of the case.

3. *Practicality:* This competence for dialectical reasoning is inherently *practical*—it focuses on the specific conditions of the situation that are relevant for taking action and enhances actions that are consistent with insight. It has to encompass a kind of practical knowledge, "knowing how." In the acquisition of such knowledge, gathering experiences with actions of this or a similar kind plays an important role.

4. *Communicability:* One significant feature of ethical reasoning is that it can and should be *shared*. As far as this reasoning is rational, other rational participants must, at least in principle, be able to comprehend the process if the rational grounds for it—theoretical, ethical, and practical assumptions—have been made explicit. If the needs and assumptions of different persons have to be considered in order to arrive at an ethically sound decision (as in every clinical situation), this possibility for sharing the reasons of one's reflection becomes imperative. Ethical reasoning in clinical practice is essentially a joint enterprise.

5. *Learnability:* Ethical competence is a *learnable and learned* ability and is best learned by theoretically informed exercising (Branch et al., 2009; Branch, 2010; Narvaez, 2006; Self & Baldwin, 1994; Sulmasy & Marx, 1997). Coping with the complexity of ethical challenges in clinical practice requires internalization not only of ethical knowledge but also of cognitive strategies, procedures, and attitudes needed for its application.

Of course this description indicates just the general structure of such an ethical competence. In clinical practice, this competence has to manifest itself in the specific tasks of ethical decision making and of providing the structural framework for making good decisions. These tasks require hermeneutical skills of articulation and interpretation, skills of establishing and maintaining an open and participatory discourse, and analytical skills of articulating arguments, balancing principles, or suggesting conclusions (for more details see Reiter-Theil, 2009).

Competence Profiles and Bedside Micro-allocation

An approach such as METAP that aims at activating and enhancing the competences of clinical team members focuses on the effort to render their own solutions as valid and practicable as possible. This will allow the caregivers to rely first on their own competence before or instead of inviting clinical ethics consultation, which is anyway an event that goes beyond everyday clinical routine. TABLE 18.2 tries to show the different profiles of clinical, moral, and ethical competence among the health care practitioners in an overview.

Regarding the fair allocation of health resources at the bedside, all competences—the clinical, the moral, and the ethical—have to work together to ensure an ethically qualified clinical practice. As in every case of *clinical*

TABLE 18.2. *Competence Profiles*

	Team member Clinical routine, METAP Level 1	Facilitator METAP Levels 2, 3	Ethics consultant METAP Level 4
Clinical Competence	Professional skills of providing good clinical care		
	Collection of necessary medical information	Collection of necessary medical information	
	Comprehensive understanding of hospital rules and procedures	Comprehensive understanding of hospital rules and procedures	Basic understanding of hospital rules and procedures
	Comprehensive understanding of the medical options	Comprehensive understanding of the medical options	Basic understanding of the medical options
Moral Competence	Sensitivity for morally salient features; moral point of view	Sensitivity for morally salient features; moral point of view	Sensitivity for morally salient features; moral point of view
	Ability to make moral judgments consistent with personal, professional, and social ethos	Ability to make moral judgments consistent with personal, professional, and social ethos	Ability to make moral judgments consistent with personal, professional, and social ethos
	Strength of character to act according to moral reasons and to deal constructively with moral feelings and distress	Strength of character to act according to moral reasons and to deal constructively with moral feelings and distress	Strength of character to act according to moral reasons and to deal constructively with moral feelings and distress
Ethical Competence	Identification of ethical issues in clinical practice	Identification of ethical issues in clinical practice	Articulation and prioritization of ethical issues in a given case
	Basic understanding and usage of concepts and principles of medical ethics	Basic understanding and usage of concepts and principles of medical ethics	Comprehensive understanding and usage of concepts and principles of medical ethics
		Moderating of ECD with the care team according to rules of discourse	Moderating and structuring interdisciplinary ECD according to rules of discourse
		Developing one's moral point of view (systematic change of perspectives)	Developing one's moral point of view (systematic change of perspectives)
		Awareness of different value systems	Awareness of different value systems
			Ethical reasoning skills to systematically analyses and weigh ethical arguments
			Critical thinking; double-check regarding error or premature agreement
			Supporting the conclusion

judgment, the care team has to examine all medical treatment options and prognoses for the patient thoroughly by collecting the relevant medical facts. The hospital rules and procedures may provide a useful framework for debating questions about the allocation of resources on the ward. To detect inequitable forms of health care, a *moral* sensitivity is required for the special vulnerability of the patient, for signs of potentially unjustified discrimination, and also for signs of time pressure as well as moral distress within the care team. In complex moral situations it may be necessary to refer explicitly to *ethical* concepts related to (un)fairness (undertreatment, overtreatment, etc.) to identify the relevant moral features. This sensitivity for forms of unfairness is linked with substantive *moral* values on the side of the team members based on their personal, professional, and social ethos. If the team members cannot articulate these moral values together with the patient's preferences in a consistent moral judgment about how to allocate the available resources, all the relevant elements of the judgment (ends, means, consequences, and attitudes) have to undergo *ethical* scrutiny. This probably requires the procedural competence of a trained facilitator that ensures, within the participative and structured process of an ECD, that the most fundamental criteria of fairness will be acknowledged, for example to avoid unequal treatment based on unjustified discrimination. More complex situations even call for the abilities of an ethics consultant, as described in TABLE 18.2. The consultant should be able to bring to the fore all criteria that METAP provides to handle fairness-sensitive issues, especially the criteria of (1) formal justice, above all to treat equal cases equally; (2) procedural justice, namely to follow the same transparent, participative, and consensually justified decision-making procedure; and (3) substantial justice, that is to consider for example the urgency of treatment, expected individual benefit, and the cost-benefit ratio (Albisser Schleger et al., 2012, pp. 184–185). For implementing the decision the team members have to be able to rely on their professional *clinical* skills. All participants involved have to rely on their *moral* strength of character (willpower, integrity, courage, etc.). A reflective *ethical* stance requires coming back to a decision if the situation changes significantly, especially concerning the state of health of the patient: in this case an ethical reevaluation will be necessary. The case examples in the next section illustrate how this works in daily practice.

▪ MORAL AND ETHICAL COMPETENCE AT WORK—CASUISTIC ILLUSTRATION

METAP in Acute Geriatric Care

Elderly patients have significant risk factors for undertreatment or unequal treatment, for example mental illness, dementia, low socioeconomic status, or terminal illness. Frequently the geriatric team faces the challenge of unclear

The Geriatric Case

A 73-year-old Spanish man came to the emergency department with a general decline in health. He was transferred to the department of acute geriatric medicine. Taking a patient history was not possible due to the patient's congenital cognitive impairment. His family members informed the care team that he had been suffering from back pain for the past month. Furthermore, he had lost a significant amount of weight and presented signs of pallor, anorexia, and oral lesions. Laboratory tests at admission revealed marked renal failure and anemia. Until now, the patient had lived in a little 2-room apartment on the 4th floor without an elevator together with his 98-year-old mother who suffered from severe dementia. The mother refused professional support for the daily routine, so the situation in this arrangement was suboptimal. Mother and son had an unusually close relationship and were not able to be separated during the hospitalization. The patient's mother was therefore simultaneously admitted to the ward.

The situation of this patient was discussed at the daily meeting of the care team. Consulting the METAP short version (*Leporello*) and applying METAP levels 1 and 2, the team realized that he had an increased risk for undercare or unequal treatment. It might have been decided not to do any diagnostic work-up because of the patient's cognitive impairment—one of the criteria of the risk profile for undercare. Eventually the team made a diagnosis of multiple myeloma with light chain deposition that was causing acute kidney failure. Based on the severity of the disease and the patient's general condition, together with the family a palliative therapy was chosen. During the course of the hospitalization, the family stated that the patient wanted to spend the remaining days of his life in Spain. After several discussions, the team realized that a transfer to Spain would be too great of a financial burden, costing around 15,000 Swiss Francs. This too seemed to confirm the risk of granting the patient less than he wished.

The care team decided to analyze the situation with the help of an "ethical case discussion" (METAP level 3). During the discussion following the METAP procedure, the team became aware of the fact that until now, the patient had never expressed *his own wishes*. A Spanish-speaking nurse who took care of the patient during the whole hospitalization period helped to answer the question of how to plan the further treatment of the patient. She stressed the fact that the patient had expressed many times that he wanted to stay in the hospital with his mother. This statement was considered a valid and accurate expression of his wishes. Due to the complex medical and nursing situation and the need for university hospital care, a transfer to a Spanish hospital was regarded too stressful for the patient.

The relatives were informed about the decision in repeated conversations and agreed finally. The patient died peacefully 6 days after the METAP discussion.

Note: In order to guarantee anonymity some details of the case have been modified. The clinicians involved have agreed to the use of the case in this publication.

medical and nursing objectives (therapeutic or palliative) due to complex and dynamic patient situations. This leads to conflicts and misunderstandings in communication within the care team, but also with the patients and their families.

On this acute geriatric ward the approaches of level 1 and 2 are routinely applied during the daily visits and reports by nurses and physicians and the staff identifies with this as a part of their professionalism. The sheet, "identi-fication of the ethical problem" is used in level 1 and 2 to localize the ethical focus of the problem or patient situation (see TABLE 18.3) and is a part of the short version as well as the manual. As a key concept for good ethical decision making, patient risk factors for inappropriate care are listed on this sheet for a quick orientation. In contrast to the daily use of levels 1 and 2, the ECDs, level 3 of METAP, are arranged on this ward whenever needed and take place approximately eight times a year. These discussions can be organized within one or two days. Two checklists support the gathering of information needed and organizing the meeting.

TABLE 18.3. *Identification of Ethical Problems*

Respect for autonomy
• Is the patient's will (direct or presumed) respected appropriately?
• Which values are meaningful for the patient?
• In the case of capacity of decision making: was the patient able to build his or her will on the basis of comprehensible information and without external pressure?
• In case of lacking capacity decision making: was the patient's presumed will explored carefully?

Beneficence/benefit
• Will the previous or planned measures be of any benefit for the patient? Will they help him or her?
• Do the previous or planned measures serve the patient's well-being?

Nonmaleficence/avoid harm and side effects	**Risk factors for overtreatment**
• Does the current situation cause disproportionate suffering/injury/side effects to the patient? • Are there any hints for possible overtreatment (see list to the right)?	• No effect of the treatment • Intervention causes a questionable proportion of physical and mental strain or pain, even when reaching the therapeutic objective • No significant improvement expected by the treatment • The treatment has an effect but will not reach the goals that are particularly important for the patient
Fairness/nondiscrimination	**Risk factors for undertreatment or unequal treatment**
• Are there any hints for possible undertreatment or unequal treatment and, if so, have they been care-fully considered (see list to the right)? • Do you have the impression that the patient is discriminated against based on personal values or one-sided economic considerations? • Does the current situation lead to unfair conse-quences for other patients?	• advanced age • female gender • low socioeconomic status • ethnic minority • single • chronic disease • multi-morbidity • high intensity of care • incompetence of judgment • mental illness • dementia • terminal illness

Perception and interaction
• Are the perceptions of the participants and persons concerned included adequately?
• Can you freely express your attitude, wishes, needs, and criticisms?

Basic information
• Is there any lack of information based on the "checklist for collection of information"?

Source: Albisser Schleger, H., Mertz, M., Meyer-Zehnder, B., & Reiter-Theil, S. (2012), p. 310.

In the case presented here, the team realized the vulnerability for undercare or potential discrimination against the patient and his mother (low socioeconomic status, chronic disease, multi-morbidity, high intensity of care, incompetence of judgment) and—despite limited prognosis—started the diagnostic process instead of prematurely reducing engagement. After having carefully gathered the diagnostic information, a palliative strategy was chosen due to the severity of the disease and the futile situation. An indication for an ECD arose because of a conflict with the relatives. The team realized that the relatives did not represent the patient's wishes but tried to impose their own preferences. Showing that the team was determined to respect the patient's wishes, the conflict with the relatives could be solved. One of the team members asserted: "Using the METAP model was the most effective way to determine what was best for the patient and avoid harm."

METAP in Operative Intensive Care

Patients in intensive care units (ICUs) sometimes are at risk for inappropriate treatment, especially prolonged overtreatment or futile treatment—issues that indicate the need for METAP procedures. This intensive care unit served as the first experimental unit for developing METAP. They have taken a very active part and also ownership in shaping its processes as an approach that would allow for enhancing staff competence rather than providing ethics consultation as the only option of improving ethical quality.

The low-threshold METAP procedures, levels 1 and 2, take place during the daily visits of the care team; however, this often happens in an implicit way. Level 3, the ethical case discussion, has been institutionalized as a weekly time window used regularly as a kind of living ethics culture on the ward. One or two days before this date, a defined staff member checks whether there is an indication for a case discussion and organizes it if necessary. In 2011, 25 ethical case discussions took place in this format. The average duration is about 45 minutes with four to eight team members present. The ECDs in the ICU include the clinical team, the surgeons, and other relevant disciplines involved in the patient's care as far as possible, since these various disciplines may have different perspectives on the best course of action. These case discussions follow the recommended structured approach and are chaired by a trained team member. First, information from the different professions is gathered and documented in a matrix (see TABLE 18.4). Ideally, this information is collected prior to the meeting and a checklist is used based on the matrix. The participants then discuss arguments for and against different options referring to ethical principles. As soon as one option is considered the best for the patient, the team plans the next steps in the treatment process. Each ethical case discussion is briefly summarized and documented for the patient chart.

The Intensive Care Case

A 75-year-old patient was hospitalized with an acute myocardial infarction. She had a severe coronary artery disease, the ventricular function was at about one-third of normal for her age, and she had severe narrowing of her aortic valve. An attempt was made to reopen the coronary vessels with stents, and she was transferred to the intensive care unit. She recovered, but her heart function did not improve. The cardiac surgeons were consulted but they refused to perform open heart surgery because the risk was too high. The plan was therefore to let her recover as much as possible and then to try an interventional aortic valve replacement. There was no doubt that the patient and her relatives were fully motivated for all these procedures.

While waiting for the aortic valve replacement, about 50 days after her initial hospitalization, the patient developed an acute abdomen. Following a CT scan the surgeons decided that she urgently needed a laparotomy, or she would die. The patient consented to the operation being aware of the high risk. After the operation the patient was again admitted to the intensive care unit. She was in shock and comatose and needed vasoactive drugs and artificial ventilation. It was clear to the intensive care team that she was at high risk of dying.

The next day, the ICU team informed the family about the poor prognosis and made clear that it was crucial that the patient showed some improvement within the next days. The nursing team thought that the family did not acknowledge the seriousness of the patient's condition, and the ICU team decided to search for more information on the patient's presumed treatment preferences by calling the family doctor. The phone call revealed that the patient had not communicated her wishes explicitly, but the doctor remembered her as a content person with a positive attitude toward life.

In this difficult situation, the team decided to assign her to the next METAP ECD date. No team member at that time had identified "an ethical problem" in this case, but the culture of the unit is that patient situations which trigger implicit questions about the sensibility of further treatment will be discussed in a structured way using a METAP ECD. At the end of this meeting, the team agreed that the patient wished for maximal therapy as long as she would qualify for open heart surgery or go home again. They also agreed that there was only a very tiny chance of reaching this goal. No observations of signs for overtreatment or undertreatment were documented. The team decided that no escalation of treatment, such as more drugs to support circulation or a further abdominal operation, should be instituted. The reasoning was that the necessity for these measures would make it extremely unlikely that the therapeutic goals of the patient would be achieved.

Over the next 3 days the patient's condition improved considerably. The tube in the trachea could be removed, and only intermittent mechanical ventilator support was necessary. Adequate contact with the patient was possible, and she made clear that she wanted treatment. The family confirmed the patient's wishes regarding treatment. Five days later the patient developed acute rectal bleeding, and it was not possible to stabilize her condition. The situation was discussed with the family and, at this time, everyone agreed that further treatment would not be in the interest of the patient because the initial goals could never be reached. Nineteen days after admission to the unit, 10 days after the METAP ECD, a palliative treatment goal was formulated and all other therapy stopped. Shortly afterwards the patient died peacefully in the presence of her family.

Note: In order to guarantee anonymity some details of the case have been modified. The clinicians involved have agreed to the use of the case in this publication.

TABLE 18.4. *Matrix—Checklist for the Collection of Information*

	Medical history / Preferences / Social environment	Problems of care / Patient's will / Structural conditions	Prognosis / Risk factors / Other information
Treatment and care	**Medical history** • What are currently the greatest medical problems? • Have all useful diagnostic procedures been carried out? • What is the therapeutic benefit of the current treatment plan? • What is the risk of complications of the treatment? • How big is the burden for the patient?	**Problems of care** • What are currently the largest problems regarding nursing care? • What kind of support does the patient need? • How much support does the patient need? • Are there specific arrangements with the family? • Is there specific information available only to employees of the therapeutic disciplines?	**Prognosis** • What is the short-term prognosis? • What is the long-term prognosis? • What is the prognosis without treatment? • What experiences have been made in similar cases? • What restrictions to independence can be expected? What is the expected quality of life?
Patient	**Preferences/way of living** • What is important for the patient? • Does he or she have any hobbies that are important to him or her? • If there is a chronic illness, how has the patient dealt with it up to now? • What is the patient's philosophy about life? • Does the patient belong to a religious community? • Is there a need for pastoral care, or are the patient and the relatives currently served by a pastor? • What was the quality of life and level of independence before the present illness?	**Patient's will** • Is the patient capable of making decisions? Is the decisional capacity limited or uncertain? • Are there any statements about the patient's will from the immediate past, for example during a preoperative discussion? • Is there an advance directive? If so, how recent is it, and is it applicable to the current situation? • Is there evidence that the patient's will has changed in the meantime? • Has the patient made any statements about his or her wishes before the current hospitalization? • How reliable is the information about the presumed will, as mentioned by the relatives? • Is there a clear distinction being made between the wishes of the patient and those of the relatives?	**Risk factors for under- or unequal treatment** • advanced age • female gender • low socioeconomic status • ethnic minority • single • chronic disease • multi-morbidity • high intensity of care • incompetence of judgment • mental illness • dementia • terminal illness **Risk factors for overtreatment** • Do you assess the situation to be at risk of overtreatment? **Other information**
Social environment and local parameters	**Social environment** • How is the social environment? • To what degree are the relatives informed? • To what degree are the relatives involved in decision-making process? • What is the attitude of the relatives? • Are there particular problems with the relatives?	**Structural conditions** • Are potential therapies offered by this hospital? • Is there currently a shortage of staff? • Are there enough time resources for potential treatment options? • Are there incentives for overtreatment during such situations?	

Source: Albisser Schleger, H., Mertz, M., Meyer-Zehnder, B., & Reiter-Theil, S. (2012), p. 311.

The case described here illustrates the importance for the team of carefully exploring the wishes of a patient, even repeatedly and by various approaches. Retrospectively, all persons involved in the case—the family, the surgeons, and the intensive care team—were satisfied that they had followed the patient's will as closely as possible. Among the care team there was no doubt that the METAP ECD, 10 days before the death of the patient, had helped to focus on the patient's needs and to communicate with the relatives in a consistent way, thus guiding the family from a position of demanding maximal therapy to one of acceptance of the dying process of their loved one.

■ CRITICAL APPRAISAL

The two cases illustrate that both clinical teams showed competence in identifying ethical concerns regarding resource micro-allocation as part of their daily routine—an achievement that is far from being trivial. Studies have documented that lack of ethics education among physicians leads them to overestimate their own competence and makes them underestimate their moral difficulties (Agledahl et al., 2010; Hurst et al., 2007). Both teams also proved their moral motivation and integrity as they strived convincingly to realize the best possible care for their respective patients despite considerable complications. Obviously, moral sensitivity and intuition provide a foundation for an interest in proper ethical decision making. However, as moral development studies suggest, ethical knowledge and skills are also required for morally good practice (Kutnick, 1986; Thoma, 1994). Did ethical competence in decision making obtained by applying METAP procedures function to appropriately assess the micro-allocation issues?

In the geriatric case, the team identified a risk of discriminating against the patient through insufficient diagnostic carefulness. Being sensitized by knowing about the risk factors summarized in the *Leporello*, they deliberately decided to invest time and effort in a thorough examination following level 2 of METAP. Their structured approach of using METAP tools (see TABLES 18.3 and 18.4) seems to have contributed to caring for a most vulnerable patient in a responsible way, avoiding any withholding of beneficial care. The team clearly showed moral sensitivity for the special—medical and social—situation of the patient given his cognitive impairment, and it displayed moral courage in deciding together with the family on a palliative treatment strategy at an early stage. The awareness that the patient's wishes (i.e., to stay with his mother) have ethical importance can be expected of the team members according to our competence profiles (see TABLE 18.2). The enquiry about the patient's will and decisional capacity is included in the *Leporello* and should thus be part of their ethical competence. However, it seems that such considerations were not a main focus of the decision-making process initially because of the cognitive disability of the patient. The ethical reflection in the ECD—with the help of a trained facilitator—revealed that the principle of respecting the patient's autonomy raised questions deserving consideration in this case. We do not know whether and how the patient's capacity was explored, although a geriatric ward is highly qualified for this, and METAP also provides procedures for this (Albisser Schleger et al., 2012, pp. 119–127). An independent ethics consultant (level 4) could have helped to ascertain that this had been done.

Given the severity of the medical condition; the fact that the patient's next of kin, especially his mother, were present at the same location; the assumed preference of the patient; and the expected costs of his transport to Spain, the health care team made a morally and ethically competent decision regarding the use of resources in this case. Working with the METAP approach not only strengthened the moral competence of the team in enhancing moral sensitivity and integrity, it also added to ethical reflection by helping to discover possible discrimination factors and drawing attention to the fact that the patient's wishes had gone almost unnoticed. Potential undertreatment and overtreatment could thus be avoided.

The rather complex treatment of the ICU patient raises further questions concerning appropriate distribution of care. In particular, the METAP approach recommends that the clinicians check the criteria of overtreatment ("futility"). If overtreatment is identified according to a list of risk factors for overtreatment (see TABLE 18.3), METAP suggests the issue should be discussed at an ECD. According to the ICU case report given here, it seems that this list had not been worked through explicitly; otherwise the team might have found more than one item suggesting futility. Because of the laudable ethics culture on this ward, the question about "sense or non-sense of further treatment" was still brought to an ECD, which supported a decision according to the procedural criteria of justice (i.e., follow the same transparent, participative, and consensually justified procedure). But what are the substantial criteria of distributive justice in a case like this, and how can they be met?

Guidance such as the METAP checklist remains too vague when it is not made explicit whether or not the patient's wish for treatment is considered as overriding suggestions or even evidence of "futility." According to our concept of ethical competence, such a list can have at most a supporting role in the decision-making process—balancing the expected individual benefit, the consequences of the treatment, and the probability of reaching the therapeutic goals must lie at its center. The team engaged in such a reflective discourse and decided, in view of the very small chances of reaching the therapeutic goal and the patient's repeatedly expressed will to seize this chance, to maintain but not to expand intensive treatment. Consistently the team decided to stop curative therapy and begin palliative treatment after deterioration in health.

This course of action lies within the procedural and normative framework of METAP.

However, the case raises further questions: Was the prognosis promising enough to justify maintaining intensive treatment at the time of the ECD? Did the value of respecting the patient's wish override considerations about effectiveness or burdens of treatment? Did the patient and her family actually realize the imbalance of the "tiny" chance for benefit and the considerable burdens for the patient? How far may—or should—health care professionals go in explaining "bad news" to ensure the understanding of the patient and his or her family (Winkler et al., 2009)? Up to which level of unfavorable prognosis would the team have agreed to maintain intensive treatment? After the ECD the patient lived another 10 days with ups and downs, during which time additional treatment to stabilize the patient proved unsuccessful. Obviously such questions defy simple and clear-cut answers, and dealing with them could exceed one's moral or ethical competence even within a discursive framework of an ECD. In such a case, the METAP approach is meant to facilitate an ethics consultant's support of the decision-making process in framing such questions from a systematic and independent point of view. The Schneiderman et al. study (2003) gave evidence that ethics consultation is able to reduce futile ICU treatment without raising mortality. The fuller range of ethical skills of an ethics consultant (see TABLE 18.2) might have helped to clarify and deepen the ethical discussion in the ICU case as well.

In both cases, METAP helped in dealing with ethical concerns related to bedside resource allocation—mainly regarding formal and procedural justice such as nondiscrimination, participation, or transparency. Regarding substantial criteria about appropriate care, it seems that the METAP procedures did not help as much as one would have wished. According to our concept of competence, such a decision has to be based on the moral competence of the persons involved in the particular situation. This acknowledges the importance of the health care professional as a person, and his or her handling of moral values—an aspect that has often been neglected in many ethics approaches (Reiter-Theil, 2009). However, the ethically challenging cases presented here require an ethical reflection of these values—and it seems that the reasoning may not have been optimally comprehensive and precise. This raises the question how ethical competence of the clinical staff could be further improved, or how the involvement of an independent ethics consultant could be promoted in such situations. More work needs to be done regarding the significance and use of ethical and evidence-based criteria, especially assessment of cost effectiveness and the balance of benefit and burden for the patient. If we move forward toward distinguishing between different problems and tasks of ethical competence, we will also be able to discover when and which forms of ethics support are "indicated" for a particular problem.

Furthermore, METAP addresses the topic of resource allocation mainly from the perspective of individual patient care. Fairness-sensitive issues in health care need also to be addressed at the meso and macro levels of the system. Experiences with clinical cases and related data should be thoroughly recorded. Their analysis, for example in case series, may provide a useful and valid basis for decision making at the institutional level where resources are being allocated.

This chapter has some limitations in that it uses only cases with end-of-life decisions in two elderly patients. However, similar conflict about appropriate treatment or disagreement could occur in patients with malignant diseases independent of age (Hauke et al., 2011). Another limitation is that we offer only some subjective evaluation of METAP. Data on more objective aspects of evaluation are currently in preparation.

■ CONCLUSIONS

Medical and clinical ethics has long focused on the competence of clinical staff to acknowledge patient rights and autonomy. While this remains a major task, fairness-sensitive issues also need to be included in ethical awareness more explicitly, with the aim of developing and supporting competence that specifically addresses ethical problems arising from undertreatment or overtreatment. Health care professionals should have—in addition to their clinical competence—moral and ethical competence. We argue that ethical competence can be learned, and existing moral competence can be strengthened, by creating favorable circumstances for careful decision-making processes in patient care. Fairness-sensitive issues, discrimination against vulnerable patients, and implicit rationing may create as much or even more ethical dilemmas than end-of-life issues. It seems that a clearly structured approach, with tools providing procedural guidance for decision making, can help to raise awareness of clinical staff and prevent escalation of problems. However, using these tools can only be conclusive when the tools give clear guidance, for example regarding cases where a patient insists on "futile" treatment. We suggest that clinical ethics support is not only valuable when it comes in the form of ethics consultation but also when it engages in lower-threshold approaches, such as those described in this chapter, that may be more accessible for implementation in daily clinical practice.

■ ACKNOWLEDGMENTS

The OPO Foundation, Zurich, Switzerland, has supported the project generously.

The last author is grateful for the excellent collaboration within the project leadership group of the Values at the Bedside study and the invitation to the Brocher Symposium that led to this publication.

Note

1. METAP is an evidence-oriented guideline providing knowledge and procedures for clinical ethics support. The project is funded by the Swiss National Science Foundation: "Between Over-Treatment and Under-Treatment: Ethical Problems of Micro-Allocation Taking Intensive and Geriatric Care as Examples—Quality Development in Medical and Nursing Care Through a Modular, Ethical Treatment Allocation Process (METAP) in Vulnerable Patient Groups," No. 3200B0-113724/1; "Fairness and Transparency. Clinical Ethics Guideline METAP—Evaluation, Methodological Foundation and Improvement," No. 3200B0-113724. Principal Investigator: Stella Reiter-Theil; Co-Investigator: Hans Pargger.

REFERENCES

Agledahl, K. M., Forde, R., & Wifstad, A. (2010). Clinical essentialising: a qualitative study of doctors' medical and moral practice. *Med Health Care Philos*, 13(2), 107–113.

Albisser Schleger, H., Pargger, H., & Reiter-Theil, S. (2008). 'Futility'—overtreatment at the end of life? Reasons for missed cessations of therapy in geriatric and critical care medicine. *Palliativmedizin*, 9(02), 67–75. [in German]

Albisser Schleger, H., Oehninger, N. R., & Reiter-Theil, S. (2011). Avoiding bias in medical ethical decision-making. Lessons to be learnt from psychology research." *Med Health Care Philos*, 14(2), 155–162.

Albisser Schleger, H., Mertz M., Meyer-Zehnder B., & Reiter-Theil S. (2012). *Klinische Ethik—METAP. Leitlinie für Entscheidungen am Krankenbett*. Berlin Heidelberg: Springer-Verlag GmbH.

Baeroe, K., & Norheim, O. F. (2011). Mapping out structural features in clinical care calling for ethical sensitivity: a theoretical approach to promote ethical competence in healthcare personel and clinical ethical support services (CESS). *Bioethics*, 25(7), 394–402.

Bartels, S., et al. (2005). How helpful are 'ethical guidelines' in the individual case? *Ethik in der Medizin*, 17(3), 191–205. [in German]

Branch, W. T. (2010). The road to professionalism: Reflective practice and reflective learning." *Patient Education and Counseling*, 80(3), 327–332.

Branch, W. T. Jr., et al. (2009). "A good clinician and a caring person: longitudinal faculty development and the enhancement of the human dimensions of care. *Academic Medicine*, 84(1), 117–125.

Clark, A. (2000). Word and Action: Reconciling Rules and Know-How in Moral Cognition. In Campbell, R., & Hunter, B.,eds. *Moral Epistemology Naturalized: Canadian Journal of Philosophy Supplement, Volume 26*. Pp. 267–290. Alberta, Canada: University of Calgary Press.

Epstein, R. M., & Hundert, E. M. (2002). Defining and assessing professional competence. *Journal of the American Medical Association*, 287(2), 226–235.

Eriksson, S., Helgesson, G., & Höglund, A. (2007). "Being, doing, and knowing: developing ethical competence in health care. *Journal of Academic Ethics*, 5(2), 207–216.

Fins, J. J., Bacchetta, M. D., & Miller, F. G. (1997). Clinical pragmatism: a method of moral problem solving." *Kennedy Institute of Ethics Journal*, 7(2), 129–145.

Gesang, B. (2010) Are moral philosophers moral experts? *Bioethics*, 24(4), 153–159.

Hauke, D., Reiter-Theil, S., et al. (2011). The role of relatives in decisions concerning life-prolonging treatment in patients with end-stage malignant disorders: informants, advocates or surrogate decision-makers? *Annals of Oncology*, 22(12), 2667–2674.

Hurst, S. A., Slowther A., Forde, R., Pegoraro, R., Reiter-Theil, S., et al. (2006), "Prevalence and determinants of physician bedside rationing: data from Europe," *J Gen Intern Med*, 21 (11), 1138–1143.

Hurst, S. A., Forde, R., Reiter-Theil, S., et al. (2007). Physicians' views on resource availability and equity in four European health care systems. *BMC Health Services Research*, 7(1), 137.

Hurst, S. A., Reiter-Theil, S., et al. (2008). Should ethics consultants help clinicians face scarcity in their practice? *Journal of Medical Ethics*, 34(4), 241–246.

Jormsri, P., et al. (2005). Moral competence in nursing practice. *Nursing Ethics*, 12(6), 582–594.

Kutnick, P. (1986). The relationship of moral judgment and moral action: Kohlberg's theory, criticism and revision. In Modgil, S., & Modgil, C., eds. *Lawrence Kohlberg: Consensus and Controversy*. pp. 125–148. Philadelphia and London: The Falmer Press.

Marcum, J. A. (2012). *The Virtuous Physician: The role of virtue in medicine*. Dordrecht, London: Springer.

Mercier, H. (2011). What good is moral reasoning? *Mind & Society*, 10(2), 131–148.

Mertz, M., Albisser, H., Meyer-Zehnder, B., & Reiter-Theil, S. (2014). Principles and discourse: an approach for the theoretical justification of ethical case discussion and ethics consultation. *Ethik in der Medizin*, 26(2), 91–104. [in German]

Miller, F. G., & Brody, H. (2001). The internal morality of medicine: an evolutionary perspective. *Journal of Medicine and Philosophy*, 26(6), 581–599.

Molewijk, A. C., Abma, T., Stolper, M., & Widdershoven, G. (2008). Teaching ethics in the clinic. The theory and practice of moral case deliberation. *Journal of Medical Ethics*, 34(2), 120–124.

Musschenga, A. W. (2008). Moral judgement and moral reasoning. In Düwell, M., Rehmann-Sutter, C., & Mieth, D., eds. *The Contingent Nature of Life*. pp. 131–146. International Library of Ethics, Law, and the New Medicine, 39: Springer Netherlands.

Musschenga, A. W. (2009). Moral intuitions, moral expertise and moral reasoning. *Journal of Philosophy of Education*, 43(4), 597–613.

Narvaez, D. (2006). Integrative ethical education. In Killen, M., & Smetana, J., eds. *Handbook of Moral Development*. pp. 703–733. Mahwah, NJ: Lawrence Earlbaum Associates.

Narvaez, D. (2010). Moral complexity. *Perspectives on Psychological Science*, 5(2), 163–181.Narvaez, D., Bock, T., & Endicott, L. (2003). Who should I become? Citizenship, goodness, human flourishing, and ethical expertise. In Wiel Veugelers, W., & Oser, F. K., eds. *Teaching in Moral and Democratic Education*. pp. 43–63. New York, Oxford, Wien: Swiss Educational Research Association.

Paxton, J. M., & Greene, J. D. (2010). Moral reasoning: hints and allegations. *Topics in Cognitive Science, 2*(3), 511–527.

Pellegrino, E. D. (2001). The internal morality of clinical medicine: a paradigm for the ethics of the helping and healing professions. *Journal of Medicine & Philosophy, 26*(6), 559–579.

Pellegrino, E. D. (2002). Professionalism, profession and the virtues of the good physician. *Mt. Sinai Journal of Medicine, 69*(6), 378–384.

Rasmussen, L. M. (2011). An ethics expertise for clinical ethics consultation. *Journal of Law and Medical Ethics, 39*(4), 649–661.

Reiter-Theil, S. (2009). Dealing with the normative dimension in clinical ethics consultation. *Cambridge Quarterly of Healthcare Ethics, 18*(4), 347–359.

Reiter-Theil, S., Mertz, M., & Meyer-Zehnder, B. (2007). The complex roles of relatives in end-of-life decision-making: an ethical analysis. *HEC Forum, 19*(4), 341–364.

Reiter-Theil, S., Mertz, M., Meyer-Zehnder, B., Albisser Schleger, H., Kressig, R. W., & Pargger, H. (2011b). Clinical ethics as partnership—or how an ethical guideline on fair resource-allocation can be developed and implemented in the clinic. *Ethik in der Medizin, 23*(2), 93–105. [in German]

Reiter-Theil, S., Mertz, M., Schürmann, J., Stingelin-Giles, N., & Meyer-Zehnder, B. (2011a). Evidence—competence—discourse: the theoretical framework of the multi-centre clinical ethics support project METAP, *Bioethics, 25*(7), 403–412.

Rest, J. R. (1994). *Moral Development in the Professions: Psychology and applied ethics*. New Jersey: Lawrence Erlbaum.

Schneiderman, L. J., Gilmer,T., Teetzel, H. D., Dugan, D. O., Blustein, J., Cranford, R., et al. (2003). Effect of ethics consultations on nonbeneficial life-sustaining treatments in the intensive care setting. *Journal of the American Medical Association, 290*(9), 1166–1172.

Self, D. J., & Baldwin, DeWitt C. (1994), Moral reasoning in medicine. In Rest, J. R., & Narváez, D., eds. *Moral Development in the Professions: Psychology and Applied Ethics.* pp. 147–162.Hillsdale, NJ: Lawrence Erlbaum Associates.

Steinkamp, N. L., Gordijn, B., & ten Have, H. A. (2008). Debating ethical expertise. *Kennedy Institute of Ethics Journal, 18*(2), 173–192.

Sulmasy, D. P., & Marx, E. S. (1997). Ethics education for medical house officers: long-term improvements in knowledge and confidence. *Journal of Medical Ethics, 23*(2), 88–92.

Thoma, S. (1994). Moral judgments and moral action. In Rest, J. R., & Narváez, D., eds. *Moral Development in the Professions: Psychology and Applied Ethics.* pp. 199–211. Hillsdale, NJ: Lawrence Erlbaum Associates.

Weinstein, B. D. (1994). The possibility of ethical expertise. *Theoretical Medicine and Bioethics, 15*(1), 61–75.

Widdershoven, G. A. M., & Abma, T. A. (2007). Hermeneutic Ethics between Practice and Theory. In Ashcroft, R. J., Dawson, A., Draper, H., & McMillan, J. R., eds. *Principles of Health Care Ethics* pp. 215–221. Chichester John Wiley & Sons, Ltd.

Winkler, E. C., Reiter-Theil, S., Lange-Riess, D., Schmahl-Menges, N., & Hiddemann, W. (2009). Patient involvement in decisions to limit treatment: the crucial role of agreement between physician and patient. *Journal of Clinical Oncology, 27*(13), 2225–2230.

19

Fair Resource Allocation in Clinical Care for Socially Disadvantaged Groups and Health Disparity Populations

Issues and Strategies

■ IRENE DANKWA-MULLAN, PAULA Y. GOODWIN, AND MATTHEW WYNIA

■ FAIR RESOURCE ALLOCATION IN AN UNFAIR WORLD

Allocation of health resources in a fair and just world would be equitable and contribute to the well-being of members of society in a nondiscriminatory manner. Physicians would authorize expenditures for services to individuals solely based on the relative benefits and risks, thereby minimizing health care costs and maximizing the delivery of high-quality healthcare. But what are the implications of allocating health care resources in contexts that are not equal or just—where individual patients have been exposed to different opportunities and experiences which potentially lead to differential health status?

Resource limitation is omnipresent in today's world of expanding medical capabilities, aging populations, and limited budgets. Rationing of health resources has always existed in various forms in every country, usually implemented through pricing, limited facilities, denial of coverage, and absence of providers (Guindo et al., 2012). Notably, each of these methods of resource allocation tends to favor the more affluent, with the result that people experiencing poverty have generally had less access to and less benefit from health care. In this chapter the question we seek to address is, what is the role of the physician in influencing the fair allocation of health resources, especially for socially disadvantaged individuals and groups, in environments where resources may be limited by bureaucracy and not a shortage of essential medical supplies (i.e., in higher-income countries with health care financing and coverage by public and private sources)?

Although fairness in general and Hippocratic principles in particular have long called on physicians to practice evenhandedly with all population groups, including people facing disadvantaged circumstances, health care delivery and other social systems have often made that mission challenging or impossible. Throughout history, the well-off have commonly had access to health care services and resources that were unavailable to the poor. Often there have simply been insufficient resources to provide adequate care to everyone. But in the various national health care systems of today, with their combinations of public and private insurance coverage, the potential for the physician to be a truly equitable arbiter of resource use is very much present. In nations where enough resources are devoted to health care to provide an adequate level of care to everyone (in theory, at least), the issue at hand is whether physicians and others responsible for resource allocation decisions are performing as equitable arbiters and, if not, how does one identify the problem and remediate it? How should physicians and the systems in which they work assure that social resources are shared fairly between those more advantaged and those less advantaged in society? When judgments must be made about clinical and financial justifications for using test X or treatment Y, physicians routinely make the call. Therefore, they must be responsible for ensuring that resources are distributed fairly and all groups treated equitably. Equitable treatment means prioritization of medical resources necessary to meet the basic needs and optimal health outcomes for socially disadvantaged groups. For example, medical interpretation services should be provided for groups with language barriers to ensure meaningful engagement with their care. In other instances, assigning a community home health nurse for continuity care should be given priority for persons with limited support and experiencing barriers (e.g., financial, transportation) in getting to the health care facility. There should be times when persons facing disadvantaged circumstances deserve and should receive more health resources needed to allow them to achieve their full health potential.

This chapter will describe how social stratification and prejudices about social groups results in unfair distribution of health care resources, placing them at further health disadvantage. We will also provide evidence from social-cognitive psychology about how stigma and stereotyping may create a culture within the medical profession leading to unconscious biases and behaviors that influence clinical decision making. A central thesis is that inequities in the provision of health care and clinical resources are often created and sustained by stereotypes that are ascribed to different social groups by the larger society and its institutions. These inequities lead to substandard quality of care and subsequent disparities in clinical outcomes, with worse health status, in the disadvantaged groups. As an example, racial and ethnic minority groups, including individuals with low or extremely low incomes, can become characterized as lacking in motivation, treatment compliance, and engagement with the health system. These perceptions can then perpetuate or worsen other prevailing adverse social circumstances and health care barriers. We will provide recommendations and strategies from emerging research to promote fair health care resource allocation and reasonable bedside rationing. This will include suggestions for reducing institutional stereotyping, stigma, and psychological biases, which can result in unfair, though inadvertent, clinical judgments even by well-intentioned professionals.

Although this chapter will focus primarily on equitable resource allocation decisions affecting individuals and groups in the context of limited, but not severely constrained, resources (i.e., in higher-income countries), we also recognize important concerns about equity that play out in very-low-income regions. Research on public health care expenditures or distribution of subsidies from government services in low-income countries indicate that such national health care services usually favor the well-off or rich (Mills et al., 2012; Ataguba & McIntyre, 2013; Gwatkin, Bhuiya, & Victora, 2004). In resource-poor and impoverished settings, a cascade of priority-setting decisions or distribution policies made at the national or government level may largely influence clinical decision making and resource allocation at the local clinic setting. That is, resource allocation in health may be influenced by macro-level constraints (such as lack of financial resources, availability of human resources for health, viable health infrastructure, and basic amenities) and by competition with other priorities (such as military, education, and infrastructure spending), leaving the heath care sector poorly funded (Asante & Zwi, 2009; Youngkong, Kapiriri, & Baltussen, 2009). Under these conditions, concerns about human rights to health are inevitable, as the denial or receipt of health care is sometimes based on social factors such as financial ability to pay, living circumstances, productive employment, patient's health literacy or level of insight into illness, level of education, criminal record, poor compliance, substance abuse, and access to treatment facilities (Moosa & Kidd, 2006).

▪ WHAT ARE SOCIALLY DISADVANTAGED PATIENT POPULATIONS AND HOW DO SOCIAL STATUS AND RELATED STEREOTYPES TRANSLATE TO HEALTH OUTCOMES?

Social inequalities, in varying degrees, exist in all societies. Individuals are hierarchically ranked in societies through a system of social stratification that may be based upon ascribed or acquired characteristics or a combination of both. Ascribed characteristics are those attributed to one by others and over which the individual typically has no control. Often they are determined at birth and cannot be changed. Examples of ascribed characteristics include race, ethnicity, gender, and some congenital anomalies/disabilities.

Acquired social characteristics, by contrast, are obtained after birth, such as occupation, education, and money (Berreman, 1972). Social stratification both arises from and reinforces the unequal distribution of resources (i.e., social inequalities), with those ranked at the bottom of the hierarchy having limited access to and control of resources that often are needed for further life success. Because of this dynamic, those on the bottom tend to experience persistent social disadvantages and fare worse than their higher-ranked counterparts on a number of indices including health status, health care access, quality of clinical encounters, and subsequent outcomes. In other words, patients who do not possess valued characteristics, are disadvantaged in society, and are not afforded equal opportunities and access to resources compared to advantaged populations.

For purposes of discussing health care, we can define socially disadvantaged populations as those groups of people who have systematically experienced greater social or economic obstacles to health based on their racial or ethnic group, nationality, religion, socioeconomic status, gender, mental health, cognitive, sensory, or physical disability, sexual orientation, geographic location, or other characteristics that have historically been linked to discrimination, bias, or exclusion (Koh, 2010; Braveman et al., 2011). Societies vary in the characteristics used to stratify individuals and groups, but most use race, ethnicity, gender, religion, social class, or some combination of these characteristics. In the United States, research has primarily focused on the social disadvantage accrued by racial and ethnic minority populations (e.g., African Americans, Hispanics, American Indians, and some Asian-American subpopulations). Numerous national reports have shown that racial and ethnic minorities in the United States have higher rates of morbidities and mortalities (Truman et al., 2011) and lower-quality health care (Smedley et al., 2003; United States. Agency for Healthcare Research and Quality, 2011.) compared to non-Hispanic white populations. European countries, although typically perceived as being more equitable with regard to health care, also exhibit health disparities related to minority ethnic status and nationality. This is especially predominant in countries marked by mass migration and racial and ethnic diversity, such as the United Kingdom, (Bhopal, 2012; Smith et al., 2000; Ahmad & Bradby, 2007), New Zealand (Harris et al., 2012), and The Netherlands (Veling et al., 2007, 2008). Social stratification in Europe has been studied primarily in relation to social class and occupational status. The existence of a socioeconomic gradient in health among European countries has been well established and indicates that the poor have worse outcomes and higher rates of mortality and morbidities than their economically advantaged counterparts (Huijts, Eikemo, & Skalicka, 2010; Kunst et al., 1998; Mackenbach et al., 2008; Mazzuco & Suhrcke, 2011).

■ HOW DO SOCIAL CATEGORIES AND STEREOTYPES SHAPE HEALTH RESOURCE ALLOCATION?

Implicit Bias Among Physicians

There are several ways in which physician's allocation of health care resources can be affected by an individual's or group's social standing. Two in particular are physician implicit biases and underrepresentation in clinical trial research. Such biases stem from messages about social groups that are created, disseminated, and sustained over time in societies via exclusionary policies and institutional cultures. Because of the pervasiveness and subtlety of these social group messages, their acceptance and the influence they have on behaviors and decisions are neither apparent nor conscious processes. It is these nonconscious attitudes and beliefs about social groups, or implicit biases, that play a role in bedside rationing. Research from the sociocognitive literature indicates that health care providers might unconsciously activate negative stereotypes about minority groups or socially disadvantaged populations in a medical setting (Burgess et al., 2007; Vendsborg, Nordentoft, & Lindhardt, 2011; Mulia et al., 2008; Zemore et al., 2011). This retrieval of information about particular social groups is referred to as *stereotype activation* and stems from repeated exposures to explicit stereotypes that have developed into subconscious beliefs (Bodenhausen, 1988). Once stereotypes are activated they are held in working memory outside of conscious awareness, where they direct subsequent cognitive, affective, and behavioral responses (Kunda & Spencer, 2003). Thus, physicians' responses dictated by unconscious or implicit stereotypes often result in implicit biases and behaviors that can affect how socially disadvantaged groups are evaluated, diagnosed, and treated (Moskowitz, Stone, & Childs, 2012).

Indeed, physicians' implicit biases have been shown to influence the allocation of resources to socially disadvantaged patients in health care settings in the United States and Europe. In the United States it has been shown that ethnic minority patients are less likely to be prescribed pain medications than white patients when they present with the same conditions (Mills et al., 2011; Green et al., 2003; Sabin & Greenwald, 2012). Even when minority patients with sickle cell disease, a disorder for which pain is a defining feature and for which African Americans are disproportionately burdened, they are often inadequately treated for pain (Green et al., 2003). There is also documented evidence of inequities in the provision of treatment to socially disadvantaged populations including angioplasty, bypass graft surgery, cardiac catheterization, thrombolysis recommendations, and renal transplantation (Lillie-Blanton et al., 2004; Schulman et al., 1999; Green et al., 2007; Malek et al., 2011).

Empirical research on the influence of physician bias in European and other countries is scant compared to the United States. Nonetheless, there is some evidence that physician biases also affect the allocation of resources to members of socially disadvantaged populations. In the United Kingdom, South Asian persons are less likely to have follow-up appointments scheduled following surgery and less likely to be offered services such as a continuity care by district nurses (Smith et al., 2000). Furthermore, similar disparities in renal transplantation rates have been found in Europe, Australia, Canada, and Japan to those that have been found in the United States, with individuals of higher socioeconomic status more likely to receive a renal transplant even after accounting for medical conditions (Vamos, Novak, & Mucsi, 2009). Mathur and colleagues, in their study on the prescribing of drugs for coronary heart disease, found that gender, ethnic, and age differences existed despite the international agreement that all groups should be prescribed coronary disease drugs (i.e., lipid-modifying drugs, beta blockers, ACE inhibitors/angiotensin receptor blockers, and low-dose aspirin) regardless of age, gender, or ethnicity (Mathur et al., 2011).

Although direct causal links to inequities between physician bias and inequities in care are still debated, evidence shows that, when other causal factors are accounted for, differences remain in the quality and type of care that is provided for socially disadvantaged populations. These findings lead to the conclusion that physician biases play a role in how health care resources are allocated.

In addition to the influence of physician biases on bedside rationing, implicit biases can also exert indirect effects on the allocation of resources via patient–provider communication and patient adherence. Discriminatory behavior on the part of clinicians (as perceived by patients) has been shown to negatively affect the communication of information by patients that allow physicians to make accurate clinical judgments (Harris et al., 2012; Dovidio & Fiske, 2012). Impaired communication between providers and patients inhibits the ability of patients to be involved in the decision-making process (Vamos, Novak, & Mucsi, 2009). This is particularly relevant for bedside rationing, since a patient's ability to articulate his or her wishes is related to the allocation of health care resources (Strech, Synofzik, & Marckmann, 2008).

Underrepresentation of Disadvantaged Patient Groups in Clinical Trials

Underrepresentation of socially disadvantaged patient groups in clinical trials and other evidence data that are used to develop clinical practice guidelines can also shape health resource allocation. Exclusion of groups from these trials may raise issues about inequities, as there is evidence that participants in certain clinical trials have better health outcomes than similar patients treated off the standard clinical trial protocol. Inclusion of underrepresented socially disadvantaged groups in clinical trials validates the generalizability of the findings to the population as a whole. It also provides further opportunities for subgroup analyses to determine if ethnic minority origin, for example, may have influenced the intervention. This is important, because when a treatment is standardized based on a clinical trial that did not include all appropriate patient groups, it may not be optimized for the actual social or cultural demographics of the patient population that were excluded but may have benefited from the trial. Therefore, when some groups are underrepresented in the evidence base, the risk of making inaccurate decisions for people from those groups increases (Karjalainen & Palva, 1989; Greil et al., 1999; Meadows et al., 1983; Davis et al., 1985; Wagner et al., 1995). Several studies have also shown the effect of inclusion in the clinical trial standard protocol, also sometimes known as an *inclusion benefit* (Lantos, 1999; Braunholtz, Edwards, & Lilford, 2001). Underrepresented groups excluded from the protocol are denied "state of the art" treatment for the disease, follow-up consultation, and closer disease monitoring and case management (Heiat, Gross, & Krumholz, 2002). In the absence of evidence of intervention efficacy for unique patient groups, due to exclusion from clinical trials, uncertainty increases, promoting the potential for practice variability. Different physicians may arrive at different answers about the utility of a screening, diagnostic test, or treatment depending on prior probabilities, values, and perhaps stereotypes. In the context of medical uncertainty, physicians more often rely on following prevailing practices, which may include those influenced by stereotypes and unconscious biases. This has particular implications for physician bedside rationing and health resource allocation.

■ SHOULD SOCIAL ADVANTAGE OR DISADVANTAGE BE CONSIDERED IN THE ALLOCATION OF CLINICAL CARE RESOURCES?

Because the ethics of medicine require care decisions not to be based on clinically irrelevant and medically inappropriate criteria, it is appealing to think that social disadvantage should play no role whatsoever in making clinical decisions. But there are several reasons for advising physicians to take a prioritarian approach in the context of making bedside clinical decisions for socially disadvantaged populations. A prioritarian model requires that physicians promote equity and justice in all resource allocation, but also give priority to providing certain uniquely useful services to populations most needy or disadvantaged. A first reason is that higher income, education, power, prestige, and social capital are among some of the most important social determinants that shape health outcomes. There is substantial evidence that a person's chances of illness, death, well-being, and life expectancy are determined by social class and opportunities. The more affluent and better educated individuals are, the healthier their lives and the longer they live. The Whitehall studies of British civil servants show that the higher you are in the organizational social status, measured by occupational class, the better your health status; the lower you are in the social or occupational strata, the worse your health is. (Marmot & Feeney, 1997; Marmot et al., 1991, 2003, 2008; Starfield, 2004; Braveman & Barclay, 2009; Braveman, 2010; Woolf & Braveman, 2011). Societal stratification results in vulnerable groups having inadequate and limited access to various types of social capital including social networks and connections. Socially advantaged groups have better health and outcomes because they have these kinds of resources available to them as a matter of course. Such differences in the degree of advantage experienced by better-off groups are reflected in research studies in their rank in measures of better health and well-being. More educated and affluent individuals are also cushioned from adversity that illness brings because of the opportunities, resources, and options available to them. When poor or vulnerable populations encounter the medical system, many attribute their poor health status to personal decisions and poor life choices when perhaps it may be the result of the rationing of public goods and unfair social policies (Woolf & Braveman, 2011). Less education and limited opportunities can lead to risky patterns of behavior, which, in turn, contribute to poor health. Therefore, giving priority to socially disadvantaged groups is a necessity for the better health and well-being enjoyed by advantaged groups. A prioritization approach to provide uniquely useful services for socially disadvantaged groups that has the potential to improve health outcomes, such as interpreter services and home visits for continuity care for those who experience health care access barriers is not merely compensation; it is meeting a basic health need.

A second reason for taking a prioritarian approach to providing care for disadvantaged groups is because the delivery of quality care includes the ability of the physician to appreciate cultural diversity and its influence on health. The health values and priorities of an individual are shaped by social, economic, physical, and political environmental conditions experienced along their life span—and medical decisions that take these factors into account will result in better outcomes for the individual patient. As described in the prior section, societal stratification often results in stereotypes that can activate implicit biases and negatively influence medical decision making. To reduce the potential for implicit stereotyping and nonconscious bias to impair clinical judgment, explicit attention should be given to this decision-making dynamic when caring for socially disadvantaged populations or stigmatized patients.

That is, *explicit* and *nondiscriminatory* attention can mitigate the effects of *implicit* biases.

A third reason for consideration of socially disadvantaged groups is the need for advocating for evidence-based medicine that focuses on effectiveness and appropriateness in allocating clinical resources for health services to all patient populations including underrepresented groups. Patient-centered care is efficient and effective and is usually informed by consideration of group social and cultural identity (Osborn & Squires, 2012; Aysola et al., 2013; Berenson et al., 2012; Grant, 2012). By considering and prioritizing care for socially disadvantaged groups, physicians will ensure and promote inclusiveness in clinical trials to improve the evidence base. Underrepresentation of socially disadvantaged groups in clinical trials that eventually determines the efficacy of interventions and their role in health care resource allocation becomes particularly salient in an era when personalized medicine is being emphasized. When resources are scarce, clinical evidence can help to make allocation decisions that minimize waste of resources on ineffective or inappropriate treatments and that maximize the use of resources. In the context of medical uncertainties, physicians would then have to rely on the prevailing practices, which may include those influenced by stereotypes and unconscious biases. Therefore, if physicians advocate for all their patients to be adequately represented in clinical trials, and facilitate their enrollment, this would help to promote fair allocation of clinical resources.

▪ GLOBAL EFFORTS PROMOTING POLICY INTERVENTIONS ON MACRO-LEVEL RESOURCE ALLOCATION

Many countries are implementing policies geared toward promoting policy to address the health of socially disadvantaged populations. In Australia, for example, studies revealing clustering of social disadvantage beginning in very early childhood associated with poorer health outcomes have prompted integration of health and social policies including targeted interventions to address indigenous groups and persons experiencing disadvantaged circumstances within the health system. (Feldman et al., 2009; Nicholson et al., 2012; Broom, 1984). In Brazil, attention has been paid to promoting equity-enhancing policy initiatives, such as conditional cash transfers, and limiting social inequalities as a means of narrowing health disparities (Guanais, 2010). In the United States, the Department of Health and Human Services has committed to reducing racial and ethnic disparities and achieving health equity. National action plans outline the goals and objectives the department will take toward that end (Koh, Graham, & Glied 2011). A Commission to End Health Care Disparities has been formed that is cochaired by leaders of the American Medical Association, the National Medical Association, and the National Hispanic Medical Association, which includes representatives from more than 70 aligned health professional organizations working toward the elimination of disparities (Commission to End Health Care Disparities, 2007). Within the European Commission, health equity has become an important component of the regional investments in economic and social development, with policy initiatives being promoted to reduce economic and social disparities. Globally, the World Health Organization (WHO) and its regional organizations have made equity a central issue on its agenda, and WHO Europe has set up a European review of "Social Determinants and the Health Divide" to provide recommendations that will feed into a new strategy for health equity for the region (Marmot et al., 2012; Bell, Taylor, & Marmot, 2010; Friel & Marmot, 2011). As evidenced by global efforts to address health disparities, social status has to be considered a priority in order to provide care that is fair and beneficial to all members of society. Thus. efforts need to be undertaken at the policy level as well as at the physician level where health resources are allocated.

■ WHAT SPECIFIC STRATEGIES CAN BE IMPLEMENTED BY PHYSICIANS TO PROMOTE EQUITABLE ALLOCATION OF RESOURCES TO MEET THE NEEDS OF SOCIALLY DISADVANTAGED POPULATIONS?

There are a number of practical strategies that can be adopted to address concerns about the ethical allocation of health care resources when caring for disadvantaged patient groups.

It is essential to consider both individual and institutional approaches, because most physicians work within organizations and systems (medical groups, government health coverage schemes, insurance companies, or managed care organizations) that provide direct guidance regarding the allocation of resources. In addition, it is important to avoid suggesting that "one size fits all" when it comes to fair allocation of resources in the care of socially disadvantaged and otherwise stigmatized populations. Even though the challenges of fair resource allocation among these populations are largely similar across all countries, there are no "magic bullets" for fair and equitable allocation of limited health care resources. The principles of accessible and affordable health care that all these countries aspire to achieve are in concert with the wider value of equal opportunity espoused in democratic societies. At the same time, however, each society, and often each community, must work to optimize use of local resources using relevant, locally available evidence including social as well as medical appropriateness criteria and evidence for improved population health that can be specific to local population groups.

The proposed strategies outlined below address general strategies for physicians as well as recommendations for ways that organizations and systems can support them. In general, physicians and their organizations should collect data on the social status and other key demographic factors of the patients they see, including race and ethnicity, especially in settings where patients are from diverse communities. In addition, they should collect data on the quality of care they deliver to every patient and use these data to track whether they are or are not, in fact, providing disparate quality care to disadvantaged individuals and groups.

Strategies for Physicians and How Their Organizations Can Support Them

The specific strategies listed below offer approaches that promote fairness in the clinical decision-making process by basing decisions on patient need and aiming to minimize or eliminate any negative influence of bias, discrimination, or stereotypes. Emphasis is given to strategies that have been shown to be effective across multiple settings, are based on evidence, and are helpful in achieving health equity for socially disadvantaged and stigmatized groups.

Strategy 1: Promote awareness of the negative consequences of stereotyping and bias within the clinical setting

Before a physician can attempt to correct negative consequences of stereotyping and biases, they must be aware that these biases exist. Physicians should be educated about the psychosocial processes of stereotyping, implicit bias, and prejudices that can promote unfair decision making and perpetuate health inequalities (Balsa & McGuire, 2003; van Ryn, 2002). This knowledge can sometimes prompt corrective action (Moskowitz, 2001; Burgess et al., 2007; Green et al., 2007). Even if the mere awareness of implicit bias is not sufficient to ensure that effective reduction efforts take place, it is a crucial starting point that can prompt physicians to seek out and implement strategies to mitigate its effects.

What physicians can do: Individual physicians can seek out information on implicit bias, including by attending training sessions that address implicit bias. Participants in these sessions can help ensure that they fully understand what implicit bias is and how it manifests in everyday decisions and behavior through active participation, asking questions or taking the Implicit Association Test (IAT) to assess their own levels of implicit bias. (Greenwald,

McGhee, & Schwartz, 1998; see Implicit Association Test: https://implicit. harvard.edu/implicit/.)

What organizations and systems can do: Medical schools, other training programs, and care delivery organizations can provide training to explain implicit bias and how it can affect medical decision making. These programs can include presenting participants with skills and strategies to use to reduce the negative effects of implicit bias. This may also include engaging them in critical thinking activities designed to help in tailoring strategies for various socially disadvantaged populations (Stone & Moskowitz, 2011).

For physicians, this type of training can be more effective if the program includes a physician as facilitator. The presence of a physician may make the discussion less threatening, and other physicians may respond more favorably when one of their colleagues advocates for an ethical position. It may also help stimulate dialogue among the physicians to figure out effective culturally and clinically relevant strategies within their own practices.

Small-group exercises and other experiential learning techniques can also make learning about implicit bias more personally relevant. In addition, training that provides illustrative examples of implicit bias across several disciplines and social situations can help participants realize the pervasiveness of the issue. Exercises that demonstrate the broad application of the phenomenon beyond social disadvantage to race, social class, age, weight, and other stigmatized categories can also be useful (Wilks & Austin, 1991).

Strategy 2: Identify and appreciate group and individual differences

In general, medical schools and health care organizations should strive to have a workforce representative of the societies they serve (Drake & Lowenstein, 1998). Several studies have shown that diversity in a medical student body is associated with preparing the students to better serve diverse populations they may encounter (Saha et al., 2008). Medical students and physicians from diverse cultural, ethnic, race, and social groups are more likely to perceive unfair treatment of patients from socially disadvantaged groups and advocate for fair allocation of resources (Wilson et al., 2004). Recognizing the potential role of stereotyping and implicit bias does not mean ignoring group and individual differences. In fact, cultivating greater awareness of and sensitivity to group and individual differences has been shown to be an effective method of reducing the negative effects of bias and stereotyping. Training seminars that acknowledge and promote an appreciation of group differences and multicultural viewpoints can help reduce implicit bias (Hickling, 2012; Teal et al., 2010; Rudman, Ashmore, & Gary, 2001).

Cultural competency and diversity training seminars in heterogeneous societies and with ethnic minorities can serve as a starting point from which the culture of the medical institution can change. When leadership actively embraces social diversity and multiculturalism, those actions can influence others (Aarts, Gollwitzer, & Hassin 2004; Wynia et al., 2006). A system-wide effort to cultivate a workplace environment that supports cultural norms, while supporting diversity, is important in reducing individual-level implicit bias. It can also affect patient experiences of care; in one study, organizations that scored higher on a cross-cultural communication measure were rated substantially higher by patients on quality of care and trust measures (Wynia et al., 2010). Culturally competent quality improvement and targeted interventions can help to reduce health disparities by differentially targeting the disadvantaged groups (Green et al., 2010). Cultural competence training programs should be pursued carefully, however, since mandatory training or other imposed pressure on physicians to comply with prioritarian standards toward a racial or ethnic group may elicit hostility and resistance from some types of individuals, failing to reduce implicit bias (Plant & Devine, 2001). In addition, concern has been raised that some methods of cultural competence training (e.g., teaching about "typical" attitudes or beliefs of ethnic minority patient groups) can actually reinforce stereotypes and prejudice (Betancourt et al., 2004; Mendoza, Gollwitzer, & Amodio, 2010; Plant & Devine, 2001).

What the physician can do: Physicians should seek out and elect to participate in diversity training and cultural competence seminars. Physicians can pursue this learning to promote an appreciation of group differences and multicultural viewpoints. Routine exposure can help physicians develop the greater social awareness needed to overcome implicit biases. In addition, using techniques like mindfulness can help physicians understand and define patients in multiple ways other than in terms of ethnicity, race, class, or occupational status, which can reduce implicit bias (Djikic, Langer, & Stapleton, 2008; Lebrecht et al., 2009; Corcoran, Hundhammer, & Mussweiler, 2009).

(a) Seek out the company of other professionals who demonstrate egalitarian goals. Surrounding oneself with other physicians who are committed to social equality will help positively influence one's own implicit beliefs and behaviors in the long run.

(b) Cultivate curiosity about different cultures and invest extra effort into identifying the unique attributes of socially disadvantaged or otherwise stigmatized groups. In particular, physicians and their medical teams should consider the factors that make individual members of socially disadvantaged groups unique—particularly from other members of the same social group. This type of conscious exercise will help reduce one's reliance on social or ethnic stereotypes when evaluating or interacting with these patients.

What the medical organization can do: In diverse societies, recruitment of a workforce that is representative of the patient population is seen as critical to meeting their health needs (Reede, 2003). Diversity is not only necessary to promote equitable care, but it is also an important part of the effort to improve quality of care. Medical organizations and systems can provide routine diversity training and continuing medical educational credits for voluntary participation in elective diversity or multiculturalism seminars. Respected senior physicians and medical educators, including those from socially disadvantaged backgrounds, could serve as role models in this context to promote prioritarian goals. Prioritarian behavior demonstrated by physician leaders can help encourage similar goals throughout the medical institution.

Strategy 3 : Address sources of ambiguity in the decision-making context by establishing standards and support tools to help guide consistent decisions while supporting shared decision making and individualized care

Ambiguity may arise for cases in which the formal guidelines or medical protocols for clinical judgment are somewhat vague (e.g., in cases of medical uncertainty, procedures that involve some degree of discretion on behalf of the physician, or when there is insufficient evidence base from clinical trials for the population group; see Corning & Bucchianeri, 2010). With sufficiently robust and structured efforts, attempts to consciously control the effects of implicit bias can be successful (Payne, 2005; Stewart & Payne, 2008). To do this, physicians must be explicitly mindful of their decision-making processes. An overt, deliberate process can help minimize stereotype activation and bias and help the physician to objectively consider the medical facts at hand instead of relying on prejudices, stereotypes, or intuition. At a minimum, for example, physicians can mitigate implicit bias by simply engaging in mental perspective-taking exercises (such as imagining themselves in the other person's situation; see Galinsky & Moskowitz, 2000).

What the physician can do: Physicians can help to promote underrepresented socially disadvantaged groups into clinical trials. There are several barriers that have been shown to hinder participation in clinical trials for disparity groups, including ethnic minorities. This includes, fear and mistrust, inappropriate exclusion criteria, sociocultural barriers, stereotypes, cultural myths, and consent issues (Ross et al., 1999; Hussain-Gambles, Atkin, & Leese, 2004). Physicians can help promote culturally sensitive research methods, materials, and data collection instruments (e.g., questionnaires) to ensure that issues such as language, education, cultural beliefs, customs, and access to health care are appropriately addressed. This knowledge will inform the design of culturally sensitive studies, enable diverse representation of eligible socially disadvantaged groups, and ensure that the benefits of the clinical trial are made available to all groups (Killien et al., 2000; Hussain-Gambles et al., 2004). In situations of clinical uncertainty, physicians could develop a structure for thoughtful clinical decision making that can help avoid being inadvertently guided by stereotypes. An example is weighing a specific set of evidence-based practices or approaches before providing a treatment plan to minimize the opportunity for implicit bias (Uhlmann & Cohen, 2005).

Physicians can also proactively commit to developing specific decision-making criteria for common clinical scenarios. Before arriving at a clinical decision context characterized by uncertainty, or in situations that permit greater discretion of clinical care, physicians could establish their own informal structure or follow suggested protocol (if instituted) to help create more objective structures in the decision-making process. Physicians could commit to these decision-making criteria before reviewing clinical cases to minimize the impact of implicit bias on the reasoning process. There are a number of decision-support tools and processes designed to promote greater deliberative (as opposed to intuitive) thinking in decision-making processes (Ali, Shah, & Tandon, 2011; Guimond et al., 2003; Anton et al., 2009; Jacobs, 1997; Kastner & Straus, 2008). These tools and processes, many of which are untested as yet, might serve as vehicles for research-based decision making and self-checking exercises that could demonstrably mitigate the impact of implicit bias. The recommendations, therefore, include the following:

(a) Use formal decision support tools, including those that facilitate shared decision making. Sharing one's reasoning process with the patient and engaging in shared decision making can also positively affect perceptions of fairness.

(b) Develop a deliberate note-taking process. When reviewing clinical evidence or forming a decision on clinical resource allocation for socially disadvantaged group members, physicians can take notes throughout the process of providing care so that they are not forced to rely on memory, which may fall more easily to biased decisions.

(c) Articulate the reasoning process for resource-allocation decisions. When physicians carefully document the reasoning behind an allocation decision in some way before implementing it, this can help them critically assess their reasoning processes for implicit bias before committing to a decision.

(d) Checklists. The use of checklists that list some "best practice" questions or exercises could prompt physicians to more systematically reflect on and scrutinize the reasoning behind any decision for possible bias. This strategy may be particularly useful after the physician has received implicit bias and diversity training. It is also probably more useful when the process is voluntary. When physicians who have not received training on implicit bias or diversity rely on a checklist, their efforts to correct for bias may be sporadic and restricted to isolated cases. Worse yet, if unwilling physicians are forced to use these checklists, the procedure could backfire, causing resentment and actually increasing biases.

What the medical organization can do: The organization could establish and institute protocols that physicians could follow to help identify sources of ambiguity and offer suggestions on how to reduce these types of clinical uncertainty in the decision-making context. There may also be a role for consultation with an expert for specific situations that are marked by uncertainty and carry the risk of implicit bias influencing decision making. However, the downside of obtaining expert consultation is that they might not have been trained in strategies to engage in deliberative thinking and other methods to reduce the impact of implicit bias on judgment. In such situations, the goal of reducing implicit bias through routine consultation with an expert who has been trained in a specific specialty might not succeed.

The organization can also develop guidance on strategies to correct for implicit bias. Research-based strategies include providing instructions to walk people through a perspective-taking exercise (Galinsky & Moskowitz, 2000), checking decisions for bias by imagining how one would evaluate the socially disadvantaged or stigmatized group, and providing a list of specific triggers to promote counter-stereotypic thoughts (Mendoza, Gollwitzer, & Amodio, 2010).

Organizations can also institute formal protocols to promote the use of decision support tools for guidance and to support shared decision making. Physician organizations could establish best-practice protocols to help their members identify and override implicit bias. These protocols could help minimize ambiguity and therefore reduce the impact implicit and unconscious bias.

Strategy 4: Identify distractions and sources of stress in the decision-making environment and remove or reduce them

Implicit biases play a larger role in decision making when decisions are made under stress, including that due to time pressure. Physicians need to have enough time and resources to thoroughly process medical information on socially disadvantaged group members to avoid relying on intuitive reasoning processes that can result in biased judgments during clinical care.

What the physician can do: The physician can allow for more time when providing care for socially disadvantaged group members or stigmatized groups in which implicit bias may be a concern. Wherever possible, physicians should prepare in advance for clinical resource decision-making situations in which socially disadvantaged or stigmatized patients are involved. Advance planning can allow physicians to devote more time during their decision-making process reviewing the facts of the particular medical case before committing to a decision. Team-based decision making might also prove useful, especially if the team itself is culturally diverse.

What the medical organization can do: An organizational review could help the medical institution evaluate whether and/or how the organization is acting to prevent bias, or to mitigate the effects of implicit bias, in clinical decision making. Part of this review should include a critical assessment of the burden on physicians and the medical team. Some environmental stressors can adversely affect physician performance and medical decision making by leading to increased physician reliance on stereotypes for decision making. This includes the demands on time with each patient (as a result of heavy caseload of patients with limited time for patient interaction and/or complex clinical cases), fatigue (as a result of long hours or other emergency situations), and distractions (as a result of multitasking, overburdened workloads). Organizations could modify procedures to allow physicians sufficient time to consider each patient case by case; for example, reorganizing the physician schedules to reduce the typical caseload, minimizing spur-of-the-moment decisions, or offering the physician flexibility to reconvene with a team when further deliberation on care is desired.

Strategy 5: Institute feedback mechanisms on potential physician biases

Providing consensus information (i.e., information that others in one's group hold similar prioritarian beliefs rather than adhere to stereotypic beliefs) and other feedback mechanisms can be powerful tools in promoting more prioritarian attitudes and behavior in a community (Sechrist & Stangor, 2001). Therefore, one way to encourage individual physicians' efforts in addressing implicit biases might be for organizations to provide physicians and other medical professionals with relevant performance feedback. As part of this process, the organization should consider the type of clinical decision-making data currently available or easily obtained that would offer physicians meaningful but nonthreatening feedback on potential biases. Transparent feedback from regular or intermittent peer reviews that raise personal awareness of biases could prompt those with prioritarian motives to do more to prevent implicit bias in future clinical decisions and actions. This feedback should include concrete suggestions on how to improve performance (Mendoza, Gollwitzer, & Amodio, 2010) and could also involve recognition of those individuals who display exceptional fairness as positive reinforcement.

Feedback tends to work best when it (a) comes from a legitimate, respected authority, (b) addresses the person's decision-making process rather than simply the decision outcome, and (c) is provided before the person commits to a decision rather than afterwards, when he or she has already committed to a particular course of action (Lerner & Tetlock, 1999). Feedback mechanisms that apply coercive pressure to comply with prioritarian standards can elicit hostility from some types of individuals and fail to mitigate implicit bias. By inciting hostility, these imposed standards may even be counterproductive to prioritarian goals, generating backlash in the form of increased explicit and implicit prejudice (Legault, Gutsell, & Inzlicht, 2011).

What the physician can do: Physicians can actively seek feedback from others. They can seek out their own informal "checks and balances" or consult with a skilled mentor or senior colleague for objective feedback on how to handle a challenging case or difficult situation.

(a) Actively seek feedback from others regarding past performance when feasible. Physicians could talk to colleagues or others to request performance feedback. This information could be helpful in determining whether a person's current efforts to control or reduce implicit bias are effective or could be improved.

(b) Articulate the reasoning process. To ensure sound reasoning in every case, physicians could choose to document or articulate the underlying logic of their decisions. Not only does this exercise afford the opportunity to critically review their clinical decision-making processes in each case, but taking it a step further—making this reasoning transparent—can have positive effects on public perceptions of fairness.

What the organization can do: Adopt a physician peer-review process. Physicians could benefit from additional feedback to help improve quality of care, and this feedback could incorporate consideration of possible implicit bias in clinical decision making. The organization could have physicians observe and provide feedback to one another on a rotating schedule. An experienced team of peer physicians could review the medical records for a few past select cases of patients from socially disadvantaged or stigmatized groups. The team would then provide performance feedback and suggestions, if necessary, for improvement. The organizational team should be trained to deliver this feedback in a constructive, nonthreatening way.

(a) ***Develop a committee dedicated to ensuring equitable care for disadvantaged patient groups.*** Physician organizations can develop a dedicated committee to oversee the informal internal grievance process that receives anonymous complaints about clinical decision making or resource allocation in the sensitive domain of socially disadvantaged groups, including complaints about racial and ethnic fairness. Similar to the peer review process mentioned above, this committee (or a select group of trained peer or mentor physicians) could review a sample of past clinical cases or observe workplace behavior and offer feedback and guidance. The group can also review hypothetical cases involving implicit bias, reveal their decisions, and discuss their reasoning for their actions frankly and candidly. This process can help physicians think more deliberatively about the possibility of implicit biases entering their decisions and offers a forum to obtain feedback from peers.

Strategy 6: Increase exposure to counter-stereotypes and reduce exposure to stereotypes of socially disadvantaged groups

Increased contact with counter-stereotypes—specifically, increased exposure to stigmatized group members that contradict social stereotypes—can help negate stereotypes, affirm counter-stereotypes, and "deactivate" the associations that underlie implicit bias. Exposure can include imagining counter-stereotypes (Blair, Ma, & Lenton, 2001), incidentally observing counter-stereotypes in the environment (Dasgupta & Greenwald, 2001; Olson & Fazio, 2006), engaging with counter-stereotypic role models (Dasgupta & Rivera, 2006, 2008; Dasgupta & Asgari, 2004), or extensive practice making counter-stereotypic associations (Kawakami et al., 2000).

In addition to promoting contact with counter-stereotypes, this strategy also involves decreased exposure to stereotypes. Certain environmental cues can automatically trigger stereotype activation and implicit bias. Images and language that are a part of any signage, pamphlets, brochures, instructional manuals, background music, or any other verbal or visual communications in the clinical environment may inadvertently activate implicit biases because they convey stereotypic information (Devine, 1989). Identifying these communications and removing them or replacing them with nonstereotypic or counter-stereotypic information can help decrease the daily exposure that physicians have with the types of social stereotypes that underlie implicit bias.

What the physician can do: The physician can imagine counter-stereotypes or seek out images of admired exemplars. To reduce the impact of implicit bias on clinical judgment, physicians could imagine or view images of admired or counter-stereotypic exemplars of the stereotyped social group before entering a decision-making scenario that could activate these social stereotypes.

(a) *Seek greater exposure or contact with counter-stereotypic role models*. Physicians who are motivated to become more egalitarian could also spend more time in the presence of socially disadvantaged group members who are counter-stereotypic role models, to mentally reinforce counter-stereotypic associations and reverse thoughts about traditional stereotypes.

(b) *Practice making counter-stereotypic associations*. Physicians who are motivated to change their automatic reactions should practice making positive associations with socially disadvantaged and stigmatized minority groups, affirming counter-stereotypes, and negating stereotypes. Implicit biases may be automatic, but corrective and deactivation strategies can also become automated with motivation and practice.

What the organization can do: The organization can seek to promote and follow equal-opportunity and affirmative action (EOAA) hiring practices. Members of stigmatized groups, when fairly represented and valued, can offer authoritative roles with opportunities to foster positive intergroup relations within the organization (Richeson & Ambady, 2003). This can also present other physicians with readily accessible counter-stereotypes that they can draw upon to reduce implicit bias.

■ THE CHALLENGES OF FAIR BEDSIDE RESOURCE ALLOCATION IN LOW-INCOME COUNTRIES

Considerations for Low-Income Countries with Impoverished Health Systems and Severe Resource Limitations

Fair bedside allocation by physicians of scarce health resources in impoverished settings is an undertaking that deserves attention well beyond the scope of this chapter. However, this section briefly introduces and acknowledges the important yet difficult challenge of assuring fairness and equity for socially disadvantaged populations in developing countries.

Addressing issues is especially important because it can potentially lead to solutions for policymaking in health care and maintain donor country interest in supporting underfunded sectors (Wikler, 2003; Youngkong, Kapiriri, & Baltussen, 2009).

Like high-income countries, low-income and impoverished regions face issues related to stereotypes, bias, and discrimination when attempting to provide equitable health care. But health care in these settings is typically provided in an environment where there are tremendous health needs and often limited resources even among those that are more socially advantaged. Often, fair priority setting in health care is made even more difficult due to political instability, inadequate social sectors, underdeveloped institutions, and the ubiquity of marked social inequalities (Kapiriri & Martin, 2007). Government expenditure in the health care sector is often so limited that even if it were fairly distributed, it would fall far short of fully financing all health needs. In addition, the human resources available for healthcare in these regions countries are significantly limited (Narasimhan et al., 2004). Given extreme health workforce shortages, many countries rely on a range of midlevel practitioners or nonphysician clinicians such as clinical officers, medical assistants, and community nurses to provide clinical care (Mullan & Frehywot, 2007; Mshana, 1993). Logistical problems in the distribution of health care services, facilities, equipment, and drugs are also pervasive, with rural settings being particularly disadvantaged. Rural facilities tend to be severely underfunded and face shortages of personnel, drugs, and equipment, while urban or central outpatient public hospitals and clinics are overcrowded. Meanwhile, investments in relatively expensive advanced technology tend to be monopolized by socially advantaged groups, as there may be no provision to subsidize the cost for the poor, while even simple, low-cost interventions and primary care for the rest of the population are limited (Gwatkin, Bhuiya, & Victora, 2004; Jayasinghe et al., 1998).

In sum, health care resource allocation in developing countries has three distinct characteristics: (1) the chronic and severe shortage of a multitude of basic resources, (2) the resulting specificity of the rationing decisions that need to be made, and (3) the very high risk that explicit and implicit rationing decisions will favor advantaged populations because of the inherent human tendency of empowered decision makers to ensure their own well-being by serving those with the ability to pay.

Can the set of strategies listed above work for physicians in developing countries with fragile health systems where the threats to fairness in clinical decision making and resource allocation are much greater? If not, or if they are not sufficient, then what additional strategies are needed for settings with severely limited resources and dramatic allocation challenges?

A human rights paradigm constitutes a widely shared foundation for addressing the effects of globalization and resource inequalities in developing countries (Backman et al., 2008; Hunt & Backman, 2008). In this paradigm, developed and developing countries alike bear responsibility for their national health plans consistent with their universal human rights obligations, which include the principles of ensuring nondiscrimination and the participation of affected communities in the development and implementation of health policies and programs. However, the challenge confronting physicians in developing countries is how to adhere to human rights principles when hunger, poverty, sometimes war, and minimal health care resources are everyday circumstances. Some physicians may have to make daily difficult decisions concerning priorities for clinical care within a very long list of critical patient needs.

Physicians in lower-income and limited-resource settings sometimes feel that resource allocation decisions are made at the national level or within their ministries of health and do not perceive themselves as "bedside rationing agents" (Johansson et al., 2011). But even so, the potential for physicians to be influenced by bias and discrimination in clinical care of patient groups exists in these nations, just as in the developed world. For example, Moosa and Kidd describe the 25-year experience of the government-requested Western Cape Committee in South Africa, composed of a renal care team that decided whether patients presenting with end-stage renal disease would be accepted or rejected for dialysis treatment. Those accepted were more often white, under 40 years old, nondiabetic, with fewer complications, and were more often employed and married with dependents. Those rejected, who were thereby relegated to dying of their disease in the near term, had more complicated diseases, were relatively more often ethnic black South Africans or nonwhite, over 40, unemployed, lived farther away from the dialysis center, and were generally socially disadvantaged (Moosa & Kidd, 2006). While the interactions between these factors are complex, not all are medically relevant or ethically appropriate criteria for decision making according to standards in the developed world. (Council on Ethical and Judicial Affairs, American Medical Association, 1994a, 1994b, 1995; Lundberg 2004; Code of ethics of the Canadian Medical Association, 1997; Kotalik, 2002). In another study of bedside rationing by practitioners in Uganda, various forms of rationing (denial, dilution, deflection, deterrence, delay, and termination) of first-line drugs and beneficial therapy were based on severity of patient's condition and ability to benefit from treatment but also on criteria like age, ability to pay, social status, and perceived potential for compliance (Kapiriri & Martin, 2006). Other studies have shown that in South Asia and sub-Saharan Africa, physicians and nurses still hold discriminatory views toward HIV-positive individuals and exhibit negative stereotypes and bias preventing them from providing optimal quality care to these patients (Ahsan Ullah, 2011). Prejudice against people with mental illness, including high rates of nontreatment, has also been documented in developing countries (Thornicroft, 2008).

What Physicians, Medical Organizations, and Systems in Developing Countries Can Do

Implicit bias and its negative effects are clearly present in low-income countries. This indicates that the previously listed strategies are relevant and might be helpful in mitigating the risk that disadvantaged populations will face additional discrimination and disadvantage when they encounter the health care system. However, these strategies must be carefully interpreted and applied in the context of the country. In the course of mitigating the effects of discrimination and bias, strategies for physicians should be tailored to societal needs and culturally relevant to the communities in question. In developing countries with extreme health workforce shortages, for example, the role of physicians—especially in the public system—may be different. As a result of their limited numbers, a larger proportion of physicians are likely to have administrative, teaching, and policy roles, on top of their clinical care roles. Each of these roles can have effects on resource-allocation decision making at the bedside. As educators and important role models, physicians have a heightened responsibility to establish and demonstrate positive attitudes toward all patients including socially disadvantaged and stigmatized groups. Finally, in many settings physicians will also play an important policy role in the allocation of public health resources and public health prevention programs such as immunization priorities, use of antiretroviral therapy, or anti-tuberculosis medications allocated to regional health centers or hospitals.

Because of the critical role of the physician elaborated above, relevant key strategies should consider the potential broad range of their responsibilities and include enhanced training that addresses issues such as the following:

(a) Selection into medicine. Medical institutions in developing countries could emphasize affirmative action for applicants from rural and socially disadvantaged backgrounds in order to train more doctors conversant with issues faced by rural, poor, and socially disadvantaged or marginalized populations.

(b) Awareness of distributional justice. During medical training, educators could teach and raise issues of medical ethics, human rights, and distributional justice in the cultural context of the country and region. Cultural competence during training could be promoted and offered in continuing education programs, especially for publicly employed physicians.

(c) Training in health policy. Medical institutions could promote knowledge of basic health policy to adequately prepare physician leaders for the policy aspects of rationing that they are going to face in low-resource settings.

(d) Establishing nondiscriminatory standards and promoting distributional justice in mission statements. In all training programs, medical organizations, and physician institutions, nondiscrimination and distributional justice could be made an essential element of the organizational mission statement.

■ CONCLUSIONS

Providing equitable care in the context of limited resources to socially disadvantaged individuals and groups can be challenging for a number of reasons. Socially disadvantaged groups are often stigmatized in a society. This stigma and ensuing prejudices result in these groups experiencing social and economic obstacles to health. When they encounter the health care system, socially disadvantaged individuals, compared to their more advantaged counterparts, are often disadvantaged because of unfair distribution of resources and subsequent outcomes of inequalities. This disadvantage can be further exacerbated when physicians have biases (implicit or explicit) regarding these groups that can affect the quality and content of the care they provide.

Even in situations where physician biases do not influence clinical decisions, socially disadvantaged groups may still be treated unfairly. Many clinical practice guidelines are developed as a result of clinical trials. When socially disadvantaged groups are underrepresented in clinical trials, the treatment and care provided to them may be inappropriate and further disadvantage them in clinical settings. Numerous strategies can be employed by both physicians and health care organizations to help ensure that socially disadvantaged groups receive fair treatment. Awareness of the consequences of stereotyping and biases can be encouraged, as well as the understanding and appreciation of individual and group differences. Developing standards to guide decision making and creating environments that minimize stress and distractions could also aid physicians in providing fair and appropriate treatment to socially disadvantaged groups.

From the most affluent to the most destitute health care settings, there exists a finite supply of health care resources that makes rationing unavoidable. However, rationing must be done in an equitable manner to the benefit of all members of society. Discriminatory or exclusionary practices leading to unequal distribution of resources are tightly linked with health equity. The social inequities in opportunities, resources, and constraints produce unequal chances in life and can impact health outcomes if these inequities are perpetuated. A prioritarian approach to clinical decision making and allocation of resources for disadvantaged groups promotes equity and justice and assures those uniquely beneficial services for health and well-being that are otherwise not available for these groups. It also assures fairness and equity. Fair bedside rationing becomes a challenge when decisions are marked by uncertainty and clinical discretion—and are therefore especially prone to influence by implicit factors, including stereotypes and bias.

The goals of this chapter were to examine the issues in fair resource allocation among socially disadvantaged groups and to suggest strategies that would help to overcome them through a prioritarian model. Even though this chapter primarily emphasized the prioritization of resources to disadvantaged groups in contexts where resources are abundant, albeit limited, it was noted that fair allocation of resources in resource-poor settings (i.e., developing countries) may be more challenging. Many of the issues that affect the fair allocation of resources to socially disadvantaged groups in developed countries also are present in developing countries (e.g., bias, discrimination, etc.). Additionally, these countries have to contend with other issues such as political instability, fragmented and underdeveloped institutions, and influences from external international donors, which can influence the fair allocation of health care resources. Overall, physicians and organizations can undertake specific actions to promote equity and prioritarianism, thereby increasing the odds that fairness in resource allocation will reduce rather than exacerbate health disparities in socially disadvantaged groups.

REFERENCES

Aarts, H., Gollwitzer, P. M., & Hassin, R. R. (2004). Goal contagion: perceiving is for pursuing. *Journal of Personality and Social Psychology*, 87 (1):23–37. doi: 10.1037/0022-3514.87.1.23.

Ahmad, W. I., & Bradby, H. (2007). "Locating ethnicity and health: exploring concepts and contexts." *Sociology of Health & Illness*, 29 (6):795–810. doi: 10.1111/j.1467-9566. 2007.01051.x.

Ahsan Ullah, A. K. (2011). "HIV/AIDS-Related Stigma and Discrimination: A Study of Health Care Providers in Bangladesh." *Journal of the International Association of Physicians in AIDS Care (Chic)*, 10 (2):97–104. doi: 10.1177/1545109710381926.

Ali, M. K., Shah, S., & Tandon, N. (2011). Review of electronic decision-support tools for diabetes care: a viable option for low- and middle-income countries? *Journal of Diabetes Science and Technology*, 5 (3):553–570.

Anton, B. B., Schafer, J. J., Micenko, A., Wolf, D. M., DiNucci, S., Donovan, P., & Jordan, B. (2009). Clinical decision support. How CDS tools impact patient care outcomes. *Journal of Healthcare Information Management*, 23 (1):39–45.

Asante, A. D., & Zwi, A. B. (2009). Factors influencing resource allocation decisions and equity in the health system of Ghana. *Public Health*, 123 (5):371–377.

Ataguba, J. E., & McIntyre, D. (2013). Who benefits from health services in South Africa? *Health Economics, Policy and Law*, 8(1):21–46.

Aysola, J., Bitton, A., Zaslavsky, A. M., & Ayanian, J. Z. (2013). Quality and equity of primary care with patient-centered medical homes: results from a national survey. *Med Care*, 51 (1):68–77.

Backman, G., Hunt, P., Khosla, R., Jaramillo-Strouss, C., Fikre, B. M., Rumble, C., et al. (2008). Health systems and the right to health: an assessment of 194 countries. *Lancet*, 372 (9655):2047–2085.

Balsa, A. I., & McGuire, T. G. (2003). Prejudice, clinical uncertainty and stereotyping as sources of health disparities. *Journal of Health Economics*, 22 (1):89–116.

Bell, R., S. Taylor, & Marmot, M. (2010). Global health governance: commission on social determinants of health and the imperative for change. *Journal of Law, Medicine & Ethics*, 38 (3):470–485.

Berenson, J., Doty, M. M., Abrams, M. K., & Shih A. (2012). Achieving better quality of care for low-income populations: the roles of health insurance and the medical home in reducing health inequities. *Issue Brief (Commonwealth Fund)*, 11:1–18.

Berreman, G. D. (1972). Race, Caste, and Other Invidious Distinctions in Social Stratification. *Race*, 13 (4):385–414.

Betancourt, J. R., Carrillo, J. E., Green, A. R., & Maina, A. (2004). Barriers to health promotion and disease prevention in the Latino population. *Clinical Cornerstone*, 6 (3):16–26; discussion 27–9.

Bhopal, R. S. (2012). The quest for culturally sensitive health-care systems in Scotland: insights for a multi-ethnic Europe. *Journal of Public Health*, 34 (1):5–11.

Blair, I. V., Ma, J. E., & Lenton, A. P. (2001). Imagining stereotypes away: the moderation of implicit stereotypes through mental imagery. *Journal of Personality and Social Psychology*, 81 (5):828–841.

Bodenhausen, G. V. (1988). Stereotypic biases in social decision making and memory: testing process models of stereotype use. *Journal of Personality and Social Psychology*, 55 (5):726–737.

Braunholtz, D. A., Edwards, S. J., & Lilford, R. J. (2001). Are randomized clinical trials good for us (in the short term)? Evidence for a "trial effect". *Journal of Clinical Epidemiology*, 54 (3):217–224.

Braveman, P. (2010). Social conditions, health equity, and human rights. *Health and Human Rights*, 12 (2):31–48.

Braveman, P. A., Kumanyika, S., Fielding, J., Laveist, T., Borrell, L. N., Manderscheid, R., & Troutman A. (2011). Health disparities and health equity: the issue is justice. *American Journal of Public Health*, 101 Suppl 1:S149–S155.

Braveman, P., & Barclay, C. (2009). Health disparities beginning in childhood: a life-course perspective. *Pediatrics*, 124 Suppl 3:S163–S175.

Broom, D. H. (1984). The social distribution of illness: is Australia more equal? *Social Science and Medicine*, 18 (11):909–917.

Burgess, D., M. van Ryn, Dovidio, J., & Saha, S. (2007). Reducing racial bias among health care providers: lessons from social-cognitive psychology. *Journal of General Internal Medicine*, 22 (6):882–887.

Code of ethics of the Canadian Medical Association. (1997). *Journal International de Bioethique*, 8 (1-2):123–125.

Commission to End Health Care Disparities. (2007). Addressing Healthcare Disparities: Goals, Guiding Principles and Key Strategies for Comprehensive Policies. Available at https://www.ama-assn.org/ama/pub/physician-resources/public-health/ eliminating-health-disparities/commission-end-health-care-disparities.page

Corcoran, K., Hundhammer, T., & Mussweiler, T. (2009). A tool for thought! When comparative thinking reduces stereotyping effects. *Journal of Experimental Social Psychology*, 45 (4):1008–1011.

Corning, A. F., & Bucchianeri, M. M. (2010). Perceiving racism in ambiguous situations: who relies on easy-to-use information? *Journal of Social Psychology*, 150 (3):258–277.

Council on Ethical and Judicial Affairs, American Medical Association. (1995). Ethical considerations in the allocation of organs and other scarce medical resources among patients. *Archives of Internal Medicine,* 155 (1):29–40.

Council on Ethical and Judicial Affairs, American Medical Association. (1994). Ethical issues in health care system reform. The provision of adequate health care. *Journal of the American Medical Association,* 272 (13):1056–1062.

Council on Ethical and Judicial Affairs, American Medical Association. (1995). Ethical issues in managed care., 273 (4):330–335.

Dasgupta, N., & Asgari, S. (2004). Seeing is believing: Exposure to counterstereotypic women leaders and its effect on the malleability of automatic gender stereotyping. *Journal of Experimental Social Psychology,* 40 (5):642–658.

Dasgupta, N., & Greenwald, A. G. (2001). On the malleability of automatic attitudes: combating automatic prejudice with images of admired and disliked individuals. *Journal of Personality and Social Psychology,* 81 (5):800–814.

Dasgupta, N., & Rivera, L. M. (2006). From automatic antigay prejudice to behavior: the moderating role of conscious beliefs about gender and behavioral control. *Journal of Personality and Social Psychology,* 91 (2):268–280.

Dasgupta, N., & Rivera, L. M. (2008). When social context matters: The influence of long-term contact and short-term exposure to admired outgroup members on implicit attitudes and behavioral intentions. *Social Cognition,* 26 (1):112–123.

Davis, S., Wright, P. W., Schulman, S. F., Hill, L. D., Pinkham, R. D., Johnson, L. P., et al. (1985). Participants in prospective, randomized clinical trials for resected non-small cell lung cancer have improved survival compared with nonparticipants in such trials. *Cancer,* 56 (7):1710–1718.

Devine, P. G. (1989). Stereotypes and Prejudice—Their Automatic and Controlled Components. *Journal of Personality and Social Psychology,* 56 (1):5–18.

Djikic, M., Langer, E. J., & Stapleton, S. F. (2008). Reducing stereotyping through mindfulness: Effects on automatic stereotype-activated behaviors. *Journal of Adult Development,* 15 (2):106–111.

Dovidio, J. F., & Fiske, S. T. (2012). Under the radar: how unexamined biases in decision-making processes in clinical interactions can contribute to health care disparities. *American Journal of Public Health,* 102 (5):945–952.

Drake, M. V., & Lowenstein, D. H. (1998). The role of diversity in the health care needs of California. *Western Journal of Medicine,* 168 (5):348–354.

Feldman, P., Warr, D., Tacticos, T., & Kelaher M. (2009). People, places and policies— trying to account for health inequalities in impoverished neighbourhoods. *Australian and New Zealand Journal of Public Health,* 33 (1):17–24.

Friel, S., & Marmot, M. G. (2011). Action on the social determinants of health and health inequities goes global. *Annual Review of Public Health,* 32:225–236.

Galinsky, A. D., & Moskowitz, G. B. (2000). Perspective-taking: Decreasing stereotype expression, stereotype accessibility, and in-group favoritism. *Journal of Personality and Social Psychology,* 78 (4):708–724.

Grant, R. (2012). A bridge between public health and primary care. *American Journal of Public Health,* 102 (Suppl 3), S304.

Green, A. R., Carney, D. R., Pallin, D. J., Ngo, L. H., Raymond, K. L., Iezzoni, L. I., & Banaji, M. R. (2007). Implicit bias among physicians and its prediction of thrombolysis decisions for black and white patients. *Journal of General Internal Medicine*, 22 (9):1231–1238.

Green, A. R., Tan-McGrory, A., Cervantes, M. C., & Betancourt, J. R. (2010). Leveraging quality improvement to achieve equity in health care. *Joint Commission Journal on Quality and Patient Safty*, 36 (10):435–442.

Green, C. R., Anderson, K. O., Baker, T. A., Campbell, L. C., Decker, S., Fillingim, R. B., et al. (2003). The Unequal Burden of Pain: Confronting Racial and Ethnic Disparities in Pain. *Pain Medicine*, 4 (3):277–294.

Greenwald, A. G., McGhee, D. E., & Schwartz, J. L. (1998). Measuring individual differences in implicit cognition: the implicit association test. *Journal of Personality and Social Psychology*, 74 (6):1464–1480.

Greil, R., Holzner, B., Kemmler, G., Kopp, M., Buchowski, A., Oberaigner, W., et al. (1999). Retrospective assessment of quality of life and treatment outcome in patients with Hodgkin's disease from 1969 to 1994. *European Journal of Cancer*, 35 (5):698–706.

Guanais, F. C. (2010). Health equity in Brazil. *British Medical Journal*, 341:c6542.

Guimond, P., Bunn, H., O'Connor, A. M., Jacobsen, M. J., Tait, V. K., Drake, E. R., et al. (2003). Validation of a tool to assess health practitioners' decision support and communication skills. *Patient Education and Counseling*, 50 (3):235–245.

Guindo, L. A., Wagner, M., Baltussen, R., Rindress, D., van Til, J., Kind, P., & Goetghebeur, M. M. (2012). From efficacy to equity: Literature review of decision criteria for resource allocation and healthcare decisionmaking. *Cost Effectiveness and Resource Allocation*, 10 (1):9.

Gwatkin, D. R., Bhuiya, A., & Victora, C. G. (2004). Making health systems more equitable. *Lancet*, 364 (9441):1273–1280.

Harris, R., Cormack, D., Tobias, M., Yeh, L. C., Talamaivao, N., Minster, J., & Timutimu R. (2012). Self-reported experience of racial discrimination and health care use in New Zealand: results from the 2006/07 New Zealand Health Survey. *American Journal of Public Health*, 102 (5):1012–1019.

Heiat, A., Gross, C. P., & Krumholz, H. M. (2002). Representation of the elderly, women, and minorities in heart failure clinical trials. *Archives of Internal Medicine*, 162 (15):1682–1688.

Hickling, F. W. (2012). Understanding patients in multicultural settings: a personal reflection on ethnicity and culture in clinical practice. *Ethnicity and Health*, 17 (1–2):203–216.

Huijts, T., Eikemo, T. A., & Skalicka, V. (2010). Income-related health inequalities in the Nordic countries: examining the role of education, occupational class, and age. *Social Science and Medicine*, 71 (11):1964–1972.

Hunt, P., & Backman, G. (2008). Health systems and the right to the highest attainable standard of health. *Health and Human Rights*, 10 (1):81–92.

Hussain-Gambles, M., Atkin, K., & Leese, B. (2004). Why ethnic minority groups are under-represented in clinical trials: a review of the literature. *Health and Society Care in the Community*, 12 (5):382–388.

Hussain-Gambles, M., Leese, B., Atkin, K., Brown, J., Mason, S., & Tovey, P. (2004). Involving South Asian patients in clinical trials. *Health Technology Assessment*, 8 (42):iii, 1–109.

Jacobs, C. M. (1997). Managing demand using clinical decision support tools. *Healthcare and Finance Management*, 51 (7):41–42.

Jayasinghe, K. S., De Silva, D., Mendis, N., & Lie, R. K. (1998). Ethics of resource allocation in developing countries: the case of Sri Lanka. *Social Science and Medicine*, 47 (10):1619–1625.

Johansson, K. A., Miljeteig, I., Kigwangalla, H., & Norheim, O. F. (2011). HIV priorities and health distributions in a rural region in Tanzania: a qualitative study. *Journal of Medical Ethics*, 37 (4):221–226.

Kapiriri, L., & Martin, D. K. (2006). Priority setting in developing countries health care institutions: the case of a Ugandan hospital. *BMC Health Services Research*, 6:127.

Kapiriri, L., & Martin, D. K. (2007). A strategy to improve priority setting in developing countries. *Health Care Analysis*, 15 (3):159–167.

Karjalainen, S., & Palva, I. (1989). Do treatment protocols improve end results? A study of survival of patients with multiple myeloma in Finland. *BMJ*, 299 (6707):1069–1072.

Kastner, M., & Straus, S. E. (2008). Clinical decision support tools for osteoporosis disease management: a systematic review of randomized controlled trials. *Journal of General Internal Medicine*, 23 (12):2095–2105.

Kawakami, K., Dovidio, J. F., Moll, J., Hermsen, S., & Russin, A. (2000). Just say no (to stereotyping): Effects of training in the negation of stereotypic associations on stereotype activation. *Journal of Personality and Social Psychology*, 78 (5):871–888.

Killien, M., Bigby, J. A., Champion, V., Fernandez-Repollet, E., Jackson, R. D., Kagawa-Singer, M., et al. (2000). Involving minority and underrepresented women in clinical trials: the National Centers of Excellence in Women's Health. *Journal of women's Health & Gender-based Medicine*, 9 (10):1061–1070.

Koh, H. K. (2010). A 2020 vision for healthy people. *New England Journal of Medicine*, 362 (18):1653–1656.

Koh, H. K., Graham, G., & Glied, S. A. (2011). Reducing racial and ethnic disparities: the action plan from the department of health and human services. *Health Affairs (Millwood)*, 30 (10):1822–1829.

Kotalik, J. F. (2002). Physician's ethical responsibilities when there is a discrepancy between demand and supply of medical services. *Annals (Royal College of Physicians and Surgeons of Canada)*, 35 (2):100–104.

Kunda, Z., & Spencer, S. J. (2003). When do stereotypes come to mind and when do they color judgment? A goal-based theoretical framework for stereotype activation and application. *Psychological Bulletin*, 129 (4):522–544.

Kunst, A. E., Groenhof, F., Mackenbach, J. P., & Health, E. W. (1998). Occupational class and cause specific mortality in middle aged men in 11 European countries: comparison of population based studies. EU Working Group on Socioeconomic Inequalities in Health. *BMJ*, 316 (7145):1636–1642.

Lantos, J. D. (1999). The "inclusion benefit" in clinical trials. *Journal of Pediatrics*, 134 (2):130–131.

Lebrecht, S., Pierce, L. J., Tarr, M. J., & Tanaka J. W. (2009). Perceptual other-race training reduces implicit racial bias. *PLoS One*, 4 (1):e4215.

Legault, L., Gutsell, J. N., & Inzlicht, M. (2011). Ironic effects of antiprejudice messages: how motivational interventions can reduce (but also increase) prejudice. *Psychological Science*, 22 (12):1472–1477.

Lerner, J. S., & Tetlock, P. E. (1999). Accounting for the effects of accountability. *Psychological Bulletin*, 125 (2):255–275.

Lillie-Blanton, M., Maddox, T. M., Rushing, O., & Mensah, G. A. (2004). Disparities in cardiac care: rising to the challenge of Healthy People 2010. *Journal of the American College of Cardiology*, 44 (3):503–508.

Lundberg, G. D. (2004). The International Code of Medical Ethics of the World Medical Association. *MedGenMed [electronic resource]*, 6 (4):37.

Mackenbach, J. P., Stirbu, I., Roskam, A. J., Schaap, M. M., Menvielle, G., Leinsalu, M., & Kunst, A. E. (2008). Socioeconomic inequalities in health in 22 European countries. *New England journal of medicine*, 358 (23):2468–2481.

Malek, S. K., Keys, B. J., Kumar, S., Milford, E., & Tullius, S. G. (2011). Racial and ethnic disparities in kidney transplantation. *Transplant International*, 24 (5):419–424.

Marmot, M., Allen, J., Bell, R., & Goldblatt, P. (2012). Building of the global movement for health equity: from Santiago to Rio and beyond. *Lancet*, 379 (9811):181–188.

Marmot, M., & Feeney, A. (1997). General explanations for social inequalities in health. *IARC Scientific Publications* (138):207–228.

Marmot, M., Friel, S. Bell, R., Houweling, T. A., & Taylor, S. (2008). Closing the gap in a generation: health equity through action on the social determinants of health. *Lancet*, 372 (9650):1661–1669.

Marmot, M. G. (2003). Understanding social inequalities in health. *Perspectives in Biology and Medicine*, 46 (3 Suppl):S9–23.

Marmot, M. G., Smith, G. D., Stansfeld, S., Patel, C., North, F., Head, J., et al. (1991). Health inequalities among British civil servants: the Whitehall II study. *Lancet*, 337 (8754):1387–1393.

Mathur, R., Badrick, E., Boomla, K., Bremner, S., Hull, S., & Robson, J. (2011). Prescribing in general practice for people with coronary heart disease; equity by age, sex, ethnic group and deprivation. *Ethnicity & Health*, 16 (2):107–123.

Mazzuco, S., & Suhrcke, M. (2011). Health inequalities in Europe: new insights from European Labour Force Surveys. *Journal of Epidemiology and Community Health*, 65 (9):757–763.

Meadows, A. T., Kramer, S., Hopson, R., Lustbader, E., Jarrett, P., & Evans. A. E. (1983. Survival in childhood acute lymphocytic leukemia: effect of protocol and place of treatment. *Cancer Investigation*, 1 (1):49–55.

Mendoza, S. A., Gollwitzer, P. M., & Amodio, D. M. (2010). Reducing the expression of implicit stereotypes: reflexive control through implementation intentions. *Personality and Social Psychology Bulletin*, 36 (4):512–523.

Mills, A., Ataguba, J. E., Akazili, J., Borghi, J., Garshong, B., Makawia, S., et al. (2012). Equity in financing and use of health care in Ghana, South Africa, and Tanzania: implications for paths to universal coverage. *Lancet*.

Mills, A. M., Shofer, F. S., Boulis, A. K., Holena, D. N., & Abbuhl. S. B. (2011). Racial disparity in analgesic treatment for ED patients with abdominal or back pain. *The American Journal of Emergency Medicine*, 29 (7):752–756.

Moosa, M. R., & Kidd, M. (2006). The dangers of rationing dialysis treatment: the dilemma facing a developing country. *Kidney International*, 70 (6):1107–1114.

Moskowitz, G. B., Stone, J., & Childs, A. (2012). Implicit stereotyping and medical decisions: unconscious stereotype activation in practitioners' thoughts about African Americans. *American Journal of Public Health*, 102 (5):996–1001.

Moskowitz, G. B. (2001). *Cognitive Social Psychology: the Princeton Symposium on the Legacy and Future of Social Cognition*. Mahwah, NJ: Lawrence Erlbaum Associates.

Mshana, E. (1993). Health centres. Good management is crucial. *HealthAction* (4):6.

Mulia, N., Ye, Y., Zemore, S. E., & Greenfield, T. K. (2008). Social disadvantage, stress, and alcohol use among black, Hispanic, and white Americans: findings from the 2005 U.S. National Alcohol Survey. *Journal of Studies on Alcohol and Drugs*, 69 (6):824–833.

Mullan, F., & Frehywot, S. (2007). Non-physician clinicians in 47 sub-Saharan African countries. *Lancet*, 370 (9605):2158–2163.

Narasimhan, V., Brown, H., Pablos-Mendez, A., Adams, O., Dussault, G., Elzinga, G., Aet al. (2004). Responding to the global human resources crisis. *Lancet*, 363 (9419):1469–1472.

Nicholson, J. M., Lucas, N. Berthelsen, D. & Wake, M. (2012). Socioeconomic inequality profiles in physical and developmental health from 0-7 years: Australian National Study. *Journla of Epidemiology and Community Health*, 66 (1):81–87.

Olson, M. A., & Fazio, R. H. (2006). Reducing automatically activated racial prejudice through implicit evaluative conditioning. *Personality and Social Psychology Bulletin*, 32 (4):421–433.

Osborn, R., & Squires, D. (2012). International perspectives on patient engagement: results from the 2011 Commonwealth Fund Survey. *Journal of Ambulatory Care Management*, 35 (2):118–128.

Payne, B. K. (2005). Conceptualizing control in social cognition: how executive functioning modulates the expression of automatic stereotyping. *Journal of Personality and Social Psychology*, 89 (4):488–503.

Plant, E. A., & Devine, P. G. (2001). Responses to other-imposed pro-black pressure: Acceptance or backlash? *Journal of Experimental Social Psychology*, 37 (6):486–501.

Reede, J. Y. (2003). A recurring theme: the need for minority physicians. *Health Affairs (Millwood)*, 22 (4):91–93.

Richeson, J. A., & Ambady. N. (2003). Effects of situational power on automatic racial prejudice. *Journal of Experimental Social Psychology*, 39 (2):177–183.

Ross, S., Grant, A., Counsell, C., Gillespie, W., Russell, I., & Prescott, R. (1999. Barriers to participation in randomised controlled trials: a systematic review. *Journal of Clinical Epidemiology*, 52 (12):1143–1156.

Rudman, L. A., Ashmore, R. D. & Gary, M. L. (2001). "Unlearning" automatic biases: the malleability of implicit prejudice and stereotypes. *Journal of Personality and Social Psychology*, 81 (5):856–868.

Sabin, J. A., & Greenwald, A. G. (2012). The Influence of Implicit Bias on Treatment Recommendations for 4 Common Pediatric Conditions: Pain, Urinary Tract Infection, Attention Deficit Hyperactivity Disorder, and Asthma. *American Journal of Public Health*, 102 (5):988–995.

Saha, S., Guiton, G., Wimmers, P. F., & Wilkerson L. (2008). Student body racial and ethnic composition and diversity-related outcomes in US medical schools. *Journal of the American Medical Association*, 300 (10):1135–1145.

Schulman, K. A., Berlin, J. A., Harless, W., Kerner, J. F., Sistrunk, S., Gersh, B. J., et al. (1999). The effect of race and sex on physicians' recommendations for cardiac catheterization. *New England Journal of Medicine*, 340 (8):618–626.

Sechrist, G. B., & Stangor, C. (2001). Perceived consensus influences intergroup behavior and stereotype accessibility. *Journal of Personality and Social Psychology*, 80 (4):645–654.

Smedley, B. D., Stith, A. Y., Nelson, A. R., and Institute of Medicine (U.S.). Committee on Understanding and Eliminating Racial and Ethnic Disparities in Health Care. (2003). *Unequal treatment: confronting racial and ethnic disparities in health care*. Washington, DC: National Academy Press.

Smith, G. D., Chaturvedi, N., Harding, S., Nazroo, J., & Williams R. 2000. Ethnic inequalities in health: A review of UK epidemiological evidence. *Critical Public Health*, 10 (4):375–408.

Starfield, B. (2004). Promoting equity in health through research and understanding. *Developing World Bioethics*, 4 (1):76–95.

Stewart, B. D., & Payne, B. K. (2008). Bringing automatic stereotyping under control: implementation intentions as efficient means of thought control. *Personality and Social Psychology Bulletin*, 34 (10):1332–1345.

Stone, J., & Moskowitz, G. B. (2011). Non-conscious bias in medical decision making: what can be done to reduce it? *Medical Education*, 45 (8):768–776.

Strech, D., Synofzik, M., & Marckmann G. (2008). How physicians allocate scarce resources at the bedside: a systematic review of qualitative studies. *Journal of Medicine and Philosophy*, 33 (1):80–99.

Teal, C. R., Shada, R. E., Gill, A. C., Thompson, B. M., Fruge, E., Villarreal, G. B., & Haidet, P. (2010). When best intentions aren't enough: helping medical students develop strategies for managing bias about patients. *Journal of General Internal Medicine*, 25 Suppl 2:S115–S118.

Thornicroft, G. (2008). Stigma and discrimination limit access to mental health care. *Epidemiologia e Psichiatria Sociale*, 17 (1):14–19.

Truman, B. I., Smith, K. C., Roy, K., Chen, Z., Moonesinghe, R., Zhu, J., et al. (2011). Rationale for regular reporting on health disparities and inequalities—United States. *MMWR Surveillance Summaries*, 60 Suppl:3–10.

Uhlmann, E., & Cohen, G. L. (2005). Constructed criteria: redefining merit to justify discrimination. *Psychological Science*, 16 (6):474–480.

United States. Agency for Healthcare Research and Quality. National healthcare disparities report 2011. In *AHRQ publication*. Rockville, MD: U.S. Dept. of Health and Human Services.

Vamos, E. P., Novak, M., & Mucsi, I. (2009). Non-medical factors influencing access to renal transplantation. *International Urology and Nephrology*, 41 (3):607–616.

van Ryn, M. (2002). Research on the provider contribution to race/ethnicity disparities in medical care. *Medical Care*, 40 (1 Suppl):I140–I151.

Veling, W., Selten, J. P., Susser, E., Laan, W., Mackenbach, J. P., & Hoek, H. W. (2007). Discrimination and the incidence of psychotic disorders among ethnic minorities in The Netherlands. *International Journal of Epidemiology*, 36 (4):761–768.

Veling, W., Susser, E., van Os, J., Mackenbach, J. P., Selten, J. P., & Hoek, H. W. (2008). Ethnic density of neighborhoods and incidence of psychotic disorders among immigrants. *American Journal of Psychiatry*, 165 (1):66–73.

Vendsborg, P., Nordentoft, M., & Lindhardt, A. (2011). [Stigmatizing of persons with a mental illness]. *Ugeskrift for Laeger*, 173 (16-17):1194–1198.

Wagner, H. P., Dingeldein-Bettler, I., Berchthold, W., Luthy, A. R., Hirt, A., Pluss, H. J., et al. (1995). Childhood NHL in Switzerland: incidence and survival of 120 study and 42 non-study patients. *Medical and Pediatric Oncology*, 24 (5):281–286.

Wikler, D. (2003. Why prioritize when there isn't enough money? *Cost Effectiveness and Resource Allocation*, 1 (1):5.

Wilks, J., & Austin, D. A. (1991). Evaluation of a strategy for changing group stereotypes of the heroin user. *Drug and Alcohol Review*, 10 (2):107–113.

Wilson, E., Grumbach, K., Huebner, J., Agrawal, J., & Bindman, A. B. (2004). Medical student, physician, and public perceptions of health care disparities. *Family Medicine*, 36 (10):715–721.

Woolf, S. H., & Braveman, P. (2011). Where health disparities begin: the role of social and economic determinants—and why current policies may make matters worse. *Health Affairs (Millwood)*, 30 (10):1852–1859.

Wynia, M. K., Johnson, M., McCoy, T. P., Griffin, L. P., & Osborn, C. Y. (2010). Validation of an organizational communication climate assessment toolkit. *American Journal of Medical Quality*, 25 (6):436–443.

Wynia, M., Matiasek, J., Johnson, M., & Jarosch, J. (2006). Promising practices for patient-centered communication with diverse populations: Lessons from 8 innovative hospitals nationwide. *Journal of General Internal Medicine*, 21:112–112.

Youngkong, S., Kapiriri, L., & Baltussen, R. (2009). Setting priorities for health interventions in developing countries: a review of empirical studies. *Tropical Medicine and International Health*, 14 (8):930–939.

Zemore, S. E., Karriker-Jaffe, K. J.,, Keithly, S., & Mulia, N. (2011). Racial prejudice and unfair treatment: interactive effects with poverty and foreign nativity on problem drinking. *Journal of Studies on Alcohol and Drugs*, 72 (3):361–370.

20 Bedside Rationing After Health Care Reform in the United States

The Emergence of Accountable Care Organizations

■ STEVEN D. PEARSON

A common criticism of health care in the United States has been that the delivery of care is fragmented. In many settings neither a single group—physicians, hospitals, or insurers—nor any integrated combination of these stakeholders takes full responsibility for guiding the health of a patient or community. As a result, care occurs across many sites without adequate integration, leading to unnecessary duplication, erratic outcomes, and higher costs.

Abetting and even encouraging this pattern of uncoordinated care has been the dominant fee-for-service payment structure adopted by most private insurers and by Medicare, the public insurer for the elderly in the United States. This approach to compensation pays individual doctors, hospitals, and other providers for each service they furnish to a patient. The more services the more payment, with very few or no questions asked regarding appropriateness of care. Fee-for-service payment provides no incentive to keep patients healthy or to seek efficiencies in care. Critics of this system have thus long contended that it creates incentives for overtreatment while undermining efforts to invest in preventive and cost-effective services (Marmor & Oberlander, 2012; Berwick, DeParle, Eddy, et al., 2003).

In an attempt to break with this entrenched pattern, recent health care reform legislation in the United States included specific measures to move away from a reliance on fee-for-service payment mechanisms. Chief among these measures are programs to encourage the formation of new "accountable care organizations" (ACOs) across the country. ACOs are combinations of hospitals and physician groups which will seek to function as integrated systems to provide all necessary care and ultimately receive from Medicare a single "global" payment for each patient for whom they care. Citing as models such highly touted health systems as the Mayo Clinic and the Geisinger Health System, advocates say that a shift toward ACOs could improve care and slow rising costs by changing the incentives that influence how doctors and hospitals deliver care (Goldsmith, 2011). In the wake of this change in payment by Medicare, private insurers are expected to fall in line and shift much of their payment structure to global payments for large provider groups as well.

Although the larger outlines of the transition toward ACOs is now evident, many questions remain about how the global payments that are envisioned going to large ACOs will affect the choices that are made regarding care delivery, including those decisions made by clinicians at the bedside. Will the financial rewards for less costly care at the organizational level lead to delay, diversion, or denial of expensive services? Will individual physicians working within ACOs seek to reduce costs, and thereby perhaps improve their own income, by withholding beneficial care from individual patients?

There is ample precedent for these concerns. In the 1990s an earlier version of global payments, then known as *capitation*, seemed in the ascendancy. Capitation was advanced with similar promises that it would reward more integrated, preventive care. But capitation agreements led to the bankruptcy of several large physician networks that were unable to meet the budgets they had negotiated with insurers. More fundamentally, even the basic idea of capitation triggered broad disaffection among clinicians and prompted prominent voices to warn that the patient–physician relationship would be undermined by distrust of physicians if they were paid more to do less (Angell, 1993; Larson, 1996). Rightly or wrongly, the specter of bedside rationing haunted every step of this earlier payment reform movement and was in no small part responsible for its demise.

Will global payments to ACOs fare differently than the capitation experiments of the 1990s? In a health care system grappling with the challenge of cost control while mired in a political environment still smoldering with claims of federal "death panels," the risks are high. How, then, can global payment agreements between insurers and ACOs be designed to achieve more cost-conscious and effective care without jeopardizing the public's trust in the integrity of physicians' decisions regarding care for individual patients?

In this chapter I will describe an analytic framework for considering this problem and delineate a set of design principles that can be used to enhance the ethical quality of physician compensation systems based on global payments. But ethical design by itself will not be enough. There are critical roles in communicating with patients and the public that can only be played by professional societies and by individual physicians. I will therefore also present an argument for how professional societies and individual physicians can address costs without losing the public's trust and how they can take the lead in demonstrating that the new world of ACOs and global payments represents our best hope for a sustainable, caring health care system for all.

■ ACOS AND THE SHIFT TO GLOBAL PAYMENTS

The US health care reform legislation passed in 2010 authorized the Medicare program to contract with ACOs through a new program launched January 1,

2012 (Patient Protection and Affordable Care Act, 2010). This program allows physician groups and hospitals that work together to coordinate care to share in any savings they achieve for the Medicare program as long as they also meet certain quality standards in the delivery of that care. The legislation stipulated that in the first two years of the program, all providers will still be paid fee-for-service by Medicare, and the cumulative expenditures of all the providers in the ACO will be compared against predicted Medicare expenditures for the group of patients cared for by that ACO. In year three of the program, those ACOs that have shown savings over the first two years compared to the benchmark of prior expenditures will be eligible to move to a global payment model, which is a per-patient per-month payment amount intended to replace some or all of the ACO's fee-for-service payments. These proposed payment mechanisms for ACOs are similar to a small number of arrangements already present in the commercial sector, such as the Alternative Quality Contract rolled out by Blue Cross Blue Shield of Massachusetts in 2009 (Mechanic, Santos, Landon, et al., 2011).

Under the health care reform law, the determination of which Medicare patients "belong" to which ACO will be done by attributing patients to ACOs on the basis of primary care use patterns. What this means is that patients will remain free to seek care from any provider, inside or outside an ACO. Only retrospectively, based on which primary care provider(s) the patient saw most, will the patient be assigned for financial accounting purposes to a particular ACO. ACOs are therefore a hybrid, perched somewhere between traditional fee-for-service Medicare and "closed" integrated health care systems, like Kaiser Permanente, that receive fully capitated payments and require their patients to seek care only within their own system. The hope is that ACOs will combine (a) the consumer appeal associated with freedom of choice with (b) the quality enhancing/cost restraining potential of limited networks paid a global amount rather than fee-for-service, thereby (c) allowing the ACO to pursue the triple aim of better care for individuals, better health for populations, and slower growth in costs.

By itself, however, the freedom to see any provider will be unlikely to assuage concerns about the risk of some form of bedside rationing by ACOs and their clinicians. In the 1990s, private health plans operating under the same kind of incentives that ACOs will have were accused of withholding necessary services through several mechanisms, including restriction of access to specialists, denial of coverage for new forms of technology, and administrative review of physicians' decisions. Critics accused insurers of using targeted recruitment efforts to "skim" for healthier enrollees in order to avoid the higher costs needed to care for some vulnerable populations. There were also significant public fears that physicians working under capitation would implicitly restrict access to the best services if these services were expensive (Woolhandler &

Himmelstein, 1995). If, as envisioned, ACOs complete their evolution toward becoming entities that receive full global capitation, then the same forces and same concerns are sure to be raised. It is essential, therefore, to understand the ethical design principles for structuring payments to ACOs and for translating those incentives down through ACOs to the individual clinician level, in order to achieve more efficient care without destroying the public's trust in physicians. To do this, the concept of "bedside rationing" will need to be addressed head on.

■ ETHICAL DESIGN PRINCIPLES

The fundamental ethical values of medicine are based on the belief that physicians are competent, are compassionate toward the sick, and will put the interests of their patients before their own (Pellegrino 1987). Conflicts of interest, however, are an inherent hazard of all compensation systems (Thompson 1993). Every method of paying physician groups and individual physicians—including fee-for-service and salary arrangements—involves incentives which influence physicians' clinical judgment and effort in ways that may compromise the care received by an individual patient. Therefore, a central ethical imperative for the ACO movement will be to integrate into the design of compensation systems safeguards that minimize, as much as possible, the potential conflicts that could lead to undertreatment.

Certain key dimensions can be useful in determining how the potential conflict of interest at the heart of global payments is managed at the organizational level and transmitted to the individual physician and patient. These dimensions can serve not only as a structure for evaluation with respect to ethics, but also as the basis for specific design principles to guide the development and operation of ethical global payment systems.

■ THE INTENSITY OF INCENTIVES

The intensity of incentives in a global payment agreement clearly affects its inherent degree of conflict of interest and thus the risk for undertreatment. Intensity is determined by four factors: (1) the scope of services included in the agreement; (2) the amount of the potential financial loss or gain; (3) the timing and structure of any bonuses or deductions ("withholds") that may be part of a global payment plan; and (4) the provision of "stop-loss" protection (a limit on the financial risk faced by physicians in caring for patients whose medical costs are unusually high). Each of these factors is described in turn below.

First, the scope of services included within a global payment agreement helps to frame the degree to which ACOs will be at financial risk. Not all ACOs will include a network of providers for every possible service patients might need. For example, some ACOs may need to rely on referrals to outside academic hospitals or specialty groups for highly specialized care. If a global payment arrangement left the ACO fully "at risk" for these highly specialized services, including those services that occur after referral and are therefore outside of their own control, the ACO may feel more pressure to reduce referral outside the organization, heightening the conflict of interest in decisions for individual patients.

The second factor that determines intensity is the actual amount that ACOs can potentially gain or lose in a global payment agreement, and this factor is of equal importance to the scope of services. In the capitation era, some physicians' groups reported income under capitation that jumped in one year to 170% of what they had earned previously while caring for the same patients under fee-for-service arrangements (Terry, 1996). Most of the time, this kind of windfall happened when the capitation agreement included special provisions offering bonuses for reducing the costs of particular tests or treatments. The risk of an equal or greater loss can also exist under global payments, and this risk can be concentrated if the global payment agreement includes "withholds" of money that will only be paid to the provider group if it achieves (reduced) utilization targets for particular tests or treatments.

The third factor that helps determine the overall intensity of incentives is the timing and structure of any bonuses or withholds that may be part of a global payment plan. Bonuses and withheld amounts that are paid out in lump sums when a specific target is attained can create especially intense conflicts of interest if a provider group is close to qualifying for the extra money near the end of a contract period. For example, consider an individual physician who, as December approaches, knows that his ACO is on the verge of qualifying for a lump-sum $1,000,000 bonus from a private insurer for meeting a specific target for reduced hospital costs. This physician may face a severe ethical test when evaluating a sick patient whose risk of death is small but who might benefit from hospitalization.

The fourth and final element that helps determine the intensity of incentives in global payment arrangements is whether there are limits on the financial risk faced by physicians in caring for patients whose medical costs are unusually high. The risk of losing money can be very real if no boundaries are placed on the absolute or percentage amount of loss that can be suffered by an ACO. In the private market these boundaries have been known as "stop-loss" provisions (Bodenheimer & Grumbach, 1996). Stop-loss insurance protects provider groups from the financial risk created by exceptionally expensive treatment by paying for health care costs once they exceed a predetermined threshold, either for an individual patient (per-patient provisions) or for all covered patients (aggregate provisions). Aggregate stop-loss insurance would protect against large decreases in an ACO's income during a contract period. Per-patient packages would ensure that an ACO cannot lose substantial income for treating a particular patient who is severely ill. Thus, only per-patient stop-loss provisions protect individual patients from being viewed as serious "money losers" for ACOs.

The intensity of incentives under global payment must be judged by looking at the interaction of all the features just discussed as they are combined in a specific global payment agreement. The ethical goal for global payment agreements is for them to present an intensity of financial risk or gain for the ACO small enough that it would not lead reasonable persons to question whether the judgments of its physicians are improperly influenced. Although in practice this principle might support many different thresholds for the intensity of incentives, the key feature is that the trust of "reasonable persons"—that is, of patients and the public—should be the guiding concept. The trust of patients and the public should be discussed openly by the government, by private insurers, by ACO leaders, and by public representatives as they decide how intense the financial incentives for ACOs should be. Whatever the budgetary goals are, maintaining trust must be not only part of the design equation but also its central and, ultimately, determining feature.

To achieve this level of trust, the amount of overall financial risk or gain based on any withholds and bonuses that may be included in global payment agreements should be small and should be structured to avoid unusually intense conflicts of interest in individual clinical decisions. In addition, bonuses and distributions from withheld surpluses should be paid out in percentages of the targets achieved, in installments, or in other ways to avoid the possibility that the entire payment will depend on the health care costs of a few patients at the end of a contract year. Finally, adequate per-patient stop-loss protection must be a core element of all global payment arrangements with ACOs.

Ultimately, further research is needed to define the optimal levels of financial risk and gain that will make physicians more conscious of cost without leading them to withhold "necessary" services. Lacking such data, previous governmental policy in the capitation era established one benchmark by focusing its concern on plans that put more than 25% of physicians' income at risk (Federal Register, 1996). In a contemporary survey of managers of health maintenance organizations, nearly half believed that physicians' decisions regarding the ordering of tests, referrals to specialists, and elective hospitalizations could be noticeably affected at individual risk levels ranging from 5% to 15% of income (Hillman, Pauly, Kerman, et al, 1991). In keeping with these views, and in the absence of empirical data, it seems reasonable to consider an aggregate risk of more than 20% for an ACO as unacceptably high. The government has determined that the first generation of ACOs will have upside potential and downside financial risks far lower than this threshold, but private contracts may approach this level, and future risk "corridors" for ACOs will be determined at a later time. It will be critical for the future of ACOs that the right balance be struck. Group incentives must be ample enough to stimulate cost-conscious practice and creative preventive strategies, but the intensity of the incentives, particularly as they are translated into payment structures for individual physicians, must not present a substantial risk for implicit bedside rationing of important medical services.

■ THE IMMEDIACY OF INCENTIVES

It is in this translation of the group incentives at the ACO level that the question of the "immediacy" of incentives comes directly into play—the extent to which incentives are perceived as related to the care of an individual patient by an individual clinician. When the financial risk or gain is spread among many patients and physicians, the effect of any single medical decision on the personal income of an individual physician is diminished, greatly reducing the potential for conflict of interest and the threat to patients' trust.

Global payment agreements with ACOs caring for small groups of patients have the potential to heighten conflicts of interest, especially since many of the counterbalances and safeguards that can be incorporated into global payment arrangements for larger groups (e.g., stop-loss provisions) become impractical to design and implement. In addition, global payment agreements involving small groups may not provide sufficient capital to stimulate groups of physicians and hospitals to hire case managers, provide weekend office hours, or otherwise restructure care.

To limit the immediacy of financial incentives, global payment should only be selected as a method of compensation for ACOs involving large numbers of patients and only if there are methods available to diffuse financial risk or gain throughout a large group of providers. How many patients are enough? How many physicians make an ACO big enough? These are difficult questions to answer in isolation from the other features of a global payment agreement, and the earliest named ACOs have all been very large integrated provider systems. But as ACOs continue to develop, there will soon come a time when lower limits of size will have to be formally established. To have a realistic chance of achieving the positive benefits of global payments, to be able to build adequate safeguards into the agreement, and to keep the apparent conflict of interest at a level low enough to maintain the public's trust, a reasonable benchmark, borrowed from recommendations during the capitation era, would be a minimum number of patients of 250 (Pearson, Sabin, & Emanuel, 1998). For similar reasons, it seems reasonable to recommend that groups of physicians purporting to function as an ACO and receiving global payments for a majority of patient care services should have 15 or more members (Hillman, 1992).

Research should determine whether these limits, or others, can meaningfully define sizes of patient and physician groups below which the immediacy of financial incentives will adversely affect physicians' decision making, clinical outcomes, and patients' trust.

■ THE BALANCING OF INCENTIVES

Specific incentives for physicians to meet positive goals can be made part of global payment agreements to balance the short-term financial incentive to reduce care expenditures. This is exactly what the preliminary ACO program does, with 30 quality measures established as minimum targets that ACOs must meet in their first 2 years in order to be able to even qualify for global payments. "Minimum quality" requirements of this type, "high-quality" targets with potential bonuses for patient satisfaction, or exceptional quality outcomes can have real financial influence and can send a clear message that ACO profits will not be increased by a solitary focus on reducing the use of services.

The government, private insurers, physicians, and patient groups should continue to work together to overcome the difficulties inherent in defining and measuring appropriate targets for these kinds of balancing incentives. These targets must address high patient turnover in health plans and physician practices, a trend that reinforces the view of the patient's health as a short-term issue.

■ THE FAIRNESS OF INCENTIVES

Incentives should be fair. If financial risk is shifted to ACOs without attempts to adjust for the clinical severity of patients' conditions and future health risks, ACOs will have a built-in incentive to attract and keep only the healthiest, and therefore the least expensive, patients.

Unfortunately, there are currently no validated, easily used methods with which to adjust for risk and severity. Using prior health care utilization by patients as a basis for estimating future health care costs is the approach being used by the first generation of ACOs, but as future patients shift from ACO to ACO this approach may not serve to eliminate the incentive to "skim" for healthier patients, much as was perceived as the *modus operandi* of the capitation era. The lack of an adequate risk adjustment methodology limits the actuarial precision of global payments, thus penalizing any ACO that cares for sicker patients and rewarding those that do not. Until robust risk-adjustment systems have been implemented across many different ACOs and judged to capture the inherent risk associated with severity of illness, comorbidities, and sociodemographic and psychosocial factors that affect health care utilization, the fairness of global compensation systems will remain a key ethical concern.

In the early days, all ACOs accepting global payments must be vigilant to buffer their individual physicians from the effects of adverse selection. It is ethically unacceptable for any system of incentives to discourage physicians from caring for the patients who are most in need.

Preliminary Conclusions

Many aspects of physician compensation systems that are based on global payment can create conflicts of interest for physicians, raise the specter of inappropriate bedside rationing, and affect patients' trust. However, there can be many morally acceptable total packages, all having strengths and weaknesses. Further research is needed to clarify how global payment affects physician–patient relationships, decision making by physicians, and clinical outcomes. Until better information is available, minimizing conflicts of interest for physicians will be the key to sustaining public trust in the integrity of physicians' clinical judgment. Reducing financial conflict of interest to zero, however, is neither possible nor even desirable. There is a delicate balance between the positive and creative power of global payment to encourage physicians to be cost conscious and the risk that it will lead to the withholding of necessary services. Innovation in the design of global payment systems is likely to continue, and it should be welcomed. As that innovation proceeds, continuing attention to the ethical distinctions that can be made among various components of these payment systems will help guide the design of payment approaches, and of ACOs, faithful to physicians' professional duties and truly worthy of public trust.

■ THE ROLE OF INDIVIDUAL PHYSICIANS AND PATIENTS: THE ACO AT THE BEDSIDE

Conceptually, global payment represents an important opportunity to change the perverse incentives inherent in the fee-for-service payment model that continues to dominate provider compensation in the United States. To be successful, however, ACOs must pass along the inherent cost-conscious incentives of global payment agreements to their member physicians, who continue to be responsible for most utilization decisions. ACOs can set organizational policies to seek cost control, such as requiring review of requests for outside referrals or selecting a limited number of parsimonious specialists as preferred providers. If, however, part of the goal of ACOs is to engage individual clinicians in becoming more cost-conscious in their everyday clinical decision making, how are we to understand the role of individual physicians in responding "professionally" to their patients' needs and preferences for health care while functioning within an organization created and financially incentivized to channel societal aims to control costs? Should physicians resist any intrusion on their approach to patient care, functioning in their individual clinical decision making as if they were blind to the goal of restraining health care costs? Or should they in some sense bring the perspective of the ACO to the bedside?

Observers of physicians' predicament have often split into two seemingly irreconcilable camps. In the first are those who believe that physicians should remain true to their traditional ethic: advocacy for each individual patient's best interest must supersede all other considerations (Levinsky, 1984; Sulmasy, 1992). In the other camp are those who believe that caring about costs at the bedside is an ethical requirement that physicians cannot and should not avoid (Morreim, 1995; Hall & Berenson, 1998). According to this latter view, even if all administrative and clinical waste were pared, the issue would remain: the health care economy must compete with other social priorities, and thus marginally beneficial care should be rationed for the overall public good.

But even physicians who endorse the philosophical reality of some form of rationing (while acknowledging that the political environment may render the term itself toxic) wonder whether patient–physician relationships could survive a frank admission of rationing at the bedside.

My experience in practice, teaching, and consulting with colleagues has led me to believe that caring about costs—the perspective of the ACO— can be brought to the bedside in a way that will sustain the trust of patients and the public. Recently published evidence from focus groups drawn from a diverse patient populations support the idea that trusting relationships can coexist with discussions of cost (Danis, Sommers, Logan, et al., 2014). Below I describe how individual physicians can exercise their instinct to fight for the interests of their patients within a framework that admits to the boundaries of responsible budgets for health care needs.

An Alternative Model of Patient Advocacy

Although it may be easy intellectually to call for a "balance" between the needs of individual patients and those of other patients and other social priorities, practicing physicians know that this concept is difficult even to imagine when caring for a real individual patient, when pain and illness call forth the deepest human instincts to care, and to care deeply, and to care without reservation. Can these honored features of the patient–physician relationship be retained within a new model of patient advocacy within ACOs that admits to the relevance of health care costs? In previous work I have described an alternative model for the patient–physician relationship that was originally named by Albert Jonsen as "proportional" advocacy (Jonsen,

1990; Pearson, 2000). In this model, the physician and patient are viewed as linked together—not as an isolated pairing seeking to maximize the patient's absolute needs, but as a pairing within a recognized group in which other physicians and other patients are also drawing from a shared pool of resources. The pressure to allocate and ration resources within acknowledged limits arises from within this balanced structure and is applied uniformly across physician–patient pairings that operate in open cooperation and collaboration. I believe this model of patient advocacy is one way to picture how to bring the ACO to the bedside in a way that will maintain physicians' integrity and patients' trust.

Proportional advocacy is not simple. It requires a critical weighing of risk and benefit in every clinical decision, a process that is both logical and ethical. But this kind of balancing of multiple considerations, with ultimate integration into a coherent assessment and plan, is not foreign to physicians. Excellent physicians can make complex clinical decisions by weighing the likelihood and quality of clinical outcomes and integrating these with patient and family values. Proportional advocacy draws upon these same time-honored skills.

One element of this model needs to be stressed: The individual physician is not seeking to ration the care of his or her individual patient blindly or alone. A physician rationing care at the bedside in isolation is far worse than a physician advocating for individual patients without concern for others. Proportional advocacy requires a true partnership with clinical colleagues—and with patients—in a common effort to define where and when it is reasonable to accept marginally less effective care options in order to make better use of available health care resources.

Putting Proportional Advocacy into Action

To put this approach into action, physicians would need to discuss with patients when beneficial care did not meet the threshold for which common resources should be used to pay for it. How might physicians and patients conduct these conversations? Specifically, what would patients need to hear from their physicians to believe that it was fair and reasonable for them *not* to receive coverage for a test or treatment that would be of some benefit?

My answer to this question is demonstrated in the hypothetical conversation between patient and physician shown below. For the example below, I have recreated a composite case from pieces of my own experience and those of many colleagues. It is the case of a general internist and his patient discussing the patient's shoulder pain, which has not improved with conservative management. The patient requests a referral to an orthopedist who is a well-known shoulder specialist—a clinician who is well regarded but not an employee of the physician's ACO. Thus, a referral to this orthopedic subspecialist would cost the ACO more money than if the patient were seen by the "regular" orthopedist who sees these kinds of patients within the ACO. The internist believes that the requested orthopedist is indeed more skilled at complex cases, but that the regular orthopedist to whom he usually refers patients is very likely to be competent to assess and treat this patient's medical needs.

> Physician: I know that the orthopedist you want to see is outstanding. On the other hand, the orthopedist I usually refer my patients to is quite good and should be able to care well for you. If I send you to the orthopedist you want, the coordination of care between us may not be as good. In addition, to be honest, the cost of your going to the other orthopedist is not covered in the payment we get as an integrated physician practice, and we feel we do a better job managing the appropriate use of tests and procedures if we work with the orthopedists we know best. How would you feel about seeing the orthopedist I usually refer to first, and seeing how you like him?

This kind of forthright language may be difficult to say, but there should be open and honest communication indicating that rationing potentially better care is on the table for the patient and clinician to discuss. Physicians should not hide behind clinical language (for example, "not indicated") to avoid the reality that they are suggesting that a choice be made that may ration something of real or potential benefit to the patient.

> Patient: I don't know, if my insurance would pay for the other orthopedist, I'd still like to understand more about why I shouldn't see him if I want to. Is this a decision that you are making by yourself?
>
> Physician: No, this really isn't just me making the decision. Our medical group has had discussions, including discussions with patient representatives, and the consensus has been that we should examine all the issues but shouldn't routinely send our patients to outside specialists in situations like yours.

Physicians should work together with patients and other representatives of the community to decide which type of services do not represent the best use of available resources. ACOs will need to do more to set up formal processes to gain broader input into these kinds of decisions. At the very least, physicians should work together within their own practice groups to discuss the appropriate threshold for the kind of "marginally" beneficial care that it would be reasonable to consider forgoing, in consultation with individual patients. Toward this larger goal of achieving a greater sense of moral community in health care, physicians have a critically important role to play as teachers and active partners with their patients.

Patient: Tell me, really, wouldn't you let a big-shot corporate executive go outside your network? Wouldn't you authorize it for yourself?

Physician: Your trust in me and in this whole process is very important to me, and I want you to know that I would make the same decision for any other patient in this situation—myself included—and I believe the other physicians in my group would also make the same decision.

As the conversation continues, the patient will want to know that the same decision not to approve the request would be made for other patients in comparable situations. Would a physician or a "VIP" patient have the same limits applied to their requests? The answer must be "yes." To buttress this claim of basic fairness, physicians should also consider whether they can claim that other physicians in their group would make the same decision. If this claim cannot be made honestly, patients will have good reason to question the legitimacy of the rationing decision.

Patient: Silence.

Physician: Does this seem reasonable to you? I can promise you that I won't abandon you if things aren't going well with my regular orthopedist, and we'll get you the care you need. (Pause) I hope you understand the reasoning behind my recommendation, but if you don't think it's right or fair, I want you to let me know. My relationship with you as a patient is very important to me, and I want to make sure you feel like we can talk about anything, especially if we disagree!

Patient: No, that's OK, Doc. I guess it makes sense... as long as you trust this other orthopedist as much as you say. Thanks for talking it through with me.

Physicians should always be aware that they may be missing something in the history or in the perspective of their patient, so it is always appropriate to assess the patient's understanding and to consider whether the vital sense of partnership in any bedside rationing decision has been maintained. Coupled with this assessment should be a restatement of the bedrock promise of proportional advocacy: that the physician is the patient's champion and will see that he gets the care he needs.

Implicit in this discussion of proportional advocacy is the idea that bedside rationing is best applied at the margins, where the potential or real benefit to the individual patient is small. The approach discussed above would therefore apply only to a subset of clinical scenarios. But the example of an orthopedic referral is meant to convey that proportional advocacy need not be relegated only to situations for which the marginal benefit is easy to dismiss as vanishingly small. I, along with other physicians I know, have agonized over just this kind of situation exactly because the benefit for the patient seems small to us—but it may not be zero, and it may not seem insignificant at all to the patient.

Patients and physicians confront choices every day that offer opportunities for the appropriate use of proportional advocacy. After a joint critical examination of the medical evidence, patients and physicians would probably find more medical care at the margin. In addition to the type of situation illustrated in the preceding section, other common examples include decisions about maximizing patient convenience in getting a test or treatment, questions about whether to order tests meant primarily to reduce the patient's anxiety, questions about using cheaper drugs with slightly less efficacy or slightly higher risk for side effects, and questions about substituting generic or other cheaper drugs for ones the patient may already be taking. In all of these situations, I believe physicians and patients could discuss their options using the precepts of proportional advocacy. At first, these conversations may feel awkward and create tension, and such discussions could be impeded by the pressure to spend less time with patients. Yet, as physician-led ACOs gain a greater foothold in the health care landscape, I believe these conversations can be held in a way that will build trust through the honesty and forthrightness with which such "difficult" topics are addressed. The appropriate exercise of proportional advocacy demands constant attention to the uniqueness of individual patients, to the relative strength of the clinical evidence, and to the maturity of the collaborative decision making that has been done to justify a recommendation to try a less expensive path. In my experience, patients can respond positively to consideration of these paths if invited in as a partner to consider the options fairly.

▪ CONCLUSION

The ACO movement represents a blend of optimism and hard-headed pragmatism. The optimism arises from the examples of creative energy and accomplishments of integrated provider networks around the United States. These health systems, including the Mayo Clinic, Intermountain Health Care, Atrius Health, HealthPartners, and others, have shown how patients can have superior outcomes when providers work together to coordinate care, to reduce unnecessary duplication of tests and treatments, and to share information with patients to engage them and their families in full partnership. The hard-headed pragmatism embedded in ACOs comes from the realization that clinicians are economic creatures too, and they will respond to financial incentives. Unsustainable financial trends in health care mandate change, and the shift toward global payment agreements to support ACOs is one of the most important experiments in the history of US health care policy.

370 PROMOTING FAIR BEDSIDE RATIONING

Whether this experiment will work is still an unanswered question. One piece of the puzzle will be the public reaction to a return to capitation-like incentives for physician groups. How will the public understand the risks of conflict of interest that their physicians will face within ACOs? What will the view be of "bedside rationing" in this new era?

I have explored in this chapter how the design principles for the global payments that will underpin ACOs can be based on an ethical analysis of the risks for conflict of interest at the bedside. There are important dimensions of global payment agreements—intensity, immediacy, balancing, and fairness—that can be crafted to minimize the potential for global payment to lead to inappropriate undertreatment. The first generation of ACO arrangements appears to be framed in a way that addresses these dimensions and will provide a framework that maintains physicians' integrity and the public trust. Whether a broader, more inclusive group of ACOs and ACO agreements, including agreements with private health insurers, will be able to meet the ethical goals described here remains to be seen.

An ethical design for any compensation system is necessary, but it will not be sufficient for sustaining trust in the patient–physician relationship. What will be needed is an active effort by physicians and policymakers to engage patients as partners in the effort to bring the ACO to the bedside: to build a bridge between cost consciousness at the group level and cost consciousness at the bedside in a way that meets the ethical standards that physicians and patients expect of the patient–physician relationship. Accomplishing this goal requires a new vision of patient advocacy on the part of individual physicians, one that is not locked in an absolute view of the patient and physician as isolated from their colleagues and their community. This vision of a proportional advocacy represents a challenge to the traditional way of viewing the role of physicians, yet it is a vision that I believe fits perfectly within the historical traditions of medicine. Central to this different form of advocacy is partnership. Physicians, whether they work in solo practices or in large provider groups, must be excellent partners with other clinicians in order to provide high-quality care in the contemporary complex health care system. Equally, if not more so, physicians must also become full partners with their patients. Physicians must work with patients and the community at a higher level in order to reach an understanding about what represents "marginal" benefit from expensive care options that would be reasonable to discuss forgoing at the bedside. In the clinical encounter itself, individual physicians will need to reach out to patients to discuss care options in full recognition and acknowledgment of the individual patient's situation and values. Ultimately, ACOs will succeed or fail on the basis of these relationships. *Within* the clinical structure of ACOs, the relationships among clinicians and between clinicians and administrators will determine whether integrated care can produce real value for patients while meeting quality and cost targets for the ACO.

Relationships *between* clinicians and patients will determine whether patients trust the ACO and experience the value of integrated care. More broadly, the relationship *between* the ACO and the community it serves can contribute to patient understanding and trust. If the shift toward ACOs and global payment can be viewed as a chance to build a new set of enduring relationships of these kinds, then the very nature of bedside rationing and its place in the national health care conversation in the United States will be transformed.

REFERENCES

Angell, M. (1993). The doctor as double agent. *Kennedy Inst Ethics J*, 3:279–286.

Berwick, D. M., DeParle, N. A., Eddy, D. M., et al. (2003). Paying for performance: Medicare should lead. *Health Aff (Millwood)*, Nov-Dec;22(6):8–10.

Bodenheimer, T. S., & Grumbach, K. (1996). Capitation or decapitation: keeping your head in changing times. *JAMA*, 276:1025–1031.

Danis M., Sommers, R., Logan J., et al. (2014). Exploring public attitudes towards approaches to discussing costs in the clinical encounter. *J Gen Intern Med*, 29 (1):223–229.

Federal Register. (1996). Requirements for physician incentive plan in prepaid health care organizations. *Fed Regist*. 61:13430, 13432–13430, 13432.

Goldsmith, J. (2011). Accountable care organizations: the case for flexible partnerships between health plans and providers. *Health Aff (Millwood)*, Jan;30(1):32–40.

Hall, M. A., & Berenson, R. A. (1998). Ethical practice in managed care: a dose of realism. *Ann Intern Med*, 128:395–402.

Hillman, A. L., Pauly, M. V., Kerman, K., et al. (1991). HMO managers' views on financial incentives and quality. *Health Aff (Millwood)*, 10:207–219.

Hillman, A. L., Welch, W. P., & Pauly, M. V. (1992). Contractual arrangements between HMOs and primary care physicians: three-tiered HMOs and risk pools. *Med Care*, 30:136–148.

Jonsen, A. R. (1990). *The New Medicine and the Old Ethics*. Cambridge, MA: Harvard University Press.

Larson, E. (1996). The soul of an HMO. *Time Magazine*, January 22, pp. 44–52.

Levinsky, N. G. (1984). The doctor's master. *N Engl J Med*, 311:1573–1575.

Marmor, T., Oberlander, J. (2012). From HMOs to ACOs: The quest for the holy grail in U.S. health policy. *J Gen Intern Med*, Sep;27(9):1215–8.

Mechanic, R. E, Santos, P., Landon, B. E., et al. (2011). Medical group responses to global payment: early lessons from the 'Alternative Quality Contract' in Massachusetts. *Health Aff (Millwood)*, 30:1734–1742.

Morreim, E. H. (1995). Moral justice and legal justice in managed care: the ascent of contributive justice. *J Law Med Ethics*, 23:247–265.

Patient Protection and Affordable Care Act. (2010). Pub. L. No. 111-148, §2702, 124 Stat. 119, 318–319.

Pearson, S. D., Sabin, J. E., & Emanuel, E. J. (1998). Ethical guidelines for physician compensation based on capitation. *New Engl J Med*, 339:689–693.

Pearson, S. D. (2000). Caring and cost: the challenge for physician advocacy. *Ann Intern Med*, 133;148–153.

372 PROMOTING FAIR BEDSIDE RATIONING

Pellegrino, E. D. (1987). Altruism, self-interest, and medical ethics. *JAMA*, 258:1939–1940.

Sulmasy, D. P. (1992). Physicians, cost control, and ethics. *Ann Intern Med*, 116:920–926.

Terry, K. (1996). Surprise! Capitation can be a boon. *Med Econ*, 73:126–138.

Thompson, D. F. (1993). Understanding financial conflicts of interest. *N Engl J Med*, 329:573–576.

Woolhandler, S., & Himmelstein, D. U. (1995). Extreme risk—the new corporate proposition for physicians. *N Engl J Med*, 333:1706–1708.

21 Priority Setting Through Clinical Practice Guidelines

Lessons Learned

■ OLE FRITHJOF NORHEIM

Clinicians make or implement priority setting decisions every day. Clinical priority setting means choosing whom to investigate and what diagnostic tests to perform, sorting the flow of patients so some are diagnosed or treated before others, allocating patients to surgery, medical treatment or watchful observation, and selecting or excluding patients for a given treatment modality (Norheim, 2008). Justice requires a fair and efficient distribution of the benefits and burdens of priority setting (Brock & Wikler, 2006; Daniels, 2008). Clinicians are concerned with two types of information: the patient's severity of disease (prognosis without the intervention) and the patient's expected outcome (prognosis with the intervention). The evidence underlying their judgment is also important. Patients too are concerned about their prognosis: how long they will live and what the quality of those life years will be. Priority setting that leads to some patients being excluded from potentially beneficial health care is commonly called *rationing* (Klein & Redmayne, 1994). It is now widely recognized that most health care systems depend on more or less explicit mechanisms for rationing potentially beneficial health care (Fleck, 1987, 2009; Hurst and Danis, 2007). To see the intricate relationship between priority setting and clinical practice guidelines, it is useful to distinguish between the levels of decision making. Levels of resource allocation involve, according to Klein, decisions about (a) the size of the total budget, (b) the allocation of resources to broad sectors or client groups, (c) the allocation of resources to specific forms of organizational provision and treatment within such broad categories, (d) the priority to be given to particular types of patients when determining access to the available services and facilities, and finally (e) the level of service to be provided to individual patients once access has been achieved (Klein, 1993). Clinical practice guidelines aim to describe the content, quality, and terms of access for the management of a particular condition. They can thus be seen as precise recommendations for priority setting at the meso level of decision making, answering such questions as what medical and personal characteristics identify the type of patients that should have access to a particular treatment, service, or facility, and what level of service should be provided once the person is selected for the service (Klein, 1993). The development of guidelines could be seen as the formalization of the informal rules defining access to and exclusion from health services (Klein et al., 1996). The use of formal and informal clinical "indications" for referral, investigation, and prescription is probably one of the most influential mechanisms of cost containment and rationing (Norheim, 1999). Practice policies or clinical guidelines can be thought of as "generic decisions—recommendations intended for a collection of patients rather than for a single patient" (Eddy, 1990). Sackett and his colleagues defined clinical practice guidelines as "user-friendly statements" for a collection of patients based on the best external evidence (Sackett et al., 1997). Eddy describes the intent of a clinical practice policy as follows: "[T]he purpose of a practice policy is to modify the behavior of practitioners to steer their decisions toward actions that the policy-makers consider desirable" (Eddy, 1990). This purpose leads to the introduction of other and legitimate stakeholders in the development of guidelines. It goes without saying that there are conflicting views about what actions are desirable among them. Grimshaw and Hutchinson argue directly that guidelines should play a role in the priority setting process: "Since the rationing of scarce resources requires a targeting of those resources to obtain best value for money, it is important to have mechanisms for assuring effective health care" (Grimshaw, 1995). The goal of effective service-provision can be achieved, the authors argue, by evidence-based clinical practice guidelines used as tools for rationing. The challenge is that guidelines might end up as instruments for unjustified and covert rationing disguised as expert recommendations (Norheim, 1999). How can this be avoided? The aim of this chapter is twofold. First, to present and examine, based on our own work, one example of priority setting through clinical practice guidelines for primary prevention of cardiovascular disease in Norway (Norheim et al., 2011). Second, to analyze and discuss the distributional impact of the recommendations in further detail than that provided in the initial report (Norheim et al., 2009). The first section presents our attempt to implement a legitimate process for guidelines development. The second section summarizes the priority relevant parts of the recommendations and their justification. The third section explores different ways to measure the potential distributional impact of the recommendations. The final section reflects on lessons learned and possible ways forward.

■ EXAMPLE: EXPLICIT GUIDELINES FOR PRIMARY PREVENTION OF CARDIOVASCULAR DISEASE IN NORWAY

General practitioners in the Nordic countries have repeatedly expressed concern that implementation of the European Society for Cardiology guidelines on prevention of cardiovascular disease in clinical practice would classify most elderly adults at high risk for cardiovascular disease and lead to widespread prescription of drugs for prevention (Graham et al., 2007; Getz et al., 2005, 2004; Hetlevik, 1999; Meland et al., 2000; Hartz, 2001). To prescribe lifelong medication for a large proportion of healthy adults raises major dilemmas, including increasing the workload for physicians and resource allocation in terms of time used and rising prescription cost. On the other hand, cardiologists and other specialists point to the overwhelming evidence supporting the use of antihypertensives, statins, and other preventive drugs to lower morbidity and premature mortality (Law et al., 2009). The Norwegian Directorate of Health invited key stakeholders to engage in a process of developing new national guidelines targeting both general practitioners and other specialists prescribing primary prevention. New guidelines, based on new principles, were published and implemented in 2009 (Norheim et al., 2009). The Norwegian primary prevention guidelines group was established in 2004 and agreed on key principles for the development of new recommendations. The group agreed that the process should be evidence based and combined with a systematic and transparent approach. To clarify disagreement, all stakeholders were asked to explain their arguments and acknowledge a diversity of reasons based on (a) medical evidence, (b) evidence on cost effectiveness, and (c) health policy and ethical concerns. Recommendations regarding treatment thresholds are arguably priority decisions and require mechanisms of accountability to achieve legitimacy (Norheim, 1999). The process of guideline development was divided in three parts. First, the Norwegian Knowledge Centre for the Health Services conducted an independent systematic review of all relevant studies with meta-analyses according to predefined endpoints suggested by the guidelines group (Fretheim et al., 2008). In addition, the center conducted a systematic review of relevant cost-effectiveness studies and developed an independent Markov model based on the meta-analyses and Norwegian data on prevalence and costs (Wisløff et al., 2008). Third, the guidelines development group used this evidence to develop recommendations by the use of GRADE—a system for grading quality of evidence and strength of recommendations (Guyatt et al., 2008). The guidelines development group had representatives from the relevant specialist groups, one representative from the Norwegian Medicines Agency, one from the Directorate of Health, and two patient-group representatives. As explained below, differentiated risk thresholds according to age were recommended, and this has ethical, health policy, and resource allocation implications. This particular aspect of the guidelines was therefore extensively discussed in the standing Norwegian Council for Priority Setting and Quality in Health Care. The Council has wide representation including citizens and health policy decision makers, and their endorsement of differentiated risk thresholds helped secure legitimacy for the recommendations. In addition, the guidelines development group conducted a wide hearing process with all possible stakeholders and revised the document accordingly. The list of stakeholders included more than 50 organizations, including patient ombudsmen, patient organizations, and university departments, as well as all relevant specialist organizations. Making all documents available on the websites of the Directorate of Health and the Priority Setting Council facilitated transparency during the hearing process. As part of the implementation strategy, a short version of the guidelines was distributed to all members of the Norwegian Medical Association. The full document and the web-based risk calculator is available on the website of the Norwegian Directorate of Health, and a series of training workshops for the target groups have been initiated and are ongoing.

■ RECOMMENDATION: DIFFERENTIATED RISK THRESHOLDS ACCORDING TO AGE

Like all recent guidelines on primary prevention, the Norwegian guidelines are based on the absolute risk approach (Jackson, 2005). Treatment recommendations are based on absolute 10-year risk of cardiovascular deaths. In collaboration with the European SCORE project (http://www.score-project.eu), a specific Norwegian risk algorithm (NORRISK) based on data from Norwegian patients was developed (Selmer et al., 2008; Lindman et al., 2007). The risk chart is used to map risk factors of healthy individuals with increased risk of premature death, such as sex, age, smoking status, serum cholesterol levels, and hypertension. Although the Norwegian SCORE-based risk chart only considers risk of cardiovascular deaths, not events, it was chosen because it enabled the use of updated national data on mortality, while national data on morbidity are lacking. As is the case with the European guidelines, we assumed that there would be a predictable relation between cardiovascular deaths and nonfatal events. In addition to a chart for risk assessment, web-based computer software for risk estimation was developed (http://rkalk.helsedir.no). Risk assessment must also take into account family history, diabetes, and other risk factors not incorporated in the risk chart. The current standard recommendation from the European Society of Cardiology (ESC) is that medication should be offered to all with an absolute 10-year risk of cardiovascular death of ≥5% Graham et al., 2007). The precise rationale for excluding patients with lower risk is not provided. In contrast, the Norwegian guidelines recommend medication for the following age and risk groups:

- 40–49 years: if 10-year risk of cardiovascular death is ≥1%
- 50–59 years: if 10-year risk of cardiovascular death is ≥5%
- 60–69 years: if 10-year risk of cardiovascular death is ≥10%

Absolute risk should be adjusted for persons with increased individual risk factors, such as a systolic blood pressure ≥160 mmHg, serum total cholesterol levels ≥8 mmol/l for men and premenopausal women, and end-organ damage. These groups should be offered targeted treatment regardless of absolute risk. The recommendations are summarized in a priority chart assigning no, normal, or high priority for medical treatment to be reimbursed. All persons with increased risk should be offered advice on changing lifestyle habits. This advice should be given before initiation of drug therapy and continued after drug therapy is started. These include interventions to quit cigarette smoking, initiate a balanced diet, and provide specific advice on increased physical activity. A new risk evaluation should be performed 3–6 months after lifestyle advice has been given. Treatment recommendations (such as choice of anti-hypertensives or statins) are, with a few exceptions, the same as in the ESC guidelines (Norheim et al., 2009).

■ JUSTIFICATION FOR DIFFERENTIATED RISK THRESHOLDS

The new principles applied for differentiated risk threshold are based on commonly accepted principles for clinical priority setting (Norheim, 2008). Since absolute risk increases with age, we found the sole use of risk to be inadequate for determining who should have priority (Bonneux, 2007). It should be noted that all previous guidelines on this topic only consider severity of risk—magnitude of health benefit and cost effectiveness is typically ignored. In addition to recommendations based on the estimated 10-year risk for cardiovascular death, we found it therefore necessary to consider the expected benefit and cost effectiveness of the treatment. For example, the Markov model estimated a gain of 2.9 undiscounted life years from treatment with a statin and two anti-hypertensives for men aged 40–49 years with 1% risk, while the gain for men aged 60–69 with 5% risk was 1.7 years (TABLE 21.1; Wisløff et al., 2008).

Considerations about the magnitude of health benefit, as well as concern for equal lifetime health (implying some priority for those with lowest lifetime health expectations), therefore lead to a lower risk threshold for the youngest and a higher risk threshold for the oldest age group. The guidelines recommended a move from absolute risk assessment to consideration of expected benefit in terms of life years gained, and the distribution of these benefits. This means that life years gained from primary medical prevention of cardiovascular disease are distributed more equally if the Norwegian guidelines are implemented, compared to a 5% risk threshold for all. All interventions for all risk levels examined (≥1%) were found to be very cost effective (Wisløff et al., 2008). Costs were therefore not important in these decisions. In addition, the risk of medicalization, namely the potential negative effects of medical treatment of healthy individuals, was considered an additional argument for the adjustment of risk thresholds (Getz et al., 2004).

■ DISTRIBUTIONAL IMPACT

To explore potential implications of our recommendations, I refer to background documents included in the Norwegian guidelines and our own calculations based on these data. The background documents include a report from a group of epidemiologists who performed a need/impact assessment of different recommendations for risk thresholds. Need was estimated from data on risk factors in a large population-based study from Tromsø, a district in the northern part of Norway, and extrapolated to the rest of the country (Hartz, 2001). Impact on undiscounted life years gained was estimated from the Markov model (Wisløff et al., 2008). TABLES 21.1 and 21.2 contain some priority relevant information from the Norwegian document that is of particular relevance here (Getz, 2004). I have, in addition, calculated the impact in inequality in estimated age at death (Gini-health), percentage of change in Gini-health, life expectancy for all at risk of cardiovascular disease, and inequality-adjusted life expectancy. Each measure will be defined and described below.[1]

TABLE 21.1 shows that, for example, the younger male age group (40–49 years) with a 1% 10-year risk of death has an expected health benefit from lifelong medication (begun at age 40–49 and taken for the rest of life) of about 2.9 years, while the oldest age group (60–69 years) with higher risk (5%) has an expected health benefit of about 1.7 years. In general, those with higher risk have higher benefits, but the youngest age group has higher benefits than the oldest. For example, if we compare the Norwegian and

TABLE 21.1. *Undiscounted Life Years Gained from Medication at Various Risk Levels*

	Age	10-year risk	Per individual
Expected Life Years Gained (Undiscounted)			
Women	40–49	1%	–*
Women	50–59	5%	3.4
Women	50–59	10%	–*
Women	60–69	5%	2.3
Women	60–69	10%	2,9
Men	40–49	1%	2.9
Men	50–59	5%	3.0
Men	50–59	10%	3.5
Men	60–69	5%	1.7
Men	60–69	10%	2.3

* = According to epidemiological studies from Norway, there were no patients (or very few) in this risk group.

TABLE 21.2. *Distribution of Life Years According to Norwegian Recommendations, European Society for Cardiology (ESC) Recommendations, or If All at Risk Are Medically Treated*

	Number of Persons Treated	Number of Life Years Saved	Gini-Health	% Change Gini	Life Expectancy for all at Risk	Inequality-adjusted life expectancy
Norwegian recommendations	198100	531000	0.011	–39	80.7	79.8
ESC recommendations	247100	539000	0.018	–4	81.3	79.9
All with >1% risk treated	276100	625000	0.016	–17	81.5	80.3
None	0	0	0.019	0	79.2	77.7

the European recommendations we see that the Norwegian guidelines exclude males and females aged 60–69 with ≤10% risk who could expect a health benefit ≤2.3 years (males) or ≤2.9 (females), while they include persons (males) aged 40–49 with ≥1% risk who could expect a health benefit ≥2.9 years (for males). The difference from other guidelines is that the Norwegian recommendation is made explicitly with reference to a clear rationale.

The potential impact is a redistribution of life expectancy from those who will or have lived longer to those who would expect a shorter life expectancy if not provided treatment. It is therefore interesting to estimate, measure, and evaluate the population impact of this recommended and intended redistribution.

TABLE 21.2 shows that the number of persons treated if the Norwegian recommendation is implemented would be considerably lower than if the European recommendation is implemented. The Norwegian recommendation is justified by the concern that the European guidelines would lead to widespread drug treatment of healthy elderly people. The Norwegian guidelines shift treatment emphasis from older to younger persons. However, we see from TABLE 21.2 that compared with the European guidelines, the total sum of life years gained is about the same (531,000 versus 529,000). What about inequality in the age at death for all those at risk?[2] I have elsewhere suggested that LeGrand's method of estimating inequality in the age at death by the Gini-coefficient is useful for the evaluation of health impact from different priority strategies (Le Grand, 1989, 1987; Norheim, 2010). The Gini applied to the distribution of life years assigns a value 0 for distributions with perfect equality and 1.0 for distributions with maximum inequality. We see from TABLE 21.2 that there is most inequality if no treatment is provided (Gini-health = 0.019), less inequality if the European guidelines are implemented (Gini-health = 0.018), and least inequality in age at death if the Norwegian guidelines are implemented (Gini-health = 0.011). If all at risk were treated, Gini-health would be 0.016. The percent change in Gini-health is illustrated in *Figure 21.1*.

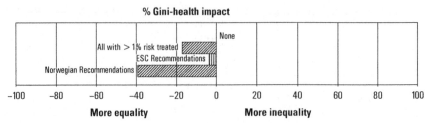

Figure 21.1 Norwegian Recommendations and Gini Health Impact.

If we accept the premise that it is an advantage to avoid medicalization of elderly healthy patients (fewer persons are treated), and that reduction in inequality is an objective for priority setting, this result may appear acceptable. However, justice does not only require a more equitable distribution of the benefits and burdens of priority setting; allocative efficiency (health maximization) is another objective. One measure of efficiency is the number of life-years saved. We saw above that the European priority strategy would save slightly more life years than the Norwegian one. So there might be a trade-off here between saving most life and reducing inequality in age at death. Another illuminating way to measure and compare health maximization is by comparing impact on life expectancy for all at risk from the two priority strategies. We see from TABLE 21.2 that the European priority strategy would yield a life expectancy of 81.3 years, while the Norwegian would yield 80.7 years—a somewhat lower life expectancy. This result illustrates a well-known trade-off involved in evaluating distributions at population level (Daniels, 2008). If we are concerned only about health maximization, the European strategy is preferable. If we are concerned only about reducing health inequality, the Norwegian strategy is preferable. If we are concerned about both objectives, we must seek the most acceptable balance between the two. Referring back to the process of the development of the Norwegian guidelines, we may say that all arguments were heard and considered by the National Council for Priority Setting, and they were directly involved in striking this balance. Reasonable people may disagree about how to balance these two concerns; hence processes that enhance legitimacy are needed. Another way to evaluate the balance is to use a measure that incorporates both a concern for health maximization and some aversion to inequality in health. Anand (2002) and Wagstaff (2002) have shown that the Gini (and other measures of health inequality) incorporate a certain degree of inequality aversion and can be combined with a measure of average health in a summary measure of population health. Put simply, such a combined "achievement index" would adjust life expectancy in a population with the degree of inequality in that population. Of two countries with the same life expectancy, the one with most inequality would get the lowest overall score. In mathematical terms, life expectancy is multiplied with 1 minus the Gini-coefficient (for more details, see Norheim, 2010, 2012; Human Development Report, 2010). The Human Development Index (IHDI) from 2010 uses this method to calculate inequality-adjusted life expectancy (Norheim, 2010). TABLE 21.2 also illustrates the combined impact of the two priority strategies by inequality-adjusted life expectancy. The Norwegian strategy yields a score of 79.8, the European strategy yields a score of 79.9, while no treatment would yield a score of 77.7. Judged by this measure the European strategy is slightly better than the Norwegian. This result can, perhaps, be explained by two factors. First, aversion to inequality may be stronger than what is captured by Gini-health. Second, and more importantly, the Norwegian strategy, developed through an explicit, open and accountable procedure, seeks to balance three objectives: (1) maximization of life expectancy, (2) reduction of inequality in age at death, and (3) minimization of treatment of the healthy elderly population. There is disagreement among reasonable people on how to strike the right balance.

▪ DISCUSSION: LESSONS LEARNED

Priority setting through clinical practice guidelines aims to guide the content, quality, and terms of access for the management of a particular medical condition. As fairly detailed and precise recommendations for priority setting at the meso level of decision making, they can be seen as an interesting arena for interchange between experience and evidence, between practice and theory, and between science and policy. The example discussed here, primary prevention of cardiovascular disease, shows that whether clinicians follow the European Society of Cardiology or the Norwegian guidelines, they implement one or another rationing policy. There is evidence for a potential medical benefit for all with >1% 10-year risk of a cardiovascular death, and both guidelines recommend withholding medical preventive treatment from some of the risk groups. This is relatively undramatic at the individual risk level but is nevertheless a good starting point for examining the impact of rationing on population-level health, because the policies affect a large number of people. Clinical guidelines of this type involve a wide range of population-level bioethics issues such the trade-off between health maximization and health inequality, whether priority to the young is acceptable, and the issue of medicalization. Another issue of relevance, but not discussed above, involves discounting of future health benefits. One important argument against our approach, mentioned by a referee to our report in the *British Medical Journal*, is that if the difference in case fatality according to age is taken into account and combined with discounting, the

apparent difference in health benefit between the young and the less young
is smaller than one would intuitively expect (Jackson et al., 2005). However,
in our model, difference in case fatality according to age is already accounted
for. Moreover, early on in our work we decided not to discount future health
gains for ethical reasons. Some economists argue that one should always discount the value of future health benefits. Most ethicists argue against this
view because it is unfair. From the societal perspective that we adopted,
it is unfair to assign lower values to health gains that occur in the future.
Life years gained now or in the future should have the same value (Broome,
1994). But again, on this issue, reasonable people disagree. The method
used in our example, with systematic review of the evidence, explicit grading of evidence and strength of recommendations, and involvement of key
stakeholders including patient representatives and the National Council for
Priority Setting, also has its limitations. For example, there was strong disagreement within the guideline development group concerning the issue of
medicalization. The primary care specialists were concerned about potential
negative effects of medical treatment for healthy individuals, as well as the
amount of time and resources spent on this group. A particular worry about
medicalization was that focus on individual prevention for people at low
risk diverts attention from (a) the resources people have that may help them
change life habits and (b) more effective population-based strategies, such
as salt reduction (NICE Public Health Guidance 25, 2010). There was also
strong support for the medicalization argument in the Council; that is, the
Council worried about excessive treatment while, interestingly, the patient
representatives on many occasions argued against that view. The organ specialists, on the other hand, were more concerned about the potential health
gains lost by increasing the risk threshold for the age group 60–69 years.
In my experience, most but not all of the initial disagreements disappeared
through the process of assessing the evidence of effectiveness. The resulting
recommendations were evidence based but not completely consensus-based
with respect to the values choices. It would be more correct to characterize the result as partly based on bargaining and compromise. Moreover, it
is unclear whether all participants in the hearing process and members of
the National Council understood, considered, and balanced all the complex
information in the same way. Since people bring different kinds of expertise to the table they pay attention to different aspects of the issue at hand,
which lies at the intersection of medical science, economics, and politics.
This holds especially for the more complex ethical issues such as the role of
discounting, the role of age, and the balancing of maximization and inequality. On a personal note, I should also say that as an ethicist initiating and
organizing the process, setting the agenda, framing the questions, and draft-
ing the final report, I am well aware that my own preferences and judgments

also shape the conclusions arrived at. Despite these shortcomings, I believe that improving the processes of developing practice guidelines can have an impact on clinical priority setting. If value choices are not made explicit, such guidelines might end up as instruments for unjustified and covert rationing disguised as expert recommendations. On the other hand, an open process makes it possible to consider, examine, and discuss a more comprehensive set of priority-setting criteria than those usually used by practitioners in the field. Recently, several groups have started to work on the role of guidelines for priority setting, and this work could help us develop better methods for efficient, fair, and legitimate decisions (Carlsen & Kjellberg, 2010; Truog et al., 2006; Cookson, 2001; Saarni & Gylling, 2004).

■ CONCLUDING REMARKS

In this chapter I have presented and examined priority setting through clinical practice guidelines for primary prevention of cardiovascular disease in Norway (Norheim et al., 2011). I have argued that the process of guidelines development is an important area of policy formation where enhanced accountability for priority setting is needed. These decisions shape the way clinicians make judgments concerning individual people and, if a process seen as legitimate backs up recommendations, they may lend support to explicit and accountable decision making also at the individual level. Gini-impact analysis adds ethically relevant information to the evaluation of the result, especially in cases involving large numbers of people with different health outcomes where intuitions concerning individual cases may mislead us—although in the end, policymaking must rely on legitimate procedures to balance complex and competing considerations.

■ ACKNOWLEDGMENTS

This chapter draws on the work of the Norwegian primary prevention guidelines development group - that included Bjørn Gjelsvik, Tor Ole Klemsdal, Steinar Madsen, Eivind Meland, Stein Olav Narvesen, Inger Njølstad, Serena Tonstad, Frøydis Ulvin, and Torbjørn Wisløff— – published as "Retningslinjer for individuell primærforebygging av hjerte- og karsykdommer" (Norheim et al., 2009, - in Norwegian) and as "New guidelines and new principles for primary prevention of cardiovascular disease in Norway: differentiated risk thresholds according to age" (Norheim et al., 2011). I want to thank each member of the group for enthusiastic participation and years of fruitful discussions about the medical, political, and ethical aspects of priorities in cardiovascular disease prevention.

Notes

1. This part of the chapter is based on my own analysis, and the views, methods, or possible errors are entirely my responsibility and were not discussed by the guidelines development group.

2. Observe that I only compare those at risk with and without medical treatment. I do not compare distributions for the extended population, namely those at risk plus those not at risk.

REFERENCES

Anand, S. (2002). The concern for equity in health. *J Epidemiol Community Health*, 56:485–487.

Bonneux, L. (2007). Cardiovascular risk models. Moral implications of models based on absolute risk could be betterunderstood BMJ, 335:107–108.

Brock, D., & Wikler, D. (2006). Ethical Issues in Resource Allocation, Research, and New Product Development. In: Jamison, D. T., Breman, J. G., Measham, A. R., Alleyne, G., Claeson, M., Evans, D. B., et al., eds. *Disease Control Priorities in Developing Countries*. 2nd Edition. pp. 259–270. New York: Oxford University Press and The World Bank.

Broome, J. (1994). Discounting the future. Philosophy & Public Affairs, 23(2):128–156.

Carlsen, B., & Kjellberg, P. K. (2010). Guidelines; from foe to friend? Comparative interviews with GPs in Norway and Denmark. *BMC Health Serv Res*, 10(17). DOI 10.1186/1472-6963-10-17.

Cookson, R., McDaid, D., & Maynard, A. Wrong SIGN, NICE mess: is national guidance distorting allocation of resources? *BMJ*, 323(7315):743–745.

Daniels, N. (2008). *Just Health: Meeting Health Needs Fairly*. Cambridge: Cambridge University Press.

Eddy, D. M. (1990). Clinical decision making: from theory to practice. Designing a practice policy. Standards, guidelines, and options. *JAMA*, 263:1839–1841.

European Society of Cardiology (2007). and other societies on cardiovascular disease prevention in clinical practice (constituted by representatives of nine societies and by invited experts). *Eur J Cardiovasc Prev Rehabil*, Sep;14 Suppl 2:S1–113.

Fleck, L. M. (1987). DRG's. Justice and the invisible rationing of health care resources. *J Med Philos*, 12:165–196.

Fleck, L. M. (2009). *Just Caring: Health Care Rationing and Democratic Deliberation*. Oxford, New York: Oxford University Press.

Fretheim, A., Håheim, L. L., Brørs, O., Kjeldsen, S. E., Kristiansen, I. S., Madsen, S., et al. (2008). *Primaerforebygging av hjerte- og karsykdom. Rapport nr 20-2008. Oslo: Nasjonalt kunnskapssenter for helsetjenesten* [Primary prevention of cardiovascular disease. Oslo: The Norwegian Knowledge Center for The Health Services].

Getz, L., Kirkengen, A. L, Hetlevik, I., et al. (2004). Ethical dilemmas arising from implementation of the European guidelines on cardiovascular disease prevention in clinical practice. A descriptive epidemiological study. *Scand J Prim Health Care*, 22:202–208.

Getz, L., Sigurdsson, J., Hetlevik, I., Kirkengen, A. L., Romundstad, S., & Holmen, J. (2005). Estimating the high risk group for cardiovascular disease in the Norwegian HUNT 2 population according to the 2003 European guidelines: modelling study. *BMJ*, 331:551–552.

Graham, I., Atar, D., Borch-Johnsen, K., Boysen, G., Burell, G., Cifkova, R., et al. (2007). European guidelines on cardiovascular disease prevention in clinical practice: full text. Fourth Joint Task Force of the European Society of Cardiology. *European Journal of Cardiovascular Prevention and Rehabilitation* 14 (Suppl 2):S1–S113.

Grimshaw, J. M., & Hutchinson, A. (1995). Clinical practice guidelines—do they enhance value for money in health care? *Br Med Bull*, 51(4):927–940.

Guyatt, G. H., Oxman, A. D., Kunz, R., Vist, G. E., Falck-Ytter, Y., & Schunemann, H. J. (2008). What is "quality of evidence" and why is it important to clinicians? *BMJ*, 336(7651):995–998.

Hartz, I., Njølstad, I., & Eggen, A. E. (2005). Does implementation of the European guidelines based on the SCORE model double the number of Norwegian adults who need cardiovascular drugs for primary prevention? The Tromsø study 2001. *Eur Heart J*, 26:2673–2680.

Hetlevik, I. (1999). The role of clinical guidelines in cardiovascular risk intervention in general practice. PhD-thesis. Trondheim: NTNU.

Hurst, S. A., & Danis, M. (2007). A framework for rationing by clinical judgment. *Kennedy Inst Ethics J*, 17(3):247–266.

Jackson, R., Lawes, C. M. M., Bennett, D. A., Milne, R. J., & Rodgers, A. (2005). Treatment with drugs to lower blood pressure and blood cholesterol based on an individual's absolute cardiovascular risk. *Lancet*, 365:434–441.

Klein, R. (1993). Rationality and rationing: diffused or concentrated decision-making? In: Tunbridge, T., ed. *Rationing of Health Care in Medicine*. pp. 73–82. London: Royal College of Physicians of London.

Klein, R., & Redmayne, S. (1994). *Patterns of Priorities. A study of the purchasing and rationing policies of health authorities*. University of Bath: Centre for the Analysis of Social Policy.

Klein, R., Day, P., & Redmayne, S. (1996). *Managing Scarcity. Priority Setting and Rationing in the National Health Service*. Buckingham: Open University Press.

Law, M. R., Morris, J. K., & Wald, N. J. (2009). Use of blood pressure lowering drugs in the prevention of cardiovascular disease: meta-analysis of 147 randomised trials in the context of expectations from prospective epidemiological studies. *BMJ*, 338:1665–1684.

Le Grand, J. (1987). Inequalities in health. *Eur Econ Rev*, 31:182–191.

Le Grand, J. (1989). An international comparison of distributions of ages-at-death. In Fox, J., ed. *Health Inequalities in European Countries*. Gower: Aldershot.

Lindman, A. S., Veierod, M. B., Pedersen, J. I., Tverdal, A., Njolstad, I., & Selmer, R. (2007). The ability of the SCORE high-risk model to predict 10-year cardiovascular disease mortality in Norway. *Eur J Cardiovasc Prev Rehabil*, 14(4):501–507.

Meland, E., Ellekjaer, H., Gjelsvik, B., Kimsaas, A., Holmen, J., & Hetlevik, I. (2000). *Medikamentell forebyggende av hjerte- og karsykdommer i allmennpraksis. Tidsskri Nor Laegeforen* [Pharmacological prevention of cardiovascular disease in general practice. *Journal of The Norwegian Medical Association*], 120:2643–2647.

National Institute of Health and Clinical Excellence [NICE]. (2010). NICE public health guidance 25: Prevention of cardiovascular disease. London: National Institute of Health and Clinical Excellence.

Norheim, O. F. (1999). Healthcare rationing—are additional criteria needed for assessing evidence based clinical practice guidelines? *BMJ*, 319(7222):1426–1429.

Norheim, O.F. (2008). Clinical priority setting. *BMJ*, Oct 9;337:a1846.

Norheim, O. F., Gjelsvik, B., Kjeldsen, S. E., Klemsdal, T. O., Madsen, S., Meland, E., et al. (2009). *Retningslinjer for individuell primaerforebygging av hjerte- og karsykdommer* [Norwegian]. Oslo: Helsedirektoratet.

Norheim, O. F. (2010). Gini impact analysis: measuring pure health inequity before and after interventions. *Public Health Ethics*, 3:282–292.

Norheim, O. F., Gjelsvik, B., Kjeldsen, S. E., Klemsdal, T. O., Madsen, S., Meland, E., et al. (2011). Norway's new principles for primary prevention of cardiovascular disease: age differentiated risk thresholds. *BMJ*,.343:d3626–3633.

Norheim, O. F. (2012). Atkinson's index applied to health: can measures of economic inequality help us understand trade-offs in health care priority setting? In Eyal, N., Hurst, S., Norheim, O. F., & Wikler, D., eds. *Inequalities in Health: Ethics and Measurement.* New York: Oxford University Press. 214–231.

Saarni, S. I., & Gylling, H. A. (2004). Evidence based medicine guidelines: a solution to rationing or politics disguised as science? *J Med Ethics*, 30:171–175.

Sackett, D. L., Richardson, W. S., Rosenberg, W., Haynes, R. B. (1997). *Evidence-based Medicine. How to Practice and Teach EBM.* New York: Churchill Livingstone.

Selmer, R., Lindman, A. S., Tverdal, A., Pedersen, J. I., Njolstad, I., & Veierod, D. M. (2008). *Modell for estimering av kardiovaskulaer risiko i Norge. Tidsskr Nor Laegeforen* [Model for estimation of cardiovascular risk in Norway. *Journal of The Norwegian Medical Association*], 128(3):286–290.

Truog, R. D., Brock, D. W., Cook, D. J., Danis, M., Luce, J. M., Rubenfeld, G. D., et al. (2006). Rationing in the intensive care unit. *Crit Care Med*, 234(4):958–963.

United Nations Development Programme UNDP. (2010). Human Development Report 2010. The Real Wealth of Nations: Pathways to Human Development. New York: UNDP.

Wagstaff, A. (2002). Inequality aversion, health inequalities and health achievement. *J Health Econ*, 21(4):627–641.

Wisløff, T., Norheim, O. F., Halvorsen, S., Selmer, R. M., & Kristiansen, I. S. (2008). *Kostnader og leveårsgevinster ved medikamentell primaerforebygging av hjertekarsykdom. Rapport nr XX 2008* [Health economic evaluation of primary prevention strategies against cardiovascular disease. Report number XX 2008. Oslo: The Norwegian Knowledge Center for The Health Services]. Oslo: Nasjonalt kunnskapssenter for helsetjenesten.

22 Physicians as Bellwethers

■ SUSAN DORR GOOLD

■ PROFESSIONAL ETHICS AND CONSTRAINED RESOURCES

Questions of distributive justice, of the tension between individual (patient) and society due to constrained resources, have confronted physicians for centuries and continue to do so in a wide variety of contemporary health systems. Traditionally, the physician's primary responsibility has been to benefit and advocate for their individual patients. This is not the only professional obligation, however; physicians have obligations to protect public health, improve access to care, and educate future physicians, and these obligations, and others, can sometimes run counter to an individual patient's interests.

What role should physicians play in controlling medical expenditures? Few would disagree that physicians should be at the forefront of efforts to identify unnecessary services and develop clinical practice guidelines. The proper role, if any, for physicians in promoting costworthy care for individual patients, however, has been challenged. On the one hand, knowledge of clinical alternatives and of patients' specific preferences and needs enable physicians to individualize recommendations, unlike decision makers who are more distant from the bedside (American Medical Association, 2012; Hall, 1994; Ubel, 1999). For example, while few would refer a young woman for laryngoscopy for hoarseness without either prolonged duration or some other worrisome symptoms, if that woman sings opera one could justify an early referral. Some argue that considering resources when caring for patients does not inherently violate physicians' duties of advocacy and beneficence. In keeping with this view it has been argued that bedside rationing is an inevitable consequence of limited resources, and thus cannot be avoided (Morreim, 1989; Ubel & Goold, 1998). While allocation decisions made on behalf of society should be transparent and open to critique and wider input (Fleck, 1990; Shaul & Mendelssohn, 1997), physicians' decisions for individual patients would generally *not* be transparent to the greater society because of the need for confidentiality.

Given the unsustainable costs of health care, it is not surprising that physicians' roles and responsibilities regarding cost containment, including but not limited to bedside rationing, are a matter of intense and pressing concern for professional organizations, practicing physicians, and patients. The Physician

Charter on Medical Professionalism authored in 2002 by the American Board of Internal Medicine Foundation, the American College of Physicians Foundation, and others, includes obligations of physicians to conserve medical resources, a position with which doctors agree in theory, if not in practice (Gruen, Campbell, & Blumenthal, 2006; Campbell et al., 2007; Blank, 2002). The American Medical Association Council on Ethical and Judicial Affairs added recommendations to the Code of Medical Ethics for physician stewardship. Recent articles in the medical literature (Orszag & Emanuel, 2010) and the lay press (Gawande, 2009) highlight this urgent and enduring issue. Medical educators, clinical leaders, and professional groups increasingly accept the idea that optimizing the care of individual patients requires clinicians to understand the systems of care in which they work and how to improve them (Whitcomb, 2007) and that failure on the part of clinicians to consider the societal costs of clinical decisions may ultimately hurt them as well as their patients.

What can physicians learn from the Values at the Bedside (VBS) study to inform professional ethical practice? In this chapter I will briefly summarize selected findings from the VBS, and then draw implications for physicians, health systems, educators and ethicists. I will propose that physicians should (and sometimes do) advocate for patients (individual patients and patients in general) to improve the fairness of the health system in which they work by taking on the role of bellwether.

■ RATIONING HAPPENS

About 60% of generalist physicians in four countries (Switzerland, Italy, Norway and the United Kingdom) reported rationing their time. A similar proportion (56%) reported that, for at least one type of service, they "personally refrain... because of cost to the system... from using [—] when it would have been the best intervention for your patient" sometime in the preceding 6 months. MRIs and screening tests were reported to be rationed more often that ICU beds or dialysis. I doubt any physician could honestly state they do not spend more time with some patients and less with others, allocating their time according to the patient's needs, for instance for more serious health issues or emotional support. Why do only 60% acknowledge this as "rationing"? Since physicians were more likely to report rationing if they agreed more strongly with rationing, this could reflect social desirability bias—refraining from reporting behavior with which they disagree—as much as actual behavior. Whatever the reason, physicians who fail to acknowledge that they consider limited resources (time, beds, cost) present the profession with an obstacle to transparent, ethically justifiable stewardship, and, of particular concern, undermine transparency with patients. While 82% of VBS respondents reported explaining to a patient at least sometimes why an expensive intervention was not used with a patient, 36% reported they sometimes did *not* inform a patient of a more expensive treatment option.

Studies in many countries over the past two decades have shown that physicians struggle with stewardship. A survey of California physicians found nearly all (95%) agreed physicians should play a role in helping to control health care costs, 88% thought physicians should consider cost effectiveness when weighing different medical interventions for their patients, yet 53% agreed that "if a medical intervention has any chance of helping the patient, it is the physician's duty to offer it" (Ginsburg, Kravitz, & Sandberg, 2000). While 78% of physicians in a US survey agreed that physicians have a professional obligation to address societal health policy issues, over half reported having a moral objection to using cost effectiveness data "to determine which treatments will be offered to patients" (Antiel, Curlin, James, & Tilburt, 2009). When physicians in Geneva completed a survey giving them a choice between a less effective test that would be accessible to all and a more effective test that would require rationing of some sort, although this was not an open-ended survey, several gave comments saying the choice was unethical or offering suggestions on how all could receive the more effective test. Only 26% favored the more effective test that would require some type of rationing (Perneger, Martin, & Bovier, 2002). Nearly all (93%) Norwegian physicians in one study reported they had experienced a conflict between the need of an individual patient and the need to manage the budget (Arnesen & Fredriksen, 1995). Canadian oncologists interviewed about restricted access to cancer drugs reported moral distress and uncomfortable discussions with patients (Berry, Hubay, Soibelman, & Martin, 2007). Choices made by physicians constrained by scarce resources reflect not only their knowledge and values, but also the environments and constraints within which they work—their practices, hospitals, health systems and the overall characteristics of the markets in which they practice (Ubel & Goold, 1998). US physicians, for instance, have been found to offer or recommend more intensive services than doctors from other countries (Koeck, Hemenway, Donelan, & Lipsitz, 1998; McKenzie, Moss, Feest, Stocking, & Siegler, 1998). The VBS found physician responses differed depending on their country, the type of service or intervention, patient resources, patient group, perceived scarcity, and perceived pressure to ration. Some considered their jobs or income at risk due to the cost of clinical decisions they made (Hurst et al., 2006; Hurst et al., 2007). In a review of 15 survey studies about physician acceptance of rationing and attitudes, Strech et al. found enormous variability; willingness to ration ranged from 94% to 9% (Strech, Persad, Marckmann, & Danis, 2009). While the accuracy of these specific proportions may suffer from self-report, social desirability, framing, and other unavoidable methodological limitations of survey research, it is safe to conclude that physicians do consider cost when making decisions and recommendations for patients. These role conflicts will intensify as aging populations and advancing technology increase medical spending, payers pressure clinicians and health care institutions to contain costs, and patients bring their expectations to the doctor–patient encounter.

■ PHYSICIANS AS BELLWETHERS

The term bellwether, from *belle* (bell) + *wether* (a ram, usually castrated), stems from the practice of putting a bell on the leader of a flock so the shepherd can more easily locate it. While being called a bellwether in the fifteenth century was somewhat insulting, and implied that those who followed you were foolish, today "bellwether" applies to things, people, or groups that indicate future developments or trends. A bellwether also can lead others, as a bellwether sheep leads the flock. Physicians can and should take on both of these roles of indicating and leading trends. By keeping alert for and bringing to the attention of others conditions that impair the consistency, flexibility and fairness of allocation, and demonstrating leadership to improve the fairness of resource distribution, they contribute to a more just health system.

The VBS adds evidence to the claim that physicians are able to and do recognize when the health system is discriminatory and/or unjust, and that they recognize that some patients are treated differently when they differ in morally irrelevant ways (type of disease or need, personal financial resources, race, ethnicity, immigrant status, and, arguably, age). For instance, while nearly all respondents in the Values at the Bedside Survey (92.8%) thought everyone in their country should have equal access to needed medical services, 44.1% thought that health care resources in their country were not distributed fairly, 23.6% considered that they were not given enough resources to treat their patients fairly, and 50.5% did not agree that everyone in their country had equal access to needed medical services. Most respondents (78.7%) also reported that at least one group of patients was more likely than others, in their health care environment, to be denied beneficial care on the basis of cost. The most frequently identified groups were patients with mental incapacitation, patients who require chronic care, illegal immigrants, and older patients. They identified some needs (e.g., for mental health care) that disproportionately go unmet, a range of adverse clinical consequences of scarcity, and differential access to services for those with difficulty paying for services, immigrants, and others. Physicians, working on the front lines, appear well placed to see the impact of differences in access to care and health status. But are their impressions accurate? While this question will require further empirical research, the disparities physician identified in the VBS are intriguingly similar to disparities identified in health policy and health services research. As Mackenbach et al. stated, "The most substantial source of health variations within coun-tries is the scale of inequalities between socioeconomic groups defined on the basis of education, occupation, or income" (Mackenbach, Karanikolos, & McKee,2013). Similarly, ethnic minorities, those with mental health needs and immigrants, even in countries with "universal access" to health care, face disproportionate financial (e.g., transportation) and nonfinancial (e.g., language, system knowledge) barriers to care (Mackenbach et al., 2008; Brattheim, Eikemo, Altreuther, Landmark, & Faxvaag, 2012; Håkonsen & Toverud, 2012; Minicozzi et al., 2012).

When physicians find themselves unable to provide what they consider to be necessary services they may "game the system," a behavior that, while hon-oring physicians' duties to patients, conflicts with professional integrity and honesty (Berry et al., 2007). Gaming the system also does little to improve the fairness of the system and may even make it worse. The bellwether role provides an alternative course of advocacy. For instance, if a primary care phy-sician finds that consultation with a pulmonologist (e.g., for a bronchoscopy) faces a prolonged wait, she might communicate with the specialist(s) to move a particular patient with urgent need ahead in the queue, *opening* the gate to care. This advocacy for urgent or necessary services needs to be justified based on judgments about clinical need and urgency; not every patient should be an exception to the routine. Obligations to other current and future patients means physicians can and should recognize the need to use constrained resources fairly, which may mean waiting one's turn absent clinical reasons to "jump the queue." When adverse outcomes become much worse or more frequent due to resource constraints, physicians as bellwethers should be the "squeaky wheels" demanding grease. If the wait time for urgent bronchosco-pies becomes a recurrent problem, the primary care physician might commu-nicate with the pulmonologist(s) and other physicians to address the reason for the profound scarcity and help to resolve it.

Physicians' clinical judgment, and their knowledge of patients' individual needs and preferences, enable them to individualize care. The tremendous variety found in medical practice makes it imperative that physicians have flexibility to meet patients' particular needs. Evidence-based guidelines, pro-tocols and other strategies to improve the quality and consistency of care must remain flexible, and open to physicians' decisions to individualize the care of their patients. Standards that put limits on the unrestrained use of resources (physician or nurse time, operating rooms use, medications, antibiotics) need to be open to appeal, and physician should recognize and alert authorities to systems and structures that constrain their ability to individualize care. For example, an internist had an elderly man report rectal bleeding and difficulty passing stool. On exam, he had a large mass in the rectosigmoid area of the colon. Although he was old and somewhat frail, he and his wife, also frail, lived independently and happily together. Since a large obstructing tumor might need removal to prevent suffering, the internist referred him for endoscopy and biopsy, procedures that are prepared for and undergone typically as an outpatient. Given the patient's frailty, however, the internist recommended these be performed in hospital, and had that approved by the necessary authorities. What if this request were denied? The physician, acting as bellwether, should advocate not just for an individual patient but also for future patients in similar circumstances.

Besides recognizing and alerting responsible parties when resource constraints compromise the standard of care, physicians should also recognize and alert authorities when they find their obligations of beneficence and advocacy are compromised. Some of the physician respondents in the VBS sensed strong pressures, such as threats to their job or substantial financial losses, and those pressures could undermine their relationships with patients, their ability to act on patients' behalf, and their ability to be honest and open with patients.

The power of physicians to advocate for individual patients' needs, and serve as bellwethers for "patient in general" must be used responsibly, credibly and honestly (Brody, 1993). Should physicians be perceived as speaking for themselves when they purport to speak for patients, they will lose credibility, and their ability to advocate for patients will suffer. Neither bellwethers nor shepherds should "cry wolf". As Croxall (1793) warned, "When we are alarmed with imaginary dangers in respect of the public, till the cry grows quite stale and threadbare, how can it be expected we should know when to guard ourselves against real ones?"

Physicians clearly recognize a responsibility to the system of care, to promoting efficiency and avoiding waste. In a US survey of physicians about professionalism, Campbell et al. found nearly all (98%) agreed that "Physicians should minimize disparities in care due to patient race or gender" while 93% agreed that "Physicians should provide necessary care regardless of the patient's ability to pay" and 86% that "Physicians should advocate legislation to assure that all people in the United States have health care insurance coverage" (Campbell et al., 2007). One quarter said that they had looked for possible disparities in their care on the basis of race or gender in their practice, clinic, hospital, or other health care setting. Serving as bellwethers, as leaders alert to front lines issues that compromise patient care, enables clinicians to combine their professional obligation to the system of care with obligations to "put the patient first" rather than pitting these obligations against each other.

REFERENCES

American Medical Assoication. (2012). *Code of Medical Ethics 2012-2013: Current Opinions with Annotations (2012)*. Chicago, IL: American Medical Association.

Antiel, R. M., Curlin, F. A., James, K. M., & Tilburt, J. C. (2009). Physicians' Beliefs and US Health Care Reform—A National Survey. *New England Journal of Medicine, 14*, e23.

Arnesen, T., & Fredriksen, S. (1995). Coping with obligations towards patient and society: an empirical study of attitudes and practice among Norwegian physicians. *Journal of medical ethics, 21*(3), 158–161.

Berry, S. R., Hubay, S., Soibelman, H., & Martin, D. K. (2007). The effect of priority setting decisions for new cancer drugs on medical oncologists' practice in Ontario: a qualitative study. *BMC health services research, 7*(1), 193.

Blank, L. (2002). Medical professionalism in the new millennium: A physician charter. *Annals of Internal Medicine, 136*(3), 243–246.

Brattheim, B. J., Eikemo, T. A., Altreuther, M. Landmark, A. D., & Faxvaag, A. (2012). Regional disparities in incidence, handling and outcomes of patients with symptomatic and ruptured abdominal aortic aneurysms in Norway. *European Journal of Vascular and Endovascular Surgery 44*(3), 267–272.

Brody, H. (1993). *The Healer's Power.*New Haven and London: Yale University Press.

Campbell, E. G., Regan, S., Gruen, R. L., Ferris, T. G., Rao, S. R., Cleary, P. D., & Blumenthal, D. (2007). Professionalism in medicine: results of a national survey of physicians. *Annals of Internal Medicine, 147*(11), 795.

Fleck, L. M. (1990). Justice, HMOs, and the invisible rationing of health care resources. *Bioethics, 4*(2), 97–120.

Gawande, A. (2009). The cost conundrum: What a Texas town can teach us about health care. *The New Yorker, 85*(16), 36–44.

Ginsburg, M. E., Kravitz, R. L., & Sandberg, W. A. (2000). A survey of physician attitudes and practices concerning cost-effectiveness in patient care. *Western Journal of Medicine, 173*(6), 390.

Gruen, R. L., Campbell, E. G., & Blumenthal, D. (2006). Public roles of US physicians. *JAMA: the journal of the American Medical Association, 296*(20), 2467–2475.

Håkonsen, H., & Toverud, E. L. (2012). Cultural influences on medicine use among first-generation Pakistani immigrants in Norway. *European Journal of Clinical Pharmacology, 68*(2), 171–178.

Hall, M. A. (1994). The problems with rule-based rationing. *Journal of Medicine and Philosophy, 19*(4), 315–332.

Hurst, S. A., Forde, R., Reiter-Theil, S., Slowther, A. M., Perrier, A., Pegoraro, R., & Danis, M. (2007). Physicians' views on resource availability and equity in four European health care systems. *BMC Health Services Research, 7*(1), 137.

Hurst, S. A., Slowther, A. M., Forde, R., Pegoraro, R., Reiter, T., S., Perrier, A.,…Danis, M. (2006). Prevalence and determinants of physician bedside rationing: data from Europe. *Journal of General Internal Medicine, 21*(11), 1138–1143.

Koeck, C., Hemenway, D., Donelan, K., & Lipsitz, S. (1998). Using a hypothetical case to measure differences in treatment aggressiveness among physicians in Canada, Germany and the United States. *Wiener Klinische Wochenschrift, 110*(22), 783.

Mackenbach, J. P., Karanikolos, M., & McKee, M. (2013). The unequal health of Europeans: successes and failures of policies. *Lancet, 381*(9872), 1125–1134.

Mackenbach, J. P., Stirbu, I., Roskam, A. J., Schaap, M., Menvielle, G., Leinsalu, M., & Kunst, A. E. and the EU Working Group on Socioeconomic Inequalities in Health. (2008) Socioeconomic Inequalities in Health in 22 European Countries. *New England Journal of Medicine, 23*, 2468–2481.

McKenzie, J. K., Moss, A. H., Feest, T. G., Stocking, C. B., & Siegler, M. (1998). Dialysis decision making in Canada, the United Kingdom, and the United States. *American Journal of Kidney Diseases, 31*(1), 12–18.

Minicozzi, P., Cirilli, C., Federico, M., Capocaccia, R., Budroni, M., Candela, P., Falcini, F., et al. (2012). Differences in stage and treatment of breast cancer across Italy point to inequalities in access to and availability of proper care. *Tumori, 98*(2), 204–209.

Morreim, E. H. (1989). Fiscal scarcity and the inevitability of bedside budget balancing. *Archives of Internal Medicine, 149*(5), 1012.

Orszag, P. R., & Emanuel, E. J. (2010). Health care reform and cost control. *New England Journal of Medicine, 363*(7), 601–603.

Perneger, T. V., Martin, D. P., & Bovier, P. A. (2002). Physicians' attitudes toward health care rationing. *Medical Decision Making, 22*(1), 65–70.

Shaul, R. Z., & Mendelssohn, D. C. (1997). Scarce Resource Allocation Decisions: Issues of Physician Conflict and Liability. *Humane Health Care International, 13*, 25–28.

Strech, D., Persad, G., Marckmann, G., & Danis, M. (2009). Are physicians willing to ration health care? Conflicting findings in a systematic review of survey research. *Health Policy (Amsterdam, Netherlands), 90*(2-3), 113.

Ubel, P. A. (1999). Physicians' duties in an era of cost containment: advocacy or betrayal? *Journal of the American Medical Association, 282*(17), 1675.

Ubel, P. A., & Goold, S. (1998). Does bedside rationing violate patients' best interests? An exploration of "moral hazard". *American Journal of Medicine, 104*(1), 64–68.

Ubel, P. A., & Goold, S. D. (1998). "Rationing" health care. Not all definitions are created equal. *Archives of Internal Medicine, 158*(3), 209–214.

Whitcomb, M. E. (2007). Professionalism in medicine. *Academic Medicine, 82*(11), 1009.

23 Moving Away from Silent Trepidation

Changing the Discussion of Rationing and Resource Allocation

■ MARION DANIS, GREER DONLEY, AND REIDUN FØRDE

The concept of rationing has been approached with great reservation across the globe. Even though many bioethicists and policy experts accept the need to set fair and explicit limits on health care to improve its financial sustainability and equity, public receptivity remains a challenge (Daniels & Sabin, 2008; Fleck, 2009; Ubel, 2001).

In this chapter, we consider why rationing has been anathema to the public and propose that by taking into account the psychology of human decision-making, discussion of rationing may become more feasible. The goal is not simply to achieve a more sustainable health care system, but also to ensure that individuals are provided transparent medical care and the opportunity to participate in the public debate regarding this sensitive topic. As such, we argue that a more explicit discussion of rationing will promote fairer rationing and serve as a prerequisite in a democratic society. We begin by briefly considering the ethical rationale for explicit discussion of rationing. We then explore strategies for more explicit discussion of resource allocation and rationing

We suggest that conversations about rationing should occur at three levels—the public arena, the institutional sphere, and the clinical encounter. At each level, different challenges need to be addressed in explicitly discussing rationing; however, conversation at all three levels will, in combination, improve public receptivity to the practice of rationing by enhancing the trustworthiness of the message. The discussion in the public arena should lay the groundwork for public understanding of the justifications for prioritizing and rationing health care as a fair strategy for allocating resources. At this level, the conversation should emphasize how fair rationing can be achieved through transparency, accountability and reasonableness. At the institutional level, the dialogue should revolve around notification and providing patients with sufficient information to help them understand the priority setting process and rationing procedures used by their organization. The language and practice of rationing in the clinical encounter should build upon patients' preferences for a trusted clinician to make appropriate decisions on their behalf. It should also nudge patients to share with their clinical provider in choosing the most cost-effective health care. Explicit acknowledgment of the costs along with the benefits of health care is warranted in all these arenas, in order to facilitate public understanding of the need for financially sustainable health care.

▪ BACKGROUND

The most commonly accepted definition of rationing in the medical and clinical ethics literature states that "rationing encompasses any explicit or implicit measures that allow people to go without beneficial healthcare" (Ubel & Goold, 1998). This definition captures a wide range of mechanisms to limit access to interventions. Based on this definition, health care rationing already exists in every country; some countries use more explicit and fair measures to ration health care, while others ration less fairly particularly on the basis of ability to pay (Ubel & Goold, 1998; Coulter & Ham, 2000). Despite the prevalence of rationing, it is a very uncomfortable topic of conversation.

At the outset we note that in European—and particularly, Nordic countries—the term *rationing* is not used as commonly as the terms *setting priorities* and *prioritization*; in these countries rationing is seen as one of many different ways of setting priorities. While we most frequently use the term rationing in this chapter, we do so as shorthand for rationing and other forms of priority setting. Occasionally, we explicitly mention both terms where there are relevant differences between them.

While laying out our approach to more explicit discussion of rationing, we will make several assumptions. First, that every country faces budgetary limits and health care costs that compete with other valued expenditures (see http://www.who.int/whosis/whostat/EN_WHS2011_Full.pdf). Second, even though there are many ways to reduce costs that ought to be pursued, we will assume that limiting utilization will inevitably be needed in comprehensive cost-containment strategies (Fleck, 2009; Ubel, 2001). It will be impossible for any society to provide every person with every possibly effective medical benefit given constrained budgets. Indeed unlimited spending on health care is unwise since it limits expenditures on health-inducing interventions outside of the health sector as well as expenditures for other valued aims. Limiting utilization in a logical and effective fashion requires making explicit decisions to prioritize particular interventions for particular indications. Some have argued that rationing will not be needed to make health care costs sustainable particularly if prices are reasonable, but we disagree that adjustments to prices alone are sufficient to create a sustainable health care system (Anderson et al., 2003).

Third, we will assume that reasonably fair rationing strategies already exist in both theory and practice (Daniels & Sabin, 2008; Fleck 2009; Coulter & Ham, 2000). The experience of rationing in a number of countries demonstrates its feasibility (Coulter & Ham, 2000). Given these assumptions, we are concerned with improving the public's understanding of rationing.

■ THE VARIED NATURE OF THE COSTS OF ILLNESS AND MEDICAL CARE ACROSS COUNTRIES

Despite the ubiquitous necessity to ration, we recognize that any argument for encouraging more explicit dialogue about rationing will need to take into account the varied nature of health care delivery and financing across borders (see http://www.who.int/whosis/whostat/EN_WHS2011_Full.pdf). High-income countries tend to have more universal health insurance than less well developed countries, although notable exceptions exist. In addition, the profile of covered benefits and the degree of out-of-pocket spending varies among countries.[1] Whether or not patients have health insurance, how much it costs, what benefits are covered, the manner in which benefits are distributed, and what is left to patients to pay personally are factors that determine the financial burden of illness faced by patients and their families. Even in nations where most of the public is insured, personal costs of illness can be quite high. In the World Health Organization's publication, *World Health Statistics 2011*, the extent to which spending on health care was financed privately and the extent to which private expenditures were paid out of pocket ranged dramatically (see http://www.who.int/whosis/whostat/EN_WHS2011_Full.pdf). While the amount of total health expenditures financed by the private sector was reported to be 38% on average in 2011, the percentages ranged from 94% in the highest ranking country to <1% in the lowest ranking country. The percentage of out-of-pocket expenditures was 50% on average, but ranged from 100% in the highest ranking countries to <1% in the lowest ranking countries (http://www.globalhealthfacts.org/data/topic/map.aspx?ind=67).

These differences in the distribution of the financial burden of illness are pertinent in any consideration about the ethics of discussing health care costs and rationing with patients and the level of comfort or aversion patients might actually have in talking about these issues.

■ THE ETHICAL IMPORTANCE OF DISCUSSING RATIONING

While the purpose of this chapter is to argue for the practical value of discussing rationing explicitly and to suggest strategies for doing so, we first briefly consider the ethical importance of explicit discussion of rationing. The major concern is that when rationing occurs without disclosure or notification, a key element of ethically sound rationing is undermined (Daniels & Sabin, 2008; Fleck, 2009). Health policy issues are a matter of great importance to the public. Health care costs, and in particular the utility-cost ratio are important considerations with profound social implications. Hence, such issues should be part of a public debate in which citizens engage directly with their elected representatives and other interested, political groups, or in which chosen representatives of the public engage in publicly accessible discussion. To the extent that governmental agencies make rationing policies, the public ought to be a part of the conversation.

At the institutional level, systematic disclosure of prevailing organizational norms and guidelines for making allocation decisions would serve to promote transparent, professional, and effective health care delivery (Young et al., 2012).

In the clinician–patient encounter, if costs influence the type of intervention recommended, there are several reasons for bringing that fact to the patient's attention. Before specifying these reasons, we want to clarify, that if a clinician believes a less expensive diagnostic or therapeutic approach is just as good in all regards as a more expensive one, the decision to use this less expensive approach should not be considered rationing. In this situation, it seems justifiable for clinicians to forgo discussion of costs despite taking costs into consideration in making such decisions. But if indeed rationing does occur, one important reason for doing so explicitly relates to the strong influence of physicians and other clinicians over the kind of care patients do or do not receive. Positioned as they are to select diagnostic and therapeutic interventions, they are in an inescapable position to determine the allocation and cost of health care resources (Crosson, 2012). Consequently, they play a role in determining whether or not medical care is distributed fairly.

Physicians make decisions about the use of resources at the bedside by three mechanisms: (1) on the basis of resource constraints such as short supplies or institutional allocation decisions that are imposed upon them, (2) by following rules of medical practice such as guidelines or triage policies, or (3) by exercising clinical judgment where the first two mechanisms do not apply (Truog et al., 2006; Hurst & Danis, 2007). Many factors influence clinicians' decisions about whether to intervene diagnostically or therapeutically including the strength of evidence, probability of effectiveness, as well as financial incentives. Given how influential physicians are with regard to making recommendations to patients and carrying out medical decisions, and in so doing, determining health care expenditures and resource distribution, it seems advisable that physicians communicate with patients about the cost of various treatments and the financial basis of their recommendations when pertinent.

Evidence suggests that when clinicians must ration, and do so implicitly, they may make choices that are not necessarily consistent with socially agreed upon priorities (Baker, 2005). Unless there are clinically justifiable reasons for doing so, this ought to be avoided whenever possible. Moreover, there are additional instrumental reasons for discussing costs with patients. Discussing pros and cons of diagnostic tools and treatment, including their costs, with well informed patients may not only lead to fewer interventions and save costs, but may in addition reduce complications and lives lost (Wennberg, 2010). To the extent that costs are borne personally by patients, explicit discussion is instrumental in allowing them to have a say regarding personal expenditures.

There are two alternatives to our recommendation about explicit clinician communication regarding resource limitations and the cost of care. One alternative is that physicians will ignore cost in medical decision making, opting simply for the treatment that is most effective (which is often the most expensive) and newest (which is often perceived to be better) regardless of the cost. This alternative is likely to contribute to persistently soaring health care costs and the lack of sustainability in a health care system. A second alternative is that clinicians will ration without mentioning this to patients. In so doing, they would practice bedside rationing without notifying patients. One might counter that the latter approach is acceptable so long as systematic notification by the health care organization is taking place. Such an approach may be appropriate in circumstances when the standard of care for a particular medical condition does not include certain interventions, and a clinician is simply following this standard. An example might be the exclusion of patients with advanced, untreatable cancers from intensive care since this approach has been endorsed in guidelines of several critical care professional organizations (ATS and ACCM). In such an instance, institutional or organizational notification about such policies might suffice. But, it may not follow that prior notification by the health care organization is adequate for informing patients about specific instances of rationing,[2] particularly when there are personal out-of-pocket costs along with shared costs (health plan or insurer costs) to consider. For this and other reasons discussion of costs in the clinical encounter may have great value. The alternative of prior notification must offer sufficient procedural fairness and respect for persons if it is to suffice.

■ AVERSION TO RATIONING: A GLOBAL PERSPECTIVE

Having argued for the merits of explicitly discussing rationing, we must confront the many reasons why it is discussed so little. The topic of rationing has been met with resistance in nearly every country (Coulter & Ham, 2000). Some factors contributing to this aversion are specific to a given country, while other factors are more universal. Clearly some cultures are more receptive to shared sacrifice than others. The initial experience with rationing of energy in Japan following the 2011 tsunami and destruction of the Fukushima nuclear power plants reflected a remarkable willingness of the Japanese to ration even in the face of public distrust of political leadership (Onishi, 2011). In other countries receptivity is less.

Historical experience with rationing plays an important role in understanding the public's aversion. Many countries share an association of rationing with wartime. During World War II for example, people predominately accepted the need for rationing policies as a sacrifice necessary to win the war (Adams, 1989; Baily, 1984; Zweiniger-Bargielowska, 1994). However, the acceptability of rationing plummeted once the war ended—rationing became viewed as a mechanism to be used only during emergencies or crises (Baily 1984; Goodin & Dryzek, 1995). This conception of rationing has deterred support of rationing as a routine means of ensuring fairness when resources are limited.

But there are psychological reactions that pose sources of aversion towards rationing that seem to supersede cultural and historic influences. For instance, people are known to irrationally value the lives of identifiable people over statistical lives (Moore, 1996). This psychological tendency has implications for rationing—identifiable, and often sick, individuals may be asked to forgo care for the sake of a greater health improvement for unidentified (and often, future) others.[3] The fact that many rationing decisions are for the sake of long term benefits, as opposed to short term gain, provides another psychological barrier to rationing; humans have generally been perceived to have a preference for immediate, over long term, rewards (though the extent to which this phenomenon exists in all circumstances is uncertain; see Frederick, 2002). Perhaps one of the more important factors in any natural reluctance to accept rationing is an inherent self-centeredness, often described as originating from evolutionary biology, which inclines humans to maximize their own gains at the expense of a group. This tendency has been portrayed in scenarios known as tragedies of the commons (see chapter 13 by Goodin; also Hardin, 1968).

These tendencies are characteristic of human judgment and decision making that often lead people to form impressions and arrive at decisions that are not internally consistent or logically coherent. Human thought processes involve judging situations, relying on mental habits, and making decisions that are likely to make it difficult for patients to choose less expensive treatment options even though these options may offer, on balance and in the long run, the potential for greater overall benefits. As Kahneman describes so lucidly in his book, *Thinking, Fast and Slow* (Kahneman, 2011), human systems of thought operate efficiently by coming to quick and automatic decisions with little voluntary thought; this automatic approach is very advantageous for promoting rapid responses to danger, and thus guarding against harm, but it often leads to shortcuts in thinking that leave little room for careful analysis of the advantages and disadvantages of the consequences of choices. Perhaps most notable among these human reactions is a general aversion to loss that likely contributes to a rather universal 'gut' reaction underlying the reluctance to ration (Ubel, 2009). Observational studies indicate that people irrationally value what they have and will therefore forgo improvement to avoid loss (Tversky, 1991; Kahneman, 2011). Only with effortful mental activity do people make careful judgments about decisions. It takes training and experience to make the kind of decisions that require careful calculation and reasoning. In TABLE 23.1 we list some of these tendencies and consider how they are likely to manifest in patients' thoughts about clinical decisions.

For all of these reasons, and perhaps others, rationing of medical care has been met with resistance. In many places, the topic of rationing has become so politically untenable that discussions promoting health care rationing are strictly avoided (Baily, 1984; Daniels & Sabin, 2008). In such political environments without public conversations supporting rationing, the public's predominate exposure to rationing becomes the often fear-inducing language used by opponents of rationing or priority-setting policies. This has been exemplified by the negative use of the term rationing during US elections and during US health care reform debates ("Obama's Senior Moment," 2009; "The Rationing Commission," 2009). In other countries it is politically feasible to have discussions at the political level. In Norway, for example, public commissions have explicitly addressed resource allocation, referring to it as *priority setting*, and ethical guidelines for doctors for nearly two decades have addressed doctors' duty to pay adequate attention to society's resources. Yet, even there, regardless of the extent to which rationing is addressed in the public arena, physicians tend to be hesitant about rationing. They tend to redefine actual rationing as doing what is beneficial and efficient in each individual decision (Skirbekk & Nortvedt, 2011). Though some physicians report considering cost when they make decisions, they often do so without communicating to patients (Sacramento Healthcare Decisions, 2001; Strech, 2008). While there are no published comparative data, it is likely that depending on the country, the reluctance to discuss costs in the clinical encounter is variably due to fear of litigation or patient backlash, a sense that such disclosure is unnecessary, or genuine opposition to rationing. Another reason may be that doctors find it morally wrong to emphasize expenses in individual patient cases (Dybwik, 2012; see also Bruun Wyller chapter 15). Unfortunately, the lack of communication between doctors and patients perpetuates the public perception that rationing and resource allocation do not occur.

Popular language and stories about rationing exacerbate aversion to it. Indeed, many human interest stories about rationing in the public media focus on adverse consequences for identifiable individuals and engender highly

TABLE 23.1. *Extrapolating from Kahneman: Characteristics of Decision Making that are Likely to Affect Reactions to Cost Conscious Medical Decisions*[7]

Decision-Making Characteristic	Explanation	Possible Implications for Medical Decision Making
Relying on lazy thinking[8]	The human mind is prone to make simple decisions automatically and quickly and require little voluntary control.	When asked to pick a highly effective treatment or a less expensive treatment that may be slightly less effective, the automatic reaction is to go for the better-chance treatment.
Making selfish choices when the mind is busy	When people must expend much energy, emotion, or self-control, they get tired, ego-depleted, and have a harder time acting virtuously.	Patients who have faced demanding situations such as illness are less likely to do well in making cognitively demanding treatment decisions. They will have a harder time making decisions that involve trade-offs in cost and benefit or forgoing benefits for the sake of others.
Jumping to conclusions	People tend to make rapid judgments; often this is an efficient use of mental energy, but it may lead to wrong conclusions.	When patients are judging options, they may quickly jump to the conclusion that the most expensive option is best
Cognitive ease	People have an easier time making decisions about which they are comfortable. Such decisions that feel familiar and effortless are more likely to be perceived as good decisions. Conversely, patients have a harder time making decisions that are unfamiliar.	If patients are unfamiliar with thinking about costs in medical decisions they will have a harder time with such decisions and are likely to find such decisions to be worse.
Tending to answer an easier question than the one asked	It may be hard to answer a question about which of two treatment regimens is the best.	A person may answer the easier question about which was the one chosen by a friend, or which is the treatment that my doctor is most familiar with. A person is likely to make a treatment choice based on answering the easier question.
Anchoring	If people are aware of the value of something, it will serve as an anchor for judging the value of other things.	If a patient knows that a hospital stay costs thousands of dollars, a medicine that costs hundreds of dollars a month may seem much more acceptable than it would otherwise. Had they been unaware of the expensive hospital cost, they might have found this expensive medicine less acceptable.
Allowing causes to trump statistics	People tend to infer causality from repeatedly observing events associated with one another.	Patients may assume that a clinical improvement was caused by a costly medical intervention, for example back pain improved after back surgery, even though studies show that statistically the intervention was not likely to have made a difference.
Trusting expert intuitions	People tend to trust the advice of a familiar, respected, and long-standing expert over newly validated scientific evidence.	Patients would prefer to rely on their doctors' advice than to follow evidence-based recommendations.

charged negative emotional reactions. Take for example stories in the media about cancer patients whose cancer medication was not be paid for by the British National Health Service ("NHS to Bruce Hardy: Drop Dead," 2008; Altaner & Rule, 2008). There are also drawbacks to the language used to discuss rationing in the academic literature. The commonly accepted definition of rationing as "any explicit or implicit measures that allow people to go without beneficial healthcare" was intended to be descriptive (Ubel & Goold, 1998) and thus lacks reference to the valuable purpose that rationing ought to serve and why it is needed. The implication of this definition, which emphasizes giving up benefit, is problematic for public acceptance of the concept. Explicit discussion of rationing that offers positive reasons both on an individual and societal level and addresses aversive reactions is warranted if fair and explicit rationing is going to take place.

■ FOSTERING DISCUSSION OF RATIONING

Having argued for the appropriateness of explicitly discussing rationing in terms that will address the worries of the public in general and patients in particular, we turn to suggesting approaches to doing so. The proposal here focuses on two aspects: (1) conducting the discussion in a way that attends to the modes of thought that people employ when they judge situations or make decisions and (2) creating a multi-tiered level of conversation in which each tier is mutually reinforcing.

■ THE LANGUAGE IN THE CONVERSATION

Given the factors that foster aversion to rationing, a key step in reducing the reluctance to discuss rationing ought to involve use of language and messages that acknowledge and address these aversions. The tendency to fear loss should be addressed with information about the gains that can be achieved through priority setting and rationing strategies. The language should be focused on a self-interested approach—namely that rationing will ensure that every individual can enjoy a health care system that will be sustainable for themselves and their children in the future. The tendency to focus on short-term gains might be addressed by evidence of immediate benefits of making medical care more affordable.

We are not suggesting that discussion of rationing be focused exclusively on its most palatable effects in a manner that is deceptive; rather, we argue that the discussion's aim should ensure that the purpose of rationing is understood and its consequences for patients are presented in a balanced manor that addresses their concerns. The best language is not likely to be uniform across countries. In Nordic countries a focus on solidarity may be better received. In these countries, the reason given for setting priorities fairly is to guarantee that the neediest get help first and that the most severe conditions with greatest negative impact on health receive attention before the treatment of more trivial conditions. The societal perspective in these countries tends to accept sacrifice of less important or pressing medical interventions so that, if an individual develops a more serious condition she is certain to get the necessary help. Again in these countries there is a sense of solidarity with others who are the worse off.

In Switzerland, on the other hand, emphasis is best framed in terms of the mutual advantage offered by rationing: "the rationing that other patients experience makes it possible for me to have access to care, and I cannot have just anything I want." In the United States, a focus on enlightened self-interest will be more consonant with prevailing political culture. The language used might thus cover both individualistic and more altruistic or enlightened motives and considerations. Yet, to the extent that the psychology of human decision transcends cultural context, there are likely to be some commonalities in the language and presentation of rationing regardless of the national context. What becomes apparent when we consider shaping the discussion about rationing to address the public's concerns is that the rationale for explicit notification and discussion of rationing that moral philosophers and medical ethicists might emphasize is necessary but not entirely sufficient to address the worries of the general public or patients. While more liberally minded individuals would be persuaded by arguments about fairness, more conservatively minded individuals would not necessarily find fairness a sufficiently complete basis for a convincing justification for rationing (Haidt, 2012). Given the broad commitments of conservatively leaning individuals to respect for authority, loyalty, and sanctity (Haidt, 2012), it seems important to explore justifications for resource allocation that acknowledge these values. Can we talk about allocating health care resources as an effort that authoritative and respected leaders might endorse? Can we talk about allocating resources as a commitment to loyalty—an effort that binds us together as a society committed to taking care of one another? Can we consider how to allocate resources in a way that is attentive rather than threatening to the sacred commitments that many people hold?

We began our argument in favor of discussing rationing with the claim that a fair rationing process includes notification. This reason for discussing rationing with patients is that the discussions provide a clear and easily understandable explanation about why rationing is needed and how it will be conducted fairly. Giving patients such an explanation is inherently part of the way rationing ought to be practiced. Proponents of rationing do not endorse all rationing mechanisms; they defend fair rationing. As moral philosophers and bioethicists might define it, fair rationing encompasses any transparent, accountable, and reasonable measures that are done for the sake of improving the efficiency and equity of the system. We would add that the explicit discussion of rationing should emphasize the positive aim underlying the need for people to go without some potentially beneficial health care—so that they and others can instead receive the most value for the cost of their health care and to foster solidarity with the worst off. We might use the term *priority setting* rather than rationing to emphasize that the task at hand is not merely about forgoing benefits but about balancing benefits. If the conversation is going to be acceptable to a public that has a wide range of moral commitments, it must also be attentive to those moral commitments.

There are many advantages to discussing the positive ends that priority setting and rationing are meant to accomplish. The first is that the definition is based on the kinds of rationing defended in scholarly works (Daniels & Sabin, 2008; Fleck, 2009). Another is that the motive of rationing policy—to improve the output and equity of the system while stabilizing costs—is included. Beyond this, the priorities of people of various persuasions can be put on the table for discussion. Presenting the trade-offs involved in rationing evenhandedly, as this definition does, may help reduce the public antipathy toward the concept when described with a sole focus on loss, harm, and fairness. The final advantage of framing discussions around fair rationing is that explicit articulation of what makes rationing fair can facilitate the lay public's judgments of whether or not actual rationing strategies are indeed fair.

The explicit discussion of rationing should facilitate public understanding that reduction of health care costs is not only a matter of shared public concern, but also a matter of immediate personal concern. Thus the discussion of rationing arguably ought to be brought up as part of a general conversation about health care costs, both those that are shared in the form of taxes and insurance premiums as well as those absorbed personally by patients. The rationale for discussing treatment priorities for the sake of controlling shared costs is that such a discussion assures fairness and due process; the justification for encouraging discussion of personal costs between clinicians and patients pertains to respect for patient autonomy, since personal health care costs pose important personal opportunity costs. Getting patients involved in talking about treatment options that range in expense will offer them the possibility of reducing personal expenses, through a personal choice to forgo care, and freeing up personal financial assets that could be spent on other expenditures that will improve their health and well-being.

But merely addressing concerns that moral philosophers and bioethicists have about the need for explicit notification about rationing in order to guarantee fairness will not suffice entirely. It will not address the problems resulting from the human tendency to make judgments and decisions that are not logically consistent and consonant with cost-effective, financially sustainable health care. If this is the case, it is ethically justifiable to utilize approaches to communication that encourage the public to resist this psychological tendency to make the kind of irrational judgments and decisions that we know people tend to make. In this sense it seems defensible and even advisable to adopt a libertarian paternalistic approach that nudges the public toward greater acceptance of rationing, while at the same time ensuring their right to participate in the dialogue. In so doing, it would help patients to understand that cost-conscious medical decisions will yield a financially sustainable health care system that is in their interest.

As Thaler and Sunstein (2008) argue, choices are never free of influence, and decisions are always constructed by a choice architect. Clinical decisions are no exception, and even the decision to avoid a discussion of rationing will shape the debate in many respects. In fact, decisions regarding medical care are exactly the kind of decisions that psychologists have argued can benefit from guidance. They are decisions that are sometimes among the most consequential to individual's health and well-being; the stakes are often high, and patients face these choices without many opportunities to practice.

Thus, health policy experts serve as choice architects who shape public views about public expenditures on health care. Professional societies who write professional guidelines shape choices about what the standard approach ought to be toward management of various clinical conditions. Clinicians, in particular, serve as the choice architects for the sort of decisions that are entirely appropriate to consciously structure in a manner that offers guidance. Of course, it is not novel to argue that clinicians ought to guide decision making with patients. But what we are suggesting is that guidance about how to factor in the cost consequences of medical decisions is reasonable and advisable. A clinician who presents a therapeutic plan, or offers a patient a set of therapeutic options to choose from, is a choice architect and as such might justifiably nudge or encourage patients through the language used to frame decisions to signal to them an accurate understanding and appreciation of the options. The failure to do so is, in fact, participating in nudging patients to avoid these needed calculations. Helping patients understand that the most cost-effective approach, the less expensive approach, or the marginally less effective but much less costly approach, in a vast array of clinical circumstances, may be the most reasonable approach to take.

Considering the sort of psychological reactions that we might expect the public and patients to have toward cost-consciousness and rationing, and the justification for nudging people to react somewhat differently, we can now consider how address these psychological tendencies in ways that might alter such reactions. The strategies that one might expect to make people more comfortable with cost-consciousness are likely to involve a series of adjustments. These include the development of more positive emotions about lowering health care costs through stories of patients who have benefited from spending less; promoting cognitive ease and skill at thinking about health care costs through practice; reducing inaccurate predictions about the consequences of rationing; and framing the reasons for resource allocation in

TABLE 23.2. *Addressing Psychological Tendencies that Could Alter Reactions to Rationing*

Strategy	Description
Alter associations with rationing to create positive emotions.	• Present stories of patients who have adopted healthy lifestyles that prevent health care spending. • Present stories of patients who have forgone some treatment they thought was necessary and have resolved their illness and/or some patients who have forgone some diagnostic test and have remained healthy, as statistics would have predicted. • Present stories of patients who have forgone some treatments and spent the money for other things of value to them.
Promote cognitive ease with the concept of rationing to make rationing more familiar and effortless. Simplify the message.	• Use resource-allocation techniques routinely so that the public is familiar with them. • Present messages about rationing that are bold, colorful, simple, and memorable.
Enhance acceptance of cost reduction in health care through reference to cost reduction in other spheres of life.	• Help patients think of many instances in which they have tried to save money in their lives.
Tame intuitive predictions that patients have about cost containment that are inaccurate.	• Intuitive predictions about the consequences of rationing are likely to be overly confident and overly extreme. Trusted clinicians may be able to assure patients that their intuitions are not accurate predictions.
Promote conditions for acquisition of the skill of cost containment.	• Create an environment that is sufficiently regular to be predictable and an opportunity to learn these regularities through practice.
Foster patient appreciation of an outside view that relies on statistics.	• Help patients become more comfortable with decisions based on practice guidelines rather than their own clinician's clinical hunches.
Find strategies for overcoming the disproportionate emotional impact of immediate gains rather than the long-term prospects of wealth and global utility. Create reference points that anchor medical expenses to less expensive alternatives.	• Use illustrative stories that give a balanced picture comparing the gains from expenditures today and expenditures tomorrow. • Encourage proactive thinking about health care costs so these decisions occur when individuals are not tired and stressed by illness.
Reduce the tendency to worry about rare events and to neglect the denominator when making choices.	• Helping the public understand true rate of problems associated with rationing may tame these impressions.

terms of a broad set of moral commitments including not only fairness but also respect for loyalty and sacredness We describe these possibilities and others in TABLE 23.2.

Some might argue that any conjecture that it would be possible to successfully nudge the public to appreciate that cost-conscious medical care, priority setting, and rationing may help to create more financially sustainable health care is folly. But there are precedents for changing public attitudes about a number of health care strategies that are pursued for greater future benefits or for the greater benefit to all. Successful efforts to change public attitudes about health-promotion strategies come to mind. For instance, it took very systematic effort to foster widespread use of cancer screening such as Pap smears and colonoscopies (Meissner, 2004). Similarly, very systematic implementation strategies have been successful in encouraging behavioral change that promotes healthy behavior including smoking cessation, adoption of physical activity, and a healthful diet (Ory et al., 2002). If we extrapolate from such efforts, it becomes apparent that while a long process of research and translation of the results may be necessary, it may be possible to change public understanding and appreciation of the need for financially sustainable medical care. In the case of rationing, the initial aversion might be stronger; however, the ultimate strategy ought to remain feasible given that in both cases provided above, an effort was made to help the public realize that the long-term benefits, both individually and societally, were worth the short-term costs, and to overcome that initial aversion.

Examples of research aimed at helping patients to choose high-value health care has begun. An experiment showing that a well designed report that presents cost data alongside easily interpretable quality information can increase the likelihood that consumers will choose high value (high quality, lower price) care (Hibbard et al., 2012). As we will describe in more detail below, we have conducted focus groups in the United States to examine what types of discussion will make patients more comfortable discussing costs with physicians. The results show that the most crucial factor is a trusting relationship with a familiar clinician (Danis, 2013).

■ FOSTERING DISCUSSION AT MANY LEVELS

Shifting from consideration of the type of language and the nature of the conversation that might address the public's aversion to rationing, we consider how the discussion at several levels including the public arena, the institutional setting, and the clinical encounter may have a useful synergistic effect in the dialogue overall. The conversation in these three settings might serve to reinforce one another. The message in the public arena should focus on the fact that rationing does occur in every society, and should emphasize how rationing strategies may contribute to fostering affordable health care. The discussion at the institutional level serves as explicit and clear notification of how rationing is practiced. The discussion in the clinical encounter involves a dialogue between the patient and clinician that is sensitive and attentive to the medical and financial concerns of each patient and family.

The Public Arena

While discussion of rationing in the public arena may be contentious, there are many factors that promote the feasibility of an open discussion of rationing. Among these is the need for austerity measures in many countries. A report from the *Economist* in 2009 about projected health care costs for European countries is illustrative:

> Across Europe, healthcare is barely managing to cover its costs. Not only are the methods for raising funds to cover its costs inadequate, but, of even greater concern, the costs themselves are set to soar. According to World Bank figures, public expenditure on healthcare in the EU could jump from 8% of GDP in 2000 to 14% in 2030 and continue to grow beyond that date. The overriding concern of Europe's healthcare sector is to find ways to balance budgets and restrain spending. Unless that is done, the funds to pay for healthcare will soon fall short of demand. (http://www.janssen-emea.com/sites/default/files/The-Future-Of-Healthcare-In-Europe.pdf.)

Broadly speaking, the public conversation about restraining health care costs will need to include the rationale and benefits of setting limits for the sake of financially sustainable health care. An effective, fair, and affordable health care system is widely considered the backbone of a humane society that attends to the welfare of its residents. For the sake of those with a broad set of moral commitments, the conversation should address the possibility that an affordable health care system can be compatible with their commitments. The public conversation would seem to be the appropriate arena to convey to the public how necessary planning, priority setting, and rationing are, and that fair, affordable, and purpose-driven resource allocation is in their interest. The conversation will include a role for many players including media, politicians, health policy experts and administrators, community leaders, religious leaders, and the public at large.

Politicians will need to be open to discussing which types of health care that they want to have prioritized and which to be rationed. In many countries, politicians who are elected officials may hesitate to discuss the cost of goods and interventions as well as the need to prioritize and possibly exclude anything. In facing their electoral public, politicians may wish to appease constituents and blame others for the problems of health care costs. But they will need to engage their constituents as active partners in deliberation about priorities if they want to work toward creating a viable and continuous solution that is ultimately in their constituents' best interests.

As we have argued, this conversation might use the sort of strategies that attend to the psychological reactions that one can anticipate. The messages might convey, for instance, how universal is the need for setting priorities and rationing, how thinking about health care costs can be similar to thinking about other living expenses, what practical steps one can take to become familiar with health care costs, and how one might become skilled at trying to cut health care costs.

The language used to communicate the need for rationing needs to deliberately address anxiety related to anticipated loss. It should consistently be stated that rationing is not exclusively about taking care away; rather, it is about choosing what matters most and ensuring that everyone gets his or her fair share at a more tolerable cost. It is also about finding alternative, less costly solutions to achieving health to which the public can contribute. We might imagine a public health campaign that depicts alternative scenarios of managing a chronic disease such as non–insulin dependent diabetes: one scenario depicts individuals who develop complications and require a great many costly medically intensive interventions; another scenario shows individuals who manage their diabetes through medications combined with more aggressive diet and exercise and avoid some complications and interventions along with avoiding higher costs (Hibbard, 2013). In so doing, such a public message combines concepts of health promotion with concepts of cutting health care costs. The message will therefore create a more positive association with cost cutting, show the role that patients can actively take in keeping costs under control, and make the matter of cost integral to other aspects of health care familiar and manageable. While these paired scenarios focus on chronic disease management, one might imagine similar paired scenarios that focus their message on a range of health circumstances from prevention to palliation.

Public deliberation about rationing would be an important component of making rationing an explicitly discussed topic in the public arena. This is in addition to the role that public deliberation may play in actually contributing to the setting of priorities and rationing decisions. Simply by opening the black box and familiarizing people with the process, the unknown becomes familiar, the reasoning becomes more routine, and the comfort level increases. Through public experience of priority setting and rationing, the intuitive reactions that people have may be replaced with more ability to reason and consider whether marginal benefits are worthwhile. With experience in thinking about rationing, they may be less likely to jump to overly simplistic conclusions about complicated choices. They may be able to appreciate that more health care is not necessarily better (Fisher, 2003; Ashton, 2003). Research shows that deliberation in small groups to prioritize covered benefits, when framed in terms of trade-offs that must be made within a constrained budget, are quite feasible (Danis et al., 2010). Using structured decision exercises for rationing, exercise participants become more cognizant of the need to pay attention to the cost of medical interventions in order to make health care affordable and become more accepting of limiting costs (Danis et al., 2007). Fleck (2009) has shown that deliberative polling provides a very explicit way of engaging the public in rationing. While Daniels (2007) has argued that the sort of deliberative polling that Fleck recommends is not practically feasible, we would suggest that this sort of engagement process, or others like it, help the public understand the need for rationing in a way that may not be possible otherwise.

The conversation in the public arena needs to foster public understanding of insurance as a shared communal resource that offers financial security by pooling their insurance premiums to cover unpredictable health care costs (Fleck, 2009). The public dialogue needs to foster understanding that we live with health care systems whose financial viability are a function of the utilization rates of everyone in the insurance pool, along with the prices for services. Failure to impose explicit limits on care creates a tragedy of the commons in which everyone tends to use resources without restraint, leading to rapidly rising costs where everyone is worse off (Fleck, 2009). The opportunity cost of unbridled expenditures in health care is the diminished availability of funds for other important needs, impacting all citizens regardless of the source of their insurance. The extent to which the public is educated about and receptive to such realities will greatly depend on the country in question.

While fair and publicly acceptable rationing will manifest differently in various countries, the concepts we have brought to bear on the discussion of rationing should be applicable in any health care system in certain regards. Given the varied nature of health care financing and delivery systems, we anticipate rationing decisions are likely to be made by all entities that have legitimate responsibility for distributing health care resources or delivering health services. These entities would include public and private insurers as they make benefit coverage decisions, as well as clinicians as they make day-to-day diagnostic and therapeutic decisions. In countries where there are more centralized systems, communication about rationing may be inherently more straightforward than more decentralized systems, but one might argue that the same logic applies. Rationing can be carried out fairly if it is consistently (a) based on evidence about comparative effectiveness and cost effectiveness, (b) practiced with attention to local constraints and the needs of the population (c) adheres to rules of fairness—transparency, relevancy, ability to appeal, and enforcement (Daniels, 2008), and (d) other features of the health care system such as pricing are reasonably arranged.[4]

The Institutional Level

The chapters in this volume about institutional efforts to promote fair rationing in Norway by Soreide, Kvinnsland, and Heggestad (chapter 16) and in Switzerland by Schurmann and colleagues (chapter 18) provide descriptions of novel efforts to create strategies to promote rationing in health care organizations. We would argue that a key element in the success of such institutional efforts to foster fair and explicit rationing at the bedside will involve the systematic notification of patients about rationing in a manner that makes patients and employees familiar and comfortable with the process. Young and colleagues (2011) take on this question in a manuscript arguing for systemic disclosure of rationing in intensive care. Notifying patients about the numerous strategies that a health care organization employs to promote fair, effective, and publicly acceptable priority setting and rationing—including explicitly explaining the institutions commitment and priorities, the use of practice guidelines, triage policies, waiting lists, and use of cost-effectiveness data—serves to familiarize patients with the systematic approach that the organization endorses and practices in delivering care to the population it serves. Notification at the institutional level plays a crucial role in setting the stage for the discussion in the clinical encounter. It serves to prepare patients to expect such a discussion in the clinical encounter. It lets them know that the discussion they have with their personal clinician is occurring on a level playing field in which other clinicians and patients are likely to be having the same sort of conversations.

The Clinical Encounter

Conversations about rationing must have a different tone during the clinical encounter than they do in the public arena or at the institutional level. These conversations require sufficient time (Jones, 2004). The clinician who faces patients who are sick or injured must be careful and considerate, taking into account how vulnerable they are when making diagnostic and therapeutic decisions. Although the tension between the physician's role as patient advocate and steward of health care resources is a pressing problem, open communication with patients about their health care choices can be compatible with caring for a patient (Gratton & Keatings, 2001; Pearson, 2000).

When aware of preventative, diagnostic, prognostic, or therapeutic interventions that are slightly less effective but much less costly than other interventions, physicians would be justified in presenting, explaining, and considering the less expensive ones. Some research suggests that patients will be particularly receptive to discussion of personal costs, as they weigh heavily on their minds (Alexander et al., 2003). To promote such an approach to clinical decision making, physicians need to have full and ready access to research on decrementally effective treatment options, which will allow them to engage responsibly and effectively in a conversation about limiting marginally more effective interventions (Nelson, Cohen, Greenberg, & Kent, 2009). Access to the results of such research is likely to become increasingly available and its use increasingly endorsed.

Doctors should communicate openly with their patients when cost is one of the factors influencing their decision. Studies on patient attitudes toward explicit rationing conducted in the United Kingdom indicate that patients prefer doctors to be open about rationing when it is occurring (Owen-Smith et al., 2009). Physicians should communicate in a way that centers the conversation on the care being offered and describes the considerations that went into their decision. In this way, fair rationing can be conveyed without focusing on the care withheld, thus mitigating a patient's loss aversion. Physicians should assure patients that they are prescribing helpful and effective interventions even though they are not prescribing the most expensive interventions.

Part of the reassurance for patients when clinicians discuss treatments is to articulate, to begin with, what they aim to achieve and how a decision that involve cost savings still achieves the intended aim. The clinician might also indicate that the standards used in choosing the treatment were reasonable and fair, if this seems to be of concern to the patient. Clinicians can convey this point by highlighting that they recommend this to all of their patients, that this is their standard approach as part of the effort to ensure that health care remains affordable for everyone. Being honest with patients regarding the motive for limiting care will be important for the discussion overall.

The discussion in the clinical encounter can be tailored to particularly address the patient's personal financial resources and how he or she would like personal finances to be taken into account in making medical decisions. As illness can be anxiety producing, the language needs to be sensitive and empathetic. This will be particularly important for very sick or terminally ill patients, as discussed below (Donley & , Danis 2001). Many physicians and patients have become familiar with a deliberative model in which they negotiate an understanding of the patient's illness and determine the best way to manage it together (Emanuel & Emanuel, 1992). Doctors ought to incorporate more of the financial ramifications as part of this deliberation. Several authors have proposed strategies for discussing costs in the clinical encounter. Hardee and colleagues (2005) suggest an empathic approach to help patients accept out-of-pocket costs, and this same strategy may be useful in talking to patients about both societal and personal costs. Similarly, Keller and Carroll (1994) have offered an approach to engaging patients in which physicians Engage, Empathize, Educate, and Enlist (the E-4 model) to facilitate such a discussion. In particular, it may be useful for the patient to receive help to clarify his or her own values and preferences.

Incorporating these approaches, a doctor might introduce the concept of costs to a patient for the first time in the following way:

> As we consider what treatment is best for you, I will mention a number of options. The treatments vary in how effective they are, how many medical side effects they have, and in how expensive they are. We will aim to find an appropriate treatment plan for you. I generally try to take this approach with all my patients. If you have any personal concerns that are important to think about while we are making these decisions, please let me know about them. I know, for example, that a

person's financial situation might be affected by the cost of medical care. If you would like, we can talk about how we can best manage your treatment in a way that is sensitive to your financial concerns.

The conversation may need to be tailored and framed differently based on the health care system in which the physician is operating. It is not clear that these strategies will necessarily be completely successful. In the focus group study done in the United States, which we discussed above, participants did not think these strategies would enhance their comfort with the prospect of discussing costs with physicians as much as a trusting relationship would (Danis, 2013).

While we have yet to identify clinical strategies that are entirely welcome on the part of patients, we have argued above that this comfort will develop over time with systematic efforts by actors across settings. Moreover, one can justifiably say that the nature of clinical discussions of cost are best if they reflect the need for fairness and concern for the patient's health, interests, and values. When costs are broached, the conversation will need to use empathetic communication strategies. When the clinician makes decisions that are in keeping with cost-conscious guidelines, this should be explained. When personal costs are at stake, physicians ought to foster joint decision making with their patients. Without reaching a decision together, patients will feel that important care was taken away from them. Patients have reported feeling that conversations regarding cost were most helpful when the physician expressed sympathy for their financial constraints, informed them about the least important medications to take, referred them to drug payment programs, asked if they could afford prescriptions, and passed along information on where to get less expensive medications (Alexander et al., 2003).

During the conversation, it is reasonable for the clinician to provide a range of therapeutic options that vary in personal and societal cost along with the probability of success, convenience, or expected duration of survival at the point of terminal illness. Some data suggests that patients would find this appealing. For example, one study with over 5,000 respondents revealed that two-thirds of patients would consider drugs that had lower effectiveness, higher chance of side effects, or higher dosing frequency if they were less expensive (Tseng et al., 2010). When physicians do discuss costs and discover that patients have cost-related concerns, clinicians need to respond to those concerns. A study of chronically ill patients has shown that approximately one-third of them underused medication because of cost concerns. While most of such patients find their doctors do respond by suggesting less expensive alternatives, as many as a third of clinicians do not do so (Piette et al., 2004). In this way, physician response to this information is vital to improvement and empty talk will not be sufficient.

■ TALKING TO PATIENTS ABOUT END-OF-LIFE COSTS

For most countries, information about the cost of health care at the end of life is not available (Blank, 2011). While information about the cost of care in the last year of life is followed carefully in the United States, the United States is unusual in this regard (Hogan, 2009). Given that higher-income countries have generally higher per capita health care expenditures and more techno-logically advanced health care systems that offer the possibility of extensive life-sustaining interventions, it is safe to surmise that they spend far more than low-income countries on end-of-life care. But even if there is such variability, worries about unsustainable costs for an aging population pertain worldwide. As the United Nations Department of Economic and Social Affairs reported in 2007, aging will be a dominant theme for development in the twenty-first century. By 2050, almost 2 billion people will be aged 60 years or over; 80% of them will live in developing countries (UN Department of Economic and Social Affairs, 2007). In European countries, where the aging of the popula-tion has already occurred, the quality and cost of end-of-life care has been a major concern (Economist Intelligence Unit, 2011).

While the sustainability of the health care system in every country is a pressing matter, the problem translates into very difficult choices for patients at the end of their lives when their chronic or terminal illnesses worsen. For instance, should a patient with widespread cancer pursue chemotherapy that costs several times their annual wages to prolong life for 2 to 3 months? Should a patient with heart failure repeatedly spend time in the intensive care unit? Should a patient with chronic obstructive lung disease repeatedly receive arti-ficial ventilation? Should families of patients with end-stage dementia choose to provide care at home, or opt for care in an institution? These choices have large financial and other ramifications for patients and families.

Because the end of a person's life is an emotionally intense time, conver-sations about the cost of end-of-life care necessarily need to be handled in a particularly thoughtful and sensitive manner; yet, we believe they can and should happen. Two strategies that clinicians might use to foster discussions of end-of-life costs with their patients are mentioned here (Donley & Danis, 2011).[5] The first is to encourage discussions of the financial ramifications of illness throughout the trajectory of a chronic illness so that attention to costs becomes routine rather than unanticipated. The second strategy is to encour-age inclusion of a financial dimension in end-of-life planning. In the United States, this would mean the inclusion of cost considerations when a patient is preparing an advance directive. Exploration and anticipation of choices before the end of life will offer patients adequate time to consider their goals and choose a strategy appropriate for them.

Discussions of cost in advance may be especially important given that many patients lack the capacity to make their own medical decisions by the time they reach the end of life (Silveira et al., 2010). In the absence of a written advance directive or verbal discussion regarding a patient's end-of-life preferences, the next of kin are often put in the position of participating in medical decisions on behalf of the patient without adequately understanding their wishes. Without prior explicit discussion about a patient's views, the spouse, partner, or children of a dying patient are likely to experience one of two conflicts when considering cost in evaluating medical decisions for someone else. Either they will have a conflict of interest regarding their inheritance, which may be negatively affected by the cost of expensive, end-of-life treatments, or they may experience an emotional conflict regarding their obligation to pursue the most aggressive care to avoid feeling (or being perceived by others as) insufficiently caring. In either case, family members may be aided in acting as surrogate decision makers if the ill family member has explicitly articulated financial concerns and goals in advance.

In suggesting that financial concerns be explicitly addressed in advance, we would make several points that apply to advance care planning in general. The first point is that while people often worry that patients will be reluctant to broach the topic of the end-of-life finances just as they have been reluctant to engage in advance care planning as a whole, we contend that when discussed in a manner that is supportive and nonthreatening, many patients will welcome the chance to discuss this topic since it is quite likely to be weighing on their minds. Second, published studies indicate that family members who have had an opportunity to have preemptive discussions of treatment preferences with patients feel more comfortable acting as surrogate decision makers.[6] Third, patients are not necessarily good at affective forecasting—knowing how they will feel at some time in the future. Some will change their minds. Thus, for those patients who remain conscious and able to participate in decisions, the opportunity to revise their previously expressed wishes should be made explicit when death approaches.

Through these strategies, clinicians can avoid abruptly and insensitively introducing financial issues at the conclusion of a person's life when one would prefer to address the painful and important issues of spiritual and existential loss that are appropriately the focus when a person is dying. Furthermore, encouraging patients to discuss the financial consequences of their illness earlier will address the financial burden that they are quite likely facing on an ongoing basis and will allow them to make trade-offs at a time when they can plan for the end of their life in a more controlled fashion.

While we have suggested that it is appropriate to discuss financial concerns about end-of-life care with patients before death is imminent, we recognize that many therapeutic decisions with potentially profound cost implications are often made close to the time of death. At this point, decisions about whether to use or forgo life-sustaining treatments are no longer abstract considerations about the future and are likely to be contingent on many factors that only crystallize as death approaches—including religious commitments, quality of life, probability of benefit from further treatment, and expected gain in survival. Patient and family religious beliefs and their inclinations to fend off death or accept it are all likely to influence treatment decisions. These decisions are made all the more difficult while families are likely to be preoccupied and vulnerable and thus hard pressed to collaborate in making carefully reasoned decisions. If costs are going to be discussed at this juncture, two points seem most salient. First, the discussion should be handled as gently and supportively as possible. Second, as we have suggested above, the introduction of the matter of cost earlier in the illness trajectory may make the discussion of cost at this point more comfortable.

■ SOME CAVEATS AND LIMITATIONS

One concern for countries where patients experience high personal health care costs is that financially disadvantaged patients may be more likely to forgo expensive care due to personal costs than wealthier patients, and consequently they may bear the brunt of the burden in reducing health care costs for all. Without systemic changes, this is likely to be the case. The opportunity costs of pursuing expensive treatments will be greater for individuals with few financial assets. The financial factors motivating poor or low-income patient to forgo expensive interventions will likely be more salient and immediate. In so far as reductions in insured costs are for the benefit of all, not for the benefit of the individual patient, it would be unjust to allow the burden to fall more heavily on one particular group, especially given that the financially less well-off already have worse health outcomes.

Addressing this inequity fully means that public and private insurers must minimize disparities in health insurance coverage. Primarily, that will entail a determination of what qualifies as a fair and decent minimum of care. That minimum ought to be covered for every beneficiary. Ideally, the amount of copays and out-of-pocket expenses ought to be an inverse function of income status, thus minimizing the disparity in the incentives for members of each group as they make treatment choices. We recognize that more fully attending to these disparities is a tall order (see chapter 19). However, conversations that explicitly address the costs of care are advisable nonetheless, since they remain likely to mitigate the burden of health care costs.

Another caveat is that significant time, resources, and information may be required for clinicians to properly discuss financial aspects of care (Nicholas, 2009). However, it need not be the case that physicians shoulder this role entirely nor do they need to be completely well versed in financial matters. Physicians should understand the need to address financial issues with patients and know to whom to refer patients and where to get financial information. Physicians ought to refer patients to other resources that might be better able to address a patient's financial needs; for instance, financial counselors or social workers. We acknowledge that more information regarding comparative effectiveness will need to be available to clinicians to allow the approach suggested here to be most effectively implemented.

A final caveat relates to the need to determine whether such conversations can be conducted in a way that is helpful to patients rather than overwhelming and confusing. Research is also needed to ensure that clinicians and patients can have such conversations in a way that does not undermine patient trust in the physician's commitment to their overall well-being.

■ CONCLUSION

Finding strategies for discussing health care costs and rationing in the clinical encounter will not be straightforward. Determining how such discussions might be incorporated into the medical conversations in a manner that will educate and engage patients in an appropriate and nonthreatening manner is important. Pursuing such discussions will be easier if the way is paved by serious public discussions on limit setting and by systematic notification about rationing strategies in health care institutions. A multi-pronged approach would prepare patients by making them familiar with the need to ration and with strategies for doing so. While we anticipate that such discussions would help patients grow accustomed to cost-conscious decision making and rationing in their personal medical care, research is needed to go beyond conjecture. We must also acknowledge that if the incentive structure for clinicians is one that induces them to provide more care, discussions among the public and between clinicians and their patients may help to increase public acceptance of the need to prioritize and ration care, but the cost of care will likely continue to rise nonetheless.

Notes

1. The WHO publication on world health statistics defines out-of-pocket expenditures on health as follows: The direct outlays of households, including gratuities and in-kind payments made to health practitioners and to suppliers of pharmaceuticals, therapeutic appliances and other goods and services. This includes household direct payments to public and private providers of health care services, nonprofit institutions, and nonreimbursable cost sharing, such as deductibles, copayments, and fees for services. Private Health Expenditure: The sum of expenditures on health by prepaid plans and risk-pooling arrangements, firms' expenditure on health, nonprofit institutions serving mainly households, and household out-of-pocket spending. See http://www.who.int/whosis/whostat/2011/en/index.html.

2. Even in this situation in which a clinician might be following established recommendations in not admitting a patient with widely metastatic cancer into the intensive care unit, it may be useful, albeit not necessarily ethically required, to discuss this decision with the patient and family as part of a larger discussion about the goals of care for such a terminally ill patient.

3. We assume few people are likely to think about rationing the way Paul Menzel would encourage them to do in chapter 14.

4. While many ways to reduce costs ought to be pursued—including, importantly, pricing—we assume that utilization rates are higher than they need to be. Indeed, while some argue that utilization rates for hospitalization are low in the United States, there is substantial overutilization of many procedures and new pharmaceuticals (Emanuel, the perfect storm of overutilization). Thus, limiting utilization will inevitably be needed in a comprehensive costs-containment strategy.

5. Much of the text here is from our prior publication on talking to patients about the costs of end-of-life care (Donley & Danis, 2010).

6. While these studies on advance directives do not explicitly involve issues of cost, we surmise that the finding might nevertheless hold true when costs enter the advance care conversation. Ultimately, family members will want to respect the wishes of their relatives, which is true whether or not cost is a part of those preferences. This is, however, in the absence or evidence, a matter of speculation.

7. We extrapolate here from the insights offered by Daniel Kahneman in *Thinking, Fast and Slow* (Kahneman, 2011) because they are likely to be helpful for improving the decision-making process for doctors and patients.

8. When Daniel Kahneman refers to lazy thinking he does not intend to be insulting of human decision making. The capacity to make efficient decisions that require little waste of time and attention is what allow humans to come to rapid necessary judgments that protect us at moments when we need to act swiftly in response to dangerous and threatening situations. Nonetheless, while thinking quickly is sometimes essential for our rapid response to dangerous situations, at other times it is likely to lead to less than the best decisions.

REFERENCES

Adams, D.P. (1989). Wartime bureaucracy and penicillin allocation: The Committee on Chemotherapeutic and Other Agents. *Journal of the History of Medicine and Allied Sciences, 44*, 196–217.

Alexander, G. C., Casalino, L.P., & Meltzer, D. O. (2003). Patient-physician communication about out-of-pocket costs. *JAMA, 290*(7), 953–958.

Altaner, D., & Rule, B. (2008). Cancer patients lose shot at longer life in U.K. cuts (update1). *Bloomberg*, November 17. Available from http://www.bloomberg.com/apps/news?pid=newsarchive&sid=aYPuCa1iuxG8.

Amos Tversky, D. K. (1991). Loss aversion in riskless choice: a reference-dependent model. *Quarterly Journal of Economics, 106*(4), 1039–1061.

Anderson, G. F., et al. (2003). It's the prices, stupid: Why the United States is so different from other countries. *Health Affairs, 22*(3), 89–105.

Ashton, C.M., et al. (2003). Hospital use and survival among Veterans Affairs beneficiaries. *New England Journal of Medicine, 349*,1637–1646.

Baily, M. A. (1984). "Rationing" and American health policy. *Journal of Health Politics,* 9(3), 489–501.

Baker, R. (1993). Visibility and the just allocation of health care: a study of age-rationing in the British National Health Service. *Health Care Analysis,* Vol. I, 139–150.

Blank, R. H. (2011). End-of-life decision making across cultures. *Journal of Law, Medicine & Ethics,* 39(2), 201–214.

Cost-Effectiveness as a Criterion for Medical and Coverage Decisions: Understanding and Responding to Community Perspectives, 2001: Sacramento. Available at: http://chcd.org/docs/vf.pdf.

Coulter, A., & Ham, C., eds. (2000). *The Global Challenge of Healthcare Rationing.* Philadelphia: Open University Press.

Crosson, F. J. (2009). Change the microenvironment: delivery system reform essential to controlling costs. *Modern Healthcare* and The Commonwealth Fund. Available at: http://www.commonwealthfund.org/Content/Publications/Commentaries/2009/Apr/Change-the-Microenvironment.aspx.

Daniels, N., & Sabin, J. E. (2008). *Setting Limits Fairly.* 2nd edition. New York: Oxford University Press.

Daniels, N. (2010). Book review of Fleck L. E., *Just Caring: Health Care Rationing and Democratic Deliberation.* Notre Dame Philosophical Reviews. Available at: http://ndpr.nd.edu/news/24413-just-caring-health-care-rationing-and-democratic-deliberation/.

Danis, M., Ginsburg, M. & Goold, S. (2010). Experiences of engaging the public in priority setting for health through structured small group decision exercises. *Journal of Ambulatory Care Management,* 33, 205–214.

Donley, G., & Danis, M. (2011). Making the case for talking to patients about the costs of end-of-life care. *Journal of Law, Medicine, and Ethics,* 39, 183–193.

Dybwik, K., Nielsen, E. W., & Brinchmann, B. S. (2012). Ethical challenges in home mechanical ventilation. A secondary analysis. *Nursing Ethics,* 19, 233–244.

Emanuel, E., & Emanuel, L. (1992). Four models of the physician-patient relationship. *Journal of the American Medical Association,* 267(16), 2221–2226.

Fisher, E.S. (2003). Medical Care—Is More Always Better? Editorial, *New England Journal of Medicine,* 349, 1665–1667.

Fleck, L. M. (2009). *Just Caring.* p. 460. New York: Oxford University Press.

Frederick, S., Loewenstein, G., & O'Donoghue, T. (2002). Time discounting and time preference: a critical review. *Journal of Economic Literature,* 40(2), 351–401.

Goodin, R. E., & Dryzek, J.S. (1995). Justice deferred: wartime rationing and postwar welfare policy. *Politics and Society,* 23(1), 49–73.

Gratton, C., & Keatings, M. (2001). Advocacy and rationing are compatible. *Healthcare Papers,* 2(2), 62–67.

Haidt, J. (2012). *The Righteous Mind: Why Good People Are Divided by Politics and Religion.* Pantheon Books: New York.

Hardee, J.T., Platt, F.W., & Kasper, I.K. (2005). Discussing health care costs with patients: an opportunity for empathic communication. *Journal of General Internal Medicine,* 20(7), 666–669.

Hardin, G. (1968). The tragedy of the commons. *Science,* 162(3859), 1243–1248.

Hibbard, J. H., Greene, J., Overton, V. (2013). Patients with lower activation associated with higher costs; delivery systems should know their patients' 'scores'. *Health Affairs (Millwood),* 32(2), 216–222.

Hogan, C., Lunney, J., Gabel, J., & Lynn, J. (2001). Medicare beneficiaries' costs of care in the last year of life. *Health Affairs,20*, 188–195.

Hurst, S.A., & Danis, M. (2007). A framework for rationing by clinical judgment. *Kennedy Institute of Ethics Journal, 17*(3), 247–266.

Jones, I. R., Berney, L., Kelly, M., Doyal, L., Griffiths, C., Feder, G., et al. (2004). Is patient involvement possible when decisions involve scarce resources? A qualitative study of decision making in primary care. *Social Science & Medicine,59*, 93–102.

Kahneman D. Thinking, Fast and Slow. New York, Farrar, Straus and Giroux. 2011.

Keller, V. F. & Carroll, J.G. (1994). A new model for physician-patient communication. *Patient Education and Counseling, 23*, 131–140.

Meissner, H. I., Smith, R. A., Rimer, B. K., Wilson, K. M., Rakowski, W., Vernon, S. W. & Briss, P. A. (2004). Promoting cancer screening: Learning from experience. *Cancer,* 101(5 Suppl), 1107–1117.

Moore, R. F. (1996). Caring for identified versus statistical lives: An evolutionary view of medical distributive justice. *Ethology and Sociobiology, 17*(6), 379–401.

"NHS to Bruce Hardy: Drop Dead" (2008). ONTD Political, December 3. Available from http://ontd-political.livejournal.com/1757751.html.

Nelson, A. L., Cohen, J. T., Greenberg, D., & Kent, D. M. (2009). Much cheaper, almost as good: decrementally cost-effective medical innovation. *Annals of Internal Medicine, 151*, 662–667.

Nicholas, J. (2009). ASCO Rx for high drug costs: doctors and patients need to talk. *Journal of the National Cancer Institute, 101*, 1441–1444.

"Obama's Senior Moment" (2009). Editorial. *Wall Street Journal,* 14 August. Available from http://online.wsj.com/article/SB1000142405297020386320457344900152168372.html.

Ory, M. G., Jordan, P. J., & Bazzarre, T. (2002). The behavior change consortium: setting the stage for a new century of health behavior-change research. *Health Education Research 2002;17,* 500–511.

Owen-Smith, A., Coast, J., & Donovan, J. (2009). Are patients receiving enough information about healthcare rationing? A qualitative study. *Journal of Medical Ethics, 36,* 88–92.

Piette, J. D., Heisler, M., Wagner, T. H. (2004). Cost-related medication underuse: do patients with chronic illnesses tell their doctors? *Archives of Internal Medicine,164*(16), 1749–1755.

Pearson, S. D. (2000). Caring and cost: the challenge for physician advocacy. *Annals of Internal Medicine, 133*(2), 148–153.

Sacramento Healthcare Decisions. (2001). *Visible Fairness: Cost-effectiveness as a criterion for medical and coverage decisions.* Available from http://chcd.org/docs/vf.pdf.

Selinger, E., & Whyte, K. P. (2011). Is there a right way to nudge? The practice and ethics of choice architecture. *Sociology Compass,* Vol. 5, No. 10, pp. 923–935. Available at SSRN: http://ssrn.com/abstract=1883243.

Silveira, M. J., Kim, S. Y. H., & Langa, K. M. (2010). Advance directives and outcomes of surrogate decision making before death. *New England Journal of Medicine, 362*(13), 1211–1218.

Skirbekk, H., & Nortvedt, P. (2011). Making a difference: a qualitative study on care and priority setting in health care. *Health Care Analysis, 19*(1), 77–88.

Strech, D., Synofzik, M., & Marckmann, G. (2008). How physicians allocate scarce resources at the bedside: a systematic review of qualitative studies. *Journal of Medicine and Philosophy, 33*, 80–99.

"The Rationing Commission" (2009). Editorial. *Wall Street Journal*. Available from http://online.wsj.com/article/SB10001424052748703792304574504020025055040.html.

Truog, R. D., Brock, D. W., Cook, D. J., Danis, M., Luce, J. M., Rubenfeld, G. D., Levy, M. M.; Task Force on Values, Ethics, and Rationing in Critical Care (VERICC). (2006). Rationing in the intensive care unit. *Critical Care Medicine, 34*(4), 958–963.

Tseng C.-W., Waitzfelder, B. E., Tierney, E. F., Gerzoff, R. B., Marrero, D. G., Piette, J. D., et al. (2010). Patients' willingness to discuss trade-offs to lower their out-of-pocket drug costs. *Archives of Internal Medicine, 170*(16), 1502–1504.

Ubel, P. A. (2009). The Cost of Human Nature. In Center, T. H., ed. *Health Care Cost Monitor*.

Ubel, P. A. (2001). *Pricing Life: Why its time for healthcare rationing*. Cambridge, MA: The MIT Press.

Ubel, P. A., & Goold, S.D. (1998). "Rationing" health care. Not all definitions are created equal. *Archives of Internal Medicine, 158*(3), 209–214.

UN Department of Economic and Social Affairs. (2007). World Economic and Social Survey 2007: Development in an Ageing World. Available at http://www.un.org/en/development/desa/policy/wess/wess_archive/2007wess.pdf

Young, M. J., Brown, S. E., Truog, R. D., & Halpern, S. D. (2012). Rationing in the intensive care unit: to disclose or disguise? *Critical Care Medicine, 40*(1), 261–266.

Zweiniger-Bargielowska, I. (1994). Rationing, austerity and the Conservative Party recovery after 1945. *The Historical Journal, 37*(1), 173–197.

24 Priority Setting As a Clinical Skill

How Do We Educate Physicians?

■ ANNE SLOWTHER
AND BENJAMIN P. BENNETT

The preceding chapters of this volume have addressed the topic of bedside rationing/priority setting from many angles. By now, it should be clear how rationing fits into broader health care contexts, why rationing is necessary, why it is morally justifiable, and how it can be implemented effectively. The contributing authors broadly agree, with the rare dissenting view, that physicians have an important and unavoidable role in decisions about how resources are allocated (rationed/prioritized) in the provision of patient care, given that overall health care budgets are finite and unlikely to be able to accommodate increasing demand for health services. This role may take many forms including contribution to development of national policy, providing clinical leadership for institutional priority setting, implementing clinical guidelines in practice, or making clinical judgments in individual cases. What is also clear is that prioritization decisions, at both the institutional and individual practitioner level, have always occurred to some extent but have been implicit rather than explicit, usually categorized under clinical judgment or improving efficiency of health care delivery. A concern with implicit prioritization is that it allows personal and professional biases to go unchallenged and is likely to lead to increased inequity in health care. There is consensus that rationing, if it is to occur, should be explicit and open to scrutiny. While there is some evidence that physicians believe bedside rationing does occur and should occur, they also report that they need support when facing these decisions (Hurst, 2008). There is also evidence that physicians resist explicit rationing measures that impact directly on them, either financially or in their relationship with their patients (Carlsen & Norheim, 2005; Tilburt et al., 2013). If physicians are not adequately equipped or motivated to engage in priority setting in the clinical setting then the arguments and suggested frameworks articulated in previous chapters will have little impact on care. To this end, this final chapter will address education of physicians with regard to priority setting.

It is important to state at the outset that fair rationing in health care will not be achieved solely by educating future and current physicians, however comprehensive and well taught a curriculum we devise. For fair rationing to become a reality we would need to see changes in a variety of cultural, political, and professional attitudes as well as changes in the structure of incentives that are beyond the reach of medical teachers (and this chapter). Educating physicians is, however, necessary for any changes we would like to see happen. As has been noted elsewhere in this book, physicians have a tremendous ability to affect the amount of money being spent in a health care system. If physicians are to influence priority setting in health care, either directly or indirectly, they have an obligation to do so fairly. And, as health care is ultimately funded by potential recipients of care (patients and the public), they have an obligation to demonstrate the fairness of the prioritization decisions that they make. Physicians should be able to justify their reasons for prioritizing some interventions "at the bedside," for complying with guidelines that prioritize resources, or indeed for acting contra to such guidelines if they choose to do so. As this is something they have not traditionally been called on to do, they will need to have appropriate training that takes account of the knowledge, skills, and attitudes required for physician priority setting and addresses the barriers that may account for the observed physician resistance to engagement in this process.

Our approach in this chapter will be to identify what we see as the key barriers or potential barriers to physician involvement in priority setting in clinical practice and to consider what education or training might be necessary to support physicians in overcoming them. In adopting this approach we hope to avoid the trap of suggesting a curriculum that is not sensitive to the experience of practicing physicians and is therefore dismissed as of marginal importance by students, learned only for the relevant examination but seen as unnecessary for actually doing the job. Where appropriate we will cross-reference to other chapters in the volume where authors suggest content, frameworks, or teaching methods that may be relevant.

We will first briefly examine the current position with regard to physician education in priority setting to provide some context on the task ahead. We will ask the question, to what extent do current medical training curricula and clinical guidelines in different countries include explicit reference to priority setting? We will then identify what we see as the training needs for future doctors to enable them to become effective and fair stewards of medical resources. Finally, we will consider some ideas for effectively integrating the relevant training into current medical curricula.

■ THE CURRENT POSITION: SCOPING THE CHALLENGE

Priority setting has not traditionally been part of medical student and physician training. However, there is some evidence that medical school and professional training curricula are beginning to recognize the need for equipping future physicians with the competencies necessary to allocate medical resources in a responsible and fair manner. In the United Kingdom, the General Medical Council (GMC) document on outcomes and standards for medical education, "Tomorrow's Doctors," has specified learning outcomes related to priority setting, although these focus on doctors' roles in management and health policy rather than in the clinical setting (GMC, 2013). The Institute of Medical Ethics has published a consensus statement on the core content of a medical ethics and law curriculum for medical schools (Stirrat et al., 2010). This includes a specific section on justice and public health which states that:

> Students should be able to demonstrate a critically reflective understanding of:
> - legal and ethical issues involved in balancing individual and community interests in accessing healthcare resources
> - local, national and international prioritization in relation to clinical decisions
> - principles and criteria for just distribution of finite healthcare resources
> - the role of the doctor as patient advocate
> - the ethical and legal considerations with respect to patient responsibility for health
> - the responsible use of resources in referral, investigations and prescribing.

This statement has been recognized by both the GMC and British Medical Association as being consistent with their guidance on undergraduate education. It would seem that curriculum developers recognize the need for students to learn to allocate resources fairly at all levels including at the bedside. However, this does not necessarily translate into effective teaching of relevant knowledge and skills in individual medical schools. A survey of UK medical schools found that 33% did not think they covered resource allocation adequately in their medical ethics teaching, although 95% reported that they covered it to some extent (Mattick & Bligh, 2006). A similar survey of North American medical schools (United States and Canada) found that 75% of participant schools reported including resource allocation in their medical ethics curricula (Lehman et al., 2004). However another North American study of US medical schools which actually reviewed the syllabi of participating schools did not identify resource allocation as a separate content area, although it may have been covered in "health care delivery" taught by 75% of schools (DuBois & Burkemper, 2002). All three of these studies commented on the lack of consistency in course content and in resources available for developing and teaching medical ethics. A similar lack of consistency in course content and structure was found in a survey of medical schools in Asia (Miyasaka et al., 1999) suggesting that this is a global phenomenon. While these studies are all at least 7 years old there is no evidence to encourage us that the situation has improved for medical ethics teaching generally and for teaching on resource allocation in particular.

If we conclude that currently medical schools are unlikely to include adequate training to equip future physicians to engage in ethically justifiable priority setting, is there evidence of the relevant education being available to practicing physicians as part of their professional training? The picture here is also one of inconsistency with some evidence of professional organizations recognizing its significance and a few examples of specific initiatives to address this deficit in physician education. In the United States the Accreditation Council for Graduate Medical Education bases its accreditation assessments on six competency areas one of which is systems based practice (ACGME, 2013a). This competency specifically includes a requirement to *"incorporate considerations of cost awareness and risk benefit analysis in patient and/or population based care as appropriate."* Under the proposed new outcome based accreditation system, specialty boards are developing detailed assessment programs for residents set against these competencies. The draft document for the Board of Family Medicine includes an example of an assessment outcome in the competency of systems based care which at its highest level requires that a resident *"role models and promotes efficient and cost-effective use of resources in the care of patients in all settings."* (AGCME, 2013b) In the United Kingdom, the curriculum for foundation program training (doctors in the first 2 years post-graduation) does not mention resource allocation or priority setting. Specialty training program curricula are the responsibility of the Royal Colleges, and some include reference to resource allocation or priority setting. The Royal College of General Practitioners (RCGP) core curriculum statement on the GP consultation includes a learning outcome that states that a GP should *"be aware of the obligation to use available healthcare resources in a prudent manner, balancing individual patient needs with fairness to other patients"*(RCGP, 2010).

There are some recent signs of movement from curriculum aims to development of specific learning resources or guidance for physicians on how to engage in rationing/priority-setting decisions. The American College of Medicine has launched a "High Value Care" initiative which aims to help physicians provide optimum care for their patients while reducing unnecessary costs. The prime focus of this initiative appears to be on increasing efficiency and reducing waste rather than priority setting, but the educational resources include a module on balancing benefits of care with harms and costs (American College of Medicine, 2013). In the United Kingdom prior to the introduction of GP Local Commissioning Groups in 2012, the RCGP published "Ethical commissioning guidance for general practitioners" (RCGP, 2011a). This document specifically addressed the ethical dimension of commissioning care for patients, providing an introduction to relevant ethical theories and frameworks and including a series of worked case scenarios to illustrate how ethical commissioning might work in practice. However, the RCGP's competencies document for clinically led commissioning does not include, in its essential skills requirements, any reference to specific knowledge or skills regarding how to make ethically justifiable priority-setting decisions (RCGP, 2011b). There seems to be a worrying mismatch between general guidance/aims and specific performance requirements. In terms of providing useful educational resources for physicians to engage in priority setting at any level of health care provision, at least in the United States and the United Kingdom, we clearly have a long way to go.

One final potential opportunity for education of physicians in relation to priority setting is in the development and implementation of clinical guidelines. If guidelines produced by accredited organizations include reference to cost effectiveness of treatment options and make recommendations based on evidence of cost as well as of effectiveness, this may have an impact on physicians' understanding of the process of priority setting and change attitudes toward priority setting in clinical practice. A study of published clinical guidance documents from US physician specialty societies from 2008–2012 found that just over half explicitly considered costs in developing their clinical guidance documents, but that of those societies who reported considering cost, only half used an explicit mechanism for integrating costs into the strength of recommendations (Schwarz & Pearson, 2013). In the United Kingdom, the National Institute for Health and Care Excellence (NICE) develops national guidance for clinicians in a range of areas. Its guideline manual specifically states that the Guideline Development Group (GDG) is required to make decisions based on the best available evidence of both clinical and cost effectiveness (NICE, 2012). Published guidance sets out the evidence for clinical and cost effectiveness underpinning the recommendations. The inclusion of cost-effectiveness considerations in clinical guidelines produced by other professional organizations in the United Kingdom is more varied. In Australia, the requirement for meeting the National Health and Medical Research Council's (NHMRC) standard for clinical practice guidelines includes as a desirable but not mandatory criterion that search strategies include search terms to identify evidence related to cost effectiveness and resource implications of practice (NHMRC, 2011). In this book, both Søreide et al. and Norheim describe the Norwegian experience of priority setting through clinical practice guidelines (chapters 16 and 21). Thus, it seems that there is some potential for changing the culture of physician practice by making explicit the need to consider cost effectiveness in making clinical decisions.

■ BARRIERS TO PHYSICIAN PRIORITY SETTING AND WHAT THEY MEAN FOR CURRICULUM DESIGN

In the following section we consider why, given the acknowledgment by physicians that there is a need for priority setting, there is a reluctance to engage in learning about how to include priority setting in health care decisions both at a macro and micro level. We identify five specific barriers to physician involvement in priority setting and the implications of these for curriculum development.

1. Bedside rationing is perceived as compromising a physician's primary duty to their patients.

Denying beneficial treatment does not, and should not, come easily to doctors. Even physicians who agree with the necessity of fair rationing struggle to reconcile this with what they see as their fundamental duty to act in their patients' best interests. From Hippocrates to the codes of contemporary physician associations and regulatory authorities, the primary ethical (and legal) obligation is that of physicians to their patients. While considerations of resources and the public good are present in current professional codes, they are presented as secondary considerations, only overriding the primary duty when the harms to others are considerable, usually life threatening. Examples that spring to mind are breaching a duty of patient confidentiality to prevent a serious harm to an identifiable other person, or triaging resources in a major disaster. In cases like these, when conflicting duties are compelling and immediate, physicians both understand the need to prioritize other persons' interests over their individual patient's and are prepared to act in such a way. Cases of bedside rationing do not provide such clearly pressing counterclaims on a physician's obligations. Other authors have considered the issue of a physician's duty of care in the context of priority setting, arguing that withholding expensive treatments of minimal benefit can both directly and indirectly benefit the patient in question; that physicians have a duty to all patients in their care and therefore must use resources in a way that is fair to each of them; and that physicians have duties to society to use public resources efficiently and fairly (see Goodin, chapter 13). The challenge for physician educators is not simply to get physicians in training to understand these arguments at an intellectual level, but to internalize them into their understanding of the concept of a duty of care and hence of their actions in clinical practice.

Implication for curriculum: A successful curriculum must justify priority setting on the basis of duty of care and must make a sufficiently compelling moral case to physicians such that it creates a change in attitude as well as understanding. Without a change in attitude, there is unlikely to be a change in behavior.

2. The knowledge required for these decisions is not seen as core to medicine.

As previous chapters have demonstrated, acceptance of the need for priority setting and the ability to implement priority setting in an ethically justifiable manner requires some understanding of health economics, political and moral philosophy, game theory, medicine, and sociology. While the core knowledge considered necessary to practice medicine (and hence to be included in a medical curriculum) has expanded in recent decades to include medical ethics and social science, even these disciplines are viewed with some skepticism by students and clinicians. A health economics text book is unlikely to feature on most medical students' reading list. However, as cost-effectiveness or cost-utility measures are increasingly used to inform clinical guidelines, physicians will need to have some grasp of these concepts if they do not want to become marginalized from policies and processes that will have a direct impact on their patients' care. Physicians who make individual patient decisions that are in part informed by the cost of the intervention will need to communicate this to their patient either to inform the patient's decision, if the patient is contributing to payment, or to justify the decision to the patient if an intervention that the patient wishes to have is not being offered.

While grappling with abstract concepts of justice, or even their practical application in health care priority setting at a national or institutional level, may be beyond the necessary core knowledge for physicians in the clinical environment, we would suggest that some understanding of the theoretical underpinning of resource-allocation decisions is a requirement for physicians in fulfilling their roles as patient advocates. If physicians wish to challenge a guideline set by a health authority on the grounds that the guideline is unfair in restricting access to an intervention for their patients, then they will need to justify their assertion of unfairness. Similarly, if physicians' individual priority-setting decisions are challenged by patients or families— for example, a decision not to admit a patient to the last available intensive care bed— then the physician's response will draw on a particular theory of justice (maximizing benefit or prioritizing need) if it is to be defensible. As with health economics, a detailed knowledge is not required; but an understanding of the basic principles is necessary to reduce arbitrariness in every day patient care. Knowledge of social determinants of health and health inequalities is now likely to be recognized as an important element of medical education. However, the institutional and cultural factors that contribute to unfair prioritization of health care resources, and specifically the implicit biases and cultural stereotyping that can lead clinicians to allocate resources inequitably, are not necessarily adequately discussed and frequently not even acknowledged (see Dankwa-Mullan, chapter 19).

Implications for curriculum: A successful curriculum should ensure that the required theoretical knowledge is linked closely to clinical practice to ensure it is integrated into clinical decision making.

3. The decisions are too complex to be made at an individual patient level

Physicians who may be persuaded that rationing/prioritizing is compatible with their duty of care may still think that physicians should not be making these decisions. They would argue that the complexity of these decisions and the reasoning processes involved, the need for consistency, and the very fact that other patients/groups need to be taken into account requires a decision process at a higher level. The clinician cannot see the bigger picture, and does not want to take responsibility for it. We have already observed that this is a somewhat disingenuous position for physicians to take, given that prioritization by clinicians already occurs implicitly, and therefore, at minimum, physicians should be prepared to make these implicit prioritization decisions explicit. Hurst and Danis provide another persuasive argument for physicians to be involved in prioritization decisions at the individual patient level; that is, the need to include respect for individual variation when considering benefits and costs and to balance this against a consistency requirement (chapter 17). Physicians are best placed to understand their individual patient's perspective and include this in the overall prioritization analysis.

Implications for curriculum: A successful curriculum should build on existing analytic skills in clinical decision making and apply these to complex ethical decisions involving conflicting values.

4. The risk of perceived and actual conflicts of interest is too great.

In countries with competitive markets and choice in physician, voluntary rationing can be bad business. Doctors may lose patient-customers if they gain a reputation for cutting corners to save money. In an era where access to medical and general knowledge is virtually unlimited, drugs and procedures are marketed directly to patients, and choice of physician is an essential feature of high-quality health insurance, patients are going to know what they want and find someone who will provide it. Even in publicly funded health care systems, while physicians might not be financially penalized by patients seeking care elsewhere, they may still be adversely affected by, for example, increased patient complaints or simply by frustration that their colleagues disregard resource constraints with little sanction. Fear of litigation can also act as a barrier to limitation of treatment on the grounds of cost; defensive medicine is usually expensive medicine. In some contexts the system may be set up to encourage use of resources; for example, in a fee-for-service system there is likely to be a financial penalty for physicians who order less interventions. Even physicians who agree with the need for rationing/prioritization are unwilling to accept system changes that may have an effect on their personal financial status (Tilburt et al., 2013). Addressing this particular barrier to physician rationing/prioritization will require more than physician education. It will also require patient education and system changes to facilitate efficient and fair use of resources.

Implications for curriculum: Current medical ethics curricula may include reflection on conflicts of interest, and this could be expanded to consider the context of prioritization. Physician communication with patients regarding cost of treatment and appropriate use of resources will be an important component of patient education. The curriculum should ensure that students develop appropriate communication skills to engage patients in conversations about cost of treatment (see chapter 23, Danis et al. and chapter 20, Pearson).

5. Medical culture is hostile to rationing.

Given the barriers identified above, it is perhaps not surprising that there is a general hostility to rationing by clinicians both within and external to the medical profession. If rationing is seen as somehow contrary to the overall goals of medicine, then for those aiming to be practitioners in this field, conforming to the norms of the profession would seem to preclude its consideration. Physicians do much of their learning on the job and model their behavior on senior role models (the hidden curriculum). The culture of the setting in which they learn, and the attitudes of those that they learn from, will largely determine their attitudes and practice later in their careers.

Implications for curriculum: The curriculum must serve to develop the skills, knowledge, and attitude necessary for rationing fairly at the bedside and to do so in a hostile climate. Students may need to challenge teachers, mentors, patients, and coworkers in an appropriate way.

■ DEVELOPING AND IMPLEMENTING A RELEVANT CURRICULUM

There may be other barriers or other ways to organize the barriers we believe exist, but our list should be sufficient for guiding an educational curriculum. The implications for curriculum development can be organized into four main domains. First, we must make a compelling moral argument for rationing that recognizes the primary moral duty of a physician to act in the best interests of their patient. Second, we must teach the relevant knowledge and analytic skills necessary for fair rationing. Third, we must teach future doctors how to communicate effectively with patients and others regarding rationing. Fourth, and perhaps the most challenging, we must facilitate a shift in attitude that allows physicians to move from intellectual understanding and acceptance of the need for bedside rationing to active engagement in the process.

It is worth saying at this point that we do not envisage, nor mean to portray, the knowledge skills and attitudes necessary for physicians to be involved in priority-setting decisions, particularly those in day-to-day clinical practice, as a discrete group of educational requirements unrelated to the traditional goals of medical education. Indeed, if they are envisaged as such they are unlikely to be fully integrated into any educational curriculum and run the risk of being dismissed as marginally important by students, learned only for the relevant examination but seen as unnecessary for actually practicing as a physician. Much of the knowledge and skills needed for engaging in priority setting are generic to medical education: ability to critically appraise evidence, applying evidence in individual cases, weighing conflicting values, awareness of ethical and legal principles, and good communication skills. The challenge for educators will be to link elements specific to priority setting to generic learning so that it is integrated into the curriculum at all levels.

Reappraising the Concept of a Duty of Care

Medical ethics is now considered a core element of most medical school and physician training curricula, and central to medical ethics is the understanding of a physician's duty of care to the patient. In exploring this concept and the other ethical obligations that are encompassed within the profession of medicine, it should be possible to make a moral case for fair prioritization of health care resources as a necessary element of a duty of care. A wider exploration of what it means to be a professional and obligations to the society that confer professional privileges could also provide an opportunity to consider the potentially conflicting duties of health professionals and how these should be resolved.

Acquiring Relevant Knowledge and Skills to Make Complex Decisions in the Clinical Setting

Evidence-based medicine (EBM) is central to medical education, and the skills necessary to practice EBM are already taught at medical school and in physician training. Evidence-based clinical guidelines now commonly include cost-effectiveness data, so familiarity with the principles of health economics can be seen as a requirement for critically appraising the evidence base for such guidance. If medical students and physicians become used to handling evidence of clinical effectiveness and cost effectiveness in an integrated fashion, then the idea of considering cost in clinical decision making will seem less alien. Theories of justice, another core element of our proposed curriculum, should already be included in a medical ethics course, although more emphasis on the individual theories and their application in clinical practice may be required. More challenging for both students and educators is the requirement for complex decision analysis skills that enable physicians to consider population-based evidence for efficacy and cost, conflicting values and perspectives, and different theories of justice to reach a decision that meets requirements of consistency and transparency necessary for fair priority setting. Medical students should become familiar with this type of decision making before they are responsible for patient care. These are complicated decisions requiring different modes of thinking, which will test ability to weigh a number of different factors. This will be easier with hypothetical cases designed to reveal specific elements of the decision-making process and where it is possible to provide enough time to think through the complexities. Clinical training already develops the ability of students and trainee physicians to make clinical management decisions, evaluating benefit and risks of treatment, and including patient preferences. Learning to integrate considerations of cost and justice into these decisions may be less of a challenge for students than for their clinical teachers, who have not habitually included these considerations in decisions about patient care. Faculty development will need to support clinical teachers in helping students to apply their classroom-based decision-making skills in the clinical setting.

Developing Communication Skills for Priority Setting

Communication skills teaching is now established as a fundamental element of medical student and physician training, often running as a longitudinal theme throughout the whole course. As Danis et al. (chapter 23) have already identified that discussing health care costs with patients is difficult and requires sensitivity, time, and a trusting relationship between patient and physician. However, there are other situations where communication is difficult and is specifically addressed in the current curricula; for example, in sessions on breaking bad news and disclosure of medical error. Teaching students how to discuss openly the cost of treatment as part of a clinical conversation about care should fit into this advanced element of communication skills teaching.

Changing Attitudes and Culture

While we have argued that medical education needs to facilitate the development of a culture where physicians are prepared to engage in discussions about the cost of the care they provide, and play their part in ensuring a fair and appropriate use of limited health care resources, we are mindful that this has significant risks. The primary role of the physician is to make the care of her patient her first concern, and we would not wish to see physicians lose sight of this by refocusing on the cost of treatment in isolation. The challenge will be to generate awareness of cost and concepts of fairness as necessary to the delivery of patient-centered care, providing the best care possible for all patients in the fairest way possible. In order to make this conceptual shift, the concept of fair use of resources and the knowledge and skills necessary to achieve it must be integrated throughout the medical curriculum. The need to train clinical faculty has already been mentioned and will be crucial given the influence of the hidden curriculum in medical education.

■ SOME SUGGESTIONS FOR HOW WE MIGHT TEACH PRIORITY SETTING

Here we offer a few suggestions for how we might engage medical students in thinking about priority setting and developing the knowledge, skills, and awareness to be able to make these decisions in clinical practice.

- Budget-holding exercises

One of the reasons physicians can be poor stewards of resources is that they lack a sense of awareness of the impact of their decisions. Even if students are provided with information about the costs of investigations or treatment, they do not usually associate their decision to order an investigation or commence a treatment with cost consequences for this or other patients unless they are responsible for their own practice budget, as in the example of UK GP fund-holding described by Allen et al. (chapter 7). Introducing a budget-holding exercise into teaching on clinical decision making could facilitate student awareness of the impact of disregarding cost. Students could be given a virtual budget and then a series of case scenarios presented for them to work through diagnosis and treatment planning, first without information about cost of investigations and treatment options, and then with cost information provided. Students would be able to see how their decisions affected their overall budget and whether their patients in the later case scenarios were denied relevant investigations or treatment because of their profligate spending in the earlier cases. Mock priority-setting forums can provide a similar experience for decision making at an institutional or population level. Students work as a group to prioritize proposed health service interventions given a specified budget and are asked to justify their decisions. Proposals cover a range of very different interventions, which may include high-cost lifesaving or life-prolonging treatment, public health interventions, treatment for chronic disease, or palliative care, requiring students to consider factors other than cost in justifying their priority-setting decisions (Tolley, 1995).

- Student debates on rationing/priority setting

Several authors of previous chapters have commented on the lack of debate on rationing/priority setting, both in the public sphere and among physicians. The barriers to physician involvement in priority setting that we have identified include issues such as the concept of a physician's duty of care, which are likely to generate conflicting views that cannot be reconciled or even addressed without open debate. The use of formal debate in a medical course can be a productive and enjoyable way of increasing understanding of controversial topics and encouraging students to investigate different perspectives on the subject. Debates on rationing could include a range of different issues, from the overarching question of whether physicians should be involved in rationing at all to more specific questions on whether to prioritize or fund a particular health care intervention. Debates also offer the opportunity for dialogue (and competition) between medical schools, which may be attractive to students.

- Developing and using guidelines

Physicians are increasingly using clinical guidelines, many of which now include evidence of cost effectiveness in their recommendations. Guidelines, however, are not rigid directives, and physicians are expected to use the guidance to make decisions that are appropriate for their individual patients taking into account the particular context and perspective of the patient in question. Students therefore need to be able to appraise clinical guidelines and understand how they are developed. Developing a clinical guideline that included evidence of clinical and cost effectiveness to support its recommendations would enable students to develop a range of skills in EBM, as well as an increased understanding of how cost and cost effectiveness already have an impact on physician decision making and patient care. For practicing physicians, taking part in the development of local guidelines will promote discussion and reflection on how different clinicians, both between and within specialties, regard interventions as high or low priority (see Søreide, chapter 16).

- Values-based practice

Values Based Practice (VBP) is a clinical skills–based approach to working with complex and conflicting values in health care (Fulford et al., 2012). Its aim is to support balanced decision making within frameworks of shared values. In the United Kingdom it was first developed for use in training mental health professionals, but it is now being applied in a range of clinical areas and more recently has informed the development of "values-based commissioning" (Heginbotham, 2012). The framework allows for and indeed requires that all relevant values should be considered when making health care decisions.

Initially introduced to ensure that patients' values and preferences were given appropriate consideration, VBP also provides a framework for physicians to include other relevant values such as cost and fairness. VBP provides a potential model for teaching medical students and physicians that incorporates considerations of fair use of resources as part of patient-centered care.

- Roleplay with simulated patients

Roleplay is a well-established teaching method for communication skills in medical student and postgraduate training (Ang, 2002; Nestel & Tierney, 2007). Scenarios could be developed where the student/trainee physician is asked to discuss diagnostic or treatment options with a patient, and to include cost consideration as part of the evidence base on which the shared decision should be made. Students could be provided with relevant guidelines or evidence of effectiveness, risks, and cost of the different interventions available. Scenarios could increase in complexity and difficulty (challenging patients) in later years or modules of the training course. Group reflection on the experience of these roleplays would enable students and physicians to articulate their concerns over having these conversations with patients and to develop appropriate strategies to make them less challenging.

■ CONCLUSION

There is increasing awareness among policymakers, the public, and physicians that resources for the provision of health care are limited and often unfairly distributed, and there is thus a need to make decisions about how these resources are prioritized at all levels within the system. There also appears to be a general consensus that physicians should be involved in priority setting at some level, and at a minimum understand the rationale for priority-setting decisions that affect their patients. Making the transition from agreement in principle to engaging in practice will require education to provide the necessary knowledge, skills, and professional culture within which priority setting can occur. The challenge for educators is to integrate these elements into more traditional medical training so that physicians can contribute to fair prioritization of health care resources while fulfilling their primary role of caring for their patients.

REFERENCES

Accreditation Council for Graduate Medical Education. (2013a). Common Programme Requirements. Available at: http://www.acgme.org/acgmeweb/Portals/0/PFAssets/ProgramRequirements/CPRs2013.pdf.

Accreditation Council for Graduate Medical Education and American Board of Family Medicine. (2013b). The Family Medicine Milestone Project. Available at: http://www. acgme-nas.org/assets/pdf/Milestones/FamilyMedicineMilestones.pdf.

American College of Medicine. (2012). High Value Care Initiative. Available at: http:// hvc.acponline.org/.

Ang, M. (2002). Advanced communication skills: conflict management and persuasion. *Acad Med*, 77(11), 1166.

Carlsen, B., & Norheim, O. F. (2005). "Saying no is no easy matter": a qualitative study of competing concerns in rationing decisions in general practice. *BMC Health Serv Res*, 5:70

DuBois, J. M., & Burkemper, J. (2002). Ethics education in U.S. medical schools: a study of syllabi. *Acad Med*, 77(5), 432–437.

Fulford, K. W. M., Peile, E., & Carroll, H. (2012). *Essentials of Values Based Practice*. Cambridge: Cambridge University Press.

General Medical Council. (2013). Tomorrow's Doctors. Available at: http://www. gmc-uk.org/TomorrowsDoctors_2009.pdf_39260971.pdf

Heginbotham, C. (2012). *Values Based Commissioning of Health and Social Care*. Cambridge: Cambridge University Press.

Hurst, S. A., Reiter-Theil, S., Slowther, A. M., Pegoraro, R., Førde, R., & Danis, M. (2008). Should ethics consultants help clinicians face scarcity in their practice? *J Med Ethics*, 34(4), 241–246.

Lehmann, L. S., Kasoff, W. S., Koch, P., & Federman, D. D. (2004). A survey of medical ethics education at U.S. and Canadian medical schools. *Acad Med*, 79(7), 682–689.

Mattick, K., & Bligh, J. (2006). Undergraduate ethics teaching: revisiting the Consensus Statement. *J Med Educ*, 40(4), 329–332.

Miyasaka, M., Kai, I., Ohi, G., & Akabayashi, A. (1999). An international survey of medical ethics curricula in Asia. *J Med Ethics*, 25(6), 514–521.

National Health and Medical Research Council. (2011). Procedures and guidance for meeting the 2011 NHMRC standards for clinical practice guidelines. Available at: http:// www.nhmrc.gov.au/_files_nhmrc/publications/attachments/cp133_nhmrc_ procedures_requirements_guidelines_v1.1_120125.pdf.

National Institute of Health and Care Excellence. (2012). The Guidelines Manual. See Chapter on process and methods guides. Available at: http://publications.nice.org.uk/ the-guidelines-manual-pmg6#the-development-process-for-clinical-guidelines.

Nestel, D., & Tierney, T. (2007). Role-play for medical students learning about communication: guidelines for maximising benefit. *J Med Educ*, Mar 2;7:3.

Royal College of General Practitioners. (2010). RCGP curriculum, the GP consultation in practice. Available at: http://www.rcgp.org.uk/gp-training-and-exams/~/ media/Files/GP-training-and-exams/Curriculum-2012/RCGP-Curriculum-2- 01-GP-Consultation-In-Practice.ashx.

Royal College of General Practitioners. (2011a). Making difficult choices: ethical commissioning guidance to general practitioners. Available at: http:// www.rcgp.org.uk/revalidation-and-cpd/~/media/Files/News/RCGP-Ethical- Commissioning-Guidance.ashx.

Royal College of General Practitioners. (2011b). Competencies for clinically led commissioning. Available at: http://www.rcgp.org.uk/revalidation-and-cpd/~/media/09BB7 5560DBB46C8B7F65E1C36C5B558.ashx.

Stirrat, G. M., Johnston, C., Gillon, R., Boyd, K. Medical Education Working Group of Institute of Medical Ethics and associated signatories. (2010). Medical ethics and law for doctors of tomorrow: the 1998 Consensus Statement updated. *J Med Ethics, 36*(1), 55–60.

Tilburt, J. C., Wynia, M. K., Sheeler, R. D., Thorsteinsdottir, B., James, K. M., Egginton, J. S., et al. (2013). Views of US physicians about controlling health care *JAMA, 310*(4), 380–388.

Tolley, K. H., & Whynes, K. (1995). The priority setting exercise: an instrument for training in health care resource allocation. *Med Teach, 17*(4), 391–398.

Any society that hopes to secure the health of its population needs to set priorities and carefully allocate resources to sustainably achieve this aspiration. This involves considering how to expend health care funds most cost effectively bearing in mind the need to distribute the benefits of these expenditures fairly.

With rare exception, the authors in this volume have argued that clinicians are and inevitably must be a part of this process. As Leonard Fleck points out, no matter how much decision making about resource allocation takes place beforehand, uncertainty will remain and clinical judgment about allocating resources will remain inescapable.

A central claim of much of the book is that resource allocation and rationing at the bedside are ethically justifiable. Reducing the use of unnecessary diagnostic and therapeutic interventions, as Howard Brody argues, is ethically straightforward. It is not only ethically permissible, it is ethically mandatory—there are no drawbacks. In contrast, limiting marginally beneficial care through bedside rationing is justifiable but only conditionally so. A number of chapters in the book thus address the necessary conditions for fair rationing at the bedside. Len Fleck explores the necessary steps that need to take place at the societal level before bedside rationing can be legitimate. Keith Syrett elucidates how important a legal framework is for creating a structure that can permit but also constrain resource allocation and rationing efforts.

Several chapters in the book explore some fundamental conceptual issues underlying the notions of resource allocation and rationing. Michael Barilan points out that since rationing entails forgoing benefits, the definition of benefit becomes crucial to the process. Paul Menzel argues that what is ordinarily called rationing in fact might better be called *priority setting* since, with the exception of absolute shortages, clinicians cannot predict with any certainty that limiting treatments for some patients for the sake of others will cause a loss of benefits to the former and gains for the latter. Robert Goodin explores the idea that managing health care resources poses a collective action problem, and he considers the implications for our analysis of rationing.

We hope it is clear in the course of reading the book that pursuing fair bedside rationing is not merely about clinicians but requires focusing on health care systems as well. The results from the Values at the Bedside study highlight that clinicians' attitudes and practices with regard to rationing vary from country to country. A number of chapters in the book are therefore focused on how various national health care systems offer different solutions.

The country-specific chapters from Norway, Italy, Switzerland and United Kingdom portray how resource allocation has played out in these particular national contexts. Additional chapters from several countries, including Thomas Allen and others' review of studies in the United Kingdom, Odd Søreide and colleagues' description of experiences in Norway, and Steve Pearson's explanation of accountable care organizations in the United States provide further insights about the practice of rationing that theoretical discussion alone cannot provide.

A key insight that we hope becomes apparent from the book is that experiences gained in one health care system can provide models from which other health systems can learn to create environments where cost effective, affordable, and fairly distributed health care can be delivered by clinicians.

Even if bedside rationing is ethically justifiable, it can only be expected to go well if clinicians are trained, experienced, and skilled at it. Thus much of the rest of the book was intended to offer clinicians strategies for practicing bedside rationing well. Samia Hurst and Marion Danis outline a framework to facilitate fair rationing by clinicians, including a closed system that offers reciprocity, attention to general concerns of justice, respect for individual variations, application of a consistent process, explicitness, and review of decisions. Jan Schurmann and colleagues show how clinical ethics consultants can help. Anne Slowther and Benjamin Bennett write about teaching clinicians in training to be capable of bedside rationing. Irene Dankwa-Mullan and others point out what clinicians need to do to avoid undue harm to patients who face disadvantages. Ole Norheim provides an example of modeling the consequences of rationing that illustrates what can be gained from repeated cycles of explicit documentation, measurement, assessment of the consequences, and improvement.

Since resource allocation and rationing have tended to be such taboo topics, we have paid some attention to ways of making the discussion of these topics more acceptable to the public. We believe that in opening the conversation as thoughtfully as possible, the public will be more understanding and accepting of the necessity of rationing.

We cannot say that we have covered all that we might have. Nor can we say that a book like this one will contribute positively to the way health care systems and clinicians prioritize care in the absence of other factors. Here are some additional issues and future challenges. First, bedside rationing is unlikely to be morally, politically, and socially acceptable unless physicians have as their dominant moral commitment the health and well-being of their patients, as opposed to having a primary commitment to the institutions to which they happen to be attached. Of worry is that the health care in the United States, for instance, is rapidly evolving in the latter direction—and that represents a potential threat to the core values of medicine. There is increasing economic competition among hospitals, health care systems, medical groups, and insurance groups. While this is supposed to have the desirable economic effect of reducing overall health care costs in the system, it may be at too high a cost to the core values of medicine if this undermines the inclination of physicians to safeguard the affordability and fair distribution of healthcare.

Second, while we have written about the need for explicit conversation about priority setting and rationing, there remains more to be said and done. Rationing judgments, guidelines, protocols, and practices must be transparent to all potentially affected by such judgments. There is much that conspires against transparency, including social divisiveness linked to the perception that one or another "disease group" is favored over others, internal professional disagreements that would otherwise require substantial conversations to achieve reasonable agreement, and worries that a focus on affordable health care will violate other moral commitments to sanctity of life and individual rights and interests. In spite of these challenges, transparency is essential to promote fairness and trust, both at the clinical level and in the health care system as a whole.

As a corollary, semi-transparency regarding rationing is not good enough. There is a strong effort to hide what are often rationing decisions behind the language of waste, inefficiency, and parsimonious care. Attention to reducing the extensive amount of wasteful and inefficient health care is certainly critically needed. But this should not be assumed to imply that there is no need to reduce access to "needed" health care, no matter how marginal the benefit, as long as there is all this waste and inefficiency in the health care system. Such an implication is a half-truth at best. There are circumstances in which care can be delivered more efficiently without diminishing at all the quality of that care; those choices are not ethically problematic, nor are they correctly described as instances of rationing. However, in the recent literature on parsimonious care, such care is sometimes defined as "no value" care and at other times as "low value" care. But there is a morally important difference between these two senses. If care is truly of "no value" then there is no ethics issue, and we have no reason to describe that as an instance of rationing. But "low value" care denied to a patient is correctly described as rationing and is in need of moral analysis and justification from the perspective of health care justice.

Third, physicians, individually and collectively as a profession, will be reluctant to endorse rationing protocols and rationing guidelines unless those protocols and guidelines have broad public legitimation. This will require, as a future challenge, creating public forums wherein public education and public deliberation regarding just rationing guidelines and protocols can occur. This is part of what is required by a commitment to transparency. These public forums need to be, and be perceived to be, scrupulously fair and objective, free from political partisanship or corruption by some ideological point of view.

Essential to this process of public education and deliberation will be creating a public capacity for discussing the problem of health care justice thoughtfully and recognizing that the most we can reasonably hope for as an outcome of that conversation will be "rough justice" because of the need to make complex trade-offs among competing justice-relevant considerations.

Fourth, physicians and the public (both while well and when sick and seeking care) must know that there is a "leak proof" system within which bedside rationing decisions are made. This was a point first emphasized by Norman Daniels. In other words, the savings achieved through making rationing decisions—denying individuals care that is excessively costly and that yields too little benefit—will be kept within the health care system or other health-promoting policy sectors and used to pay for higher-priority, more just health care needs as opposed to "leaking out" of the system in the form of profits to shareholders or bonuses to executives or physicians. This is essential for building and maintaining trust in a system for controlling health care costs more justly. This is also essential for creating the legal protections that physicians would need in these circumstances.

Fifth, given the nature of medicine and often the complexity and uncertainty associated with possible medical treatments, some degree of flexibility and respect for clinical judgment must be built into rationing guidelines. The challenge is to create mechanisms for monitoring and assessing that judgment in practice in order to preserve the justness intended by the guidelines without creating burdensome bureaucratic processes and reporting requirements.

Sixth, accessible and efficient appeal mechanisms in the system are needed and should be applied fairly. If laws are passed with a very strong emphasis on patient rights, they may have some inadvertent unjust consequences that should be anticipated and addressed carefully. In the setting of limited health care budgets, rights-based supply of health care services may all too likely be given first to those who are able to fight for their rights at the expense of the less privileged who will have their health care rationed without being able to complain. Sick patients may thus require assistance in asserting their rights to treatments. In such cases there is a tension between the emphasis on patients' rights and considerations of fairness in the distribution of resources.

Finally the challenge remains, unaddressed here, of considering how to pursue bedside rationing in nations with far fewer resources than the countries we have focused on in most of this book. The clinical task is far more daunting in resource-poor settings. We will only be able to tackle the issue well when we collaborate with colleagues who have faced the issues and studied them carefully.

■ INDEX

Aaron, Henry 29
Aaron & Schwartz, The Painful
　　Prescription 129
absolute clinical freedom 129
absolute risk approach 376
Accreditation Council for Graduate
　　Medical Education (ACGME) 426
accountable care organizations
　　(ACOs) 238
accountable care organizations (ACOs)
　　and bedside rationing 356, 358–59
　　and ethical design principles 359–64,
　　　370–71
　　and global payment mechanisms
　　　357–59, 362–63
　　and threat to physician loyalty to
　　　patients 356–57, 362–63, 370–71
accountable care organizations (ACOs) and
　　global payment mechanisms 357–64
　　and limits on financial risks 360–62
　　risks of great gains/great losses 360
　　and role of physicians 365
　　and scope of services 360
　　timing and structure of bonuses 360
accountable care organizations (ACOs)
　　and patient advocacy 365–69
　　and conversations with
　　　colleagues 366–67
　　and conversations with
　　　patients 366–70
　　and proportional advocacy 366–70
　　and threshold for marginally beneficial
　　　care 368, 370
accountable care organizations (ACOS)
　　and physician compensation
　　　incentives 359
　　and balancing of incentives 363
　　and conflicts of interest 359, 362–64,
　　　366, 370–71
　　and fairness of incentives 363–64
　　and immediacy of incentives 362–63

and intensity of incentives 359–62
and risk of adjustment methodology 363
accountability for reasonableness
　　model 142, 251 (*See also* Daniels,
　　Norman)
adhesion contracts 147
Affordable Care Act 174, 179, 358
Agency for Healthcare Research and
　　Quality (AHRQ) 212
aging of the population 146
Alternative Quality Contract 358
American Board of Internal Medicine
　　Foundation 388
American College of Physicians 174, 207
　　and high value care 426
　　and parsimonius care 207
American College of Physicians
　　Foundation 388
American Medical Association 142
American Medical Association Council
　　on Ethical and Judicial Affairs 388
ankylosing spondylitis 182, 195
aporia 152
Area Health Authorities (ASLs) 90
　　(*See also* Italian Health Care System)
Aristotelian tradition 260
Aristotle 258, 261
Arrow, Kenneth 161
ascribed characteristics, defined 325–26
Atrius Health 369
Australia, National Health and Medical
　　Research Council 427
Australian Pharmaceutical Benefits
　　Scheme 234
autologous bone marrow transplant 205
　　and breast cancer 205

barriers to physician priority setting 424,
　　428
　　compromise of physician's duty to
　　　patient 428

barriers to physician priority setting (*Cont.*)
  cost effectiveness and priority
    setting not seen as core to medical
    practice 429
  decisions seen as too complex to be
    made at individual patient level 430
  medical culture as hostile to
    rationing 431
  risk of conflict of interest is too
    great 430–31
basic need, distinct from objective
  need 150, 159–60
  reasonable health care needs 160–61
bedside rationing
  acceptance by physicians 21–24, fig. 1
  accountable public deliberation versus
    personal choice 155–57, 162–64
  and administration 173
  and basic needs 159
  best applied at the margins 368–69
  as a collective action problem 225–27
  cost-effectiveness 171, 197
  criteria for 27, 172
  and deliberative agreement in
    Norway 37
  doctor must calculate risk-benefit
    ratio 154
  and ethics of proximity 257–58
  and exercise of clinical
    judgment 285–87
  and framework for fair rationing
    285–92, 439–40
  and freedom to use resources 32–33,
    37–38
  frequency of 20–22
  highest in Switzerland 53
  and insurance schemes 147
  justification required by physicians 428
  and limits of loyal patient
    advocacy 178–79, 183–93
  and loyalty owed patients 238
  must be done fairly by
    physicians 424–27
  must be explicit 285, 287–89, 291,
    423–24
  necessity of 172, 174–75
  need for explicit discussion 21–23

  need for physician flexibility of
    judgment 179–80, 183–93, 288
  need for public legitimacy 134–36,
    139–41, 154, 159, 176–77, 179–80,
    182–83, 219–20, 247–49, 251,
    281–82, 285, 370, 374–75, 382
  need for transparent judgments 197
    (*See also* transparency)
  New Public Management 255
  normative political choices 255
  not morally possible fairly 258–59
  physician practices 20–24
  and physician resistance to explicit
    rationing 423–24
  physician's perspective and patient's
    interests 146–47
  and pressure to deny resources 33–34,
    37–38
  principles of 145
  pure distributive justice, brutal
    consequences of 258
  respect for autonomy and gaming the
    system 153, 158, 163
  role of physician as impartial
    advisor 165
  role of physicians 284–85, 294–96
  and stewardship 254–55
  and Swiss physicians 21–24, 37–38
  and third party interests 256–57
  thought experiments 150–51
  and three conditions for success 163–64
  ubiquity in health systems 30
  unavoidable role for physicians 423, 428
  and virtue ethics 257–58
  when morally justified 172, 197–99,
    359–64, 370–71
bedside rationing and Accountable Care
    Organizations (ACOs) 356, 358–59
  and ethical design principles 359–64,
    370–71
  and global payment mechanisms 357–61
  and threat to physician loyalty to
    patients 357, 360, 369–71
bedside rationing by physicians 398
  based on clinical judgment 398
  based on practice guidelines 398
  based on resource constraints 398

and end-of-life costs 415–17
financial ramifications for
    patients 412–414, 417–418
need for prior public deliberation 418
and need to discuss with patients 399,
    403–07, 412–414
and problem of implicit rationing 399
bedside resource allocation 301–02
    and considerations of futility 302
    and METAP (Modular, Ethical
        Treatment decisions, Allocation of
        resources at the micro-level, Process)
        Project 302–04, 308, 311–16
bellwethers of rationing 13, 387, 390–92
benchmarks of efficiency 217–220
Bentham, Jeremy 232
Bergen Hospital Trust 269–270
Bevan, Aneurin 61
Bismarckian model of insurance
    coverage 126
Bobbit, Phillip 175
Brazil 141
breaking bad news 433
British Medical Association (BMA) 425
budget-holding and GPs 7–8, 105–12,
    119–20
    exercises 434
    GPs as gatekeepers 107
    practice-based commissioning 106
    research on fundholding 107–12
burdens of judgment 180, 190 (See also
    Rawls, John)
Burke, Leslie case 187–88, 195–96

Calabresi and Bobbitt 175 (See also tragic
    choices)
Calabresi, Guido 175
Campbell, Stephen, et al. 115, 118
capitation 357
capitation-like incentives 370
Central Birmingham Health
    Authority 134
Choosing Wisely campaign 204, 207–09,
    217
    and shared decision making 208
clinical autonomy and allocative
    choices 134–36, 141–42

and interpretation of guidelines 136–38
and reasoned justifications for
    allocative choices 140
clinical competence 304–06, 308–09
clinicians as choice architects 406
    (See also nudging)
collective action problems 9, 224–26
    and GP fundholder scheme 235
    indifference to the health of
        others 229–230
    particular interests versus common
        good 226–27, 230–31
    patients as moral agents 227–29
    patients seeking comparative
        advantage 228–29
    physicians as agents for patients 231–33
    and Primary Care Trusts 235
    professions as representatives of all
        patients 230–35
Commission to End Health Care
    Disparities 331–32
commitment devices 153, 164–65
common law systems 127
complex decision analysis skills 432–33
concepts of justice 429
consequence of rationing guidelines 13
Consumers Union 217
cookbook medicine 137
Council of Civil Service Unions v Minister for
    the Civil Service [1985]132
cream-skimming by GP
    fundholders 109–110
cultural competency 334–35
cultural stereotyping 429
curricular design and bedside
    rationing 428–31
    need for communication skills and
        priority setting 431–33
    need to integrate clinical effectiveness
        and cost effectiveness 432–33

Daniels, Norman 149, 152
    and leakproof system 442
Daniels and Sabin 140
    Accountability for Reasonableness 287
Danis, Marion 4, 198
"death panels" 358

democratic deliberation 150, 152, 154,
    157–59, 165, 176–78, 180, 182, 194
Diaz, Angel case 188
disclosure of medical error 433
discontinuum model 205
discrimination against vulnerable patient
    groups 12
disparities in health insurance coverage 417
distinction between *is* and *ought* 254
distinction between law and ethics 136–39
distributive justice 175–80, 182–84, 188,
    192, 194–95, 211, 217–18, 253–54,
    287–92, 301, 307–08, 310, 317–18,
    332, 342–44, 373, 378–81, 387, 425,
    429, 432–33, 439, 441–42
    and efficiency 254
diversity training seminars 334–35
Doran, Tim 113, 117

economic sustainability 2–3
Eddy, David 136, 177
efficiency versus inefficiency 211–220
    benchmarks of efficiency 217–219
    definitions of 212–13
    harms of inefficiency 214–215
    problem of inconsistency and
        non-compliance 219–220
    rationing versus inefficiency 214,
        216–18
    role of physicians in managing XII 3–8
Engage, Empathize, Educate, Enlist
    (the E-4 model) 413
enzyme replacement therapy 189–90
ethical competence 306–11, 319
    and communicability 308
    as dialectical 307
    and individual cases 307
    as inherently practical 307
    and learnability 308
    nature of 306–307
    reflective versus intuitive 307–10
ethically justified clinical judgment 306–07
ethics of proximity 259–61
European Observatory on Health Systems
    and Policies 2
European Society of Cardiology
    (ESC) 189, 374, 376, 381

European strategy and health
    maximization 380–81
evidence-based clinical guidelines 432–33
evidence-based medicine 273, 289–90,
    294, 391–92, 432–33
excessive pricing 2
explicit rationing 131, 134–36, 139
    and "meso" level 135, 139
    and rationing by guideline 134–40
    and transparency 139 (*See also*
        transparency)
    versus implicit rationing 191

fair allocation of health resources 323, 325
    and low income countries 342–45
    no "magic bullets" 332
    and physicians 323–24, 327
    and practical strategies 332–42
    and reasonable bedside rationing 325
    and the socially disadvantaged
        323–25, 341–42
fair and decent minimum of care 417
fair rationing 176, 197–98, 215–17, 253,
    258–59, 296, 396–97, 404–06,
    410–11, 424, 427–28, 431
    libertarian paternalistic approach 406
    and need for nudging 407–08
fair resource allocation in an unfair
    world 323
fairness 152
fairness by country 33 fig. 3, 37–38
fee-for-service payment 13, 356
fetal scan screening 83
financial burden of illness 398–99
fiscal sustainability 2–3
Fleck, Leonard 410–11
Forde, Reidun 5
formal justice 312
functionalist approach to law 130

gaming the system 391
Gawande, Atul 173
Geisinger Health System 357
General Medical Council 425
Gini-coefficient 379, 381
Gini-health 378
Gini-impact analysis 380–81

global budgets 9
global payment mechanisms and ACOs
    13, 359–64 (*See also* ACOs)
    and limits on financial risks 360–62
    risks of great gains/great losses 361
    and role of physician 364–66
    and scope of services 359–60
    timing and structure of bonuses 360–63
Good Samaritan 260–61
Good Stewardship Working Group 212,
    214–18
Goodwin, Nick 109–10
GP consortia 8
GP fundholder scheme 235
GP Local Commissioning Groups 8,
    426–27
guidelines, developing and using 435

Hall, Mark 165
Havighurst, Clark 147
Health and Social Care Act of 201–266
health care costs 146
health care need 148–51
health care rationing
    explicit in NHS 66–67
    and law 8
Health Care Service Reform and Health
    Professionals Act 59
health care services, three categories
    151–54, 159
health inequalities 429
Health Partners 369
health policy experts as choice architects
    234–35, 406 (*See also* nudging)
health technology assessment 53 (*See also*
    National Institute of Health and
    Clinical Excellence)
    and Norway 273–74
hegemony of modernity 257
high value care 426
Hippocratic Oath 129
Hippocratic principles 323, 428
Human Development Index (IHDI) 381
human dignity 145–46, 151, 159–60
Hunter Syndrome 189–90, 196–97
Hurst, Samia 5, 198
Hurst and Danis 198, 430

identifiable versus statistical lives 10, 238
    and breast cancer screening 239–40
    and clinical practice 247–49
    Kantian perspective 239
    and macro-allocation 246
    and practice guidelines 247–48
    pricelessness of human life
        objection 245
    rationing versus prioritizing 246–48
    recipients versus beneficiaries 241–44
    refining the distinction 241–44
    in relation to prevention 239–40
    statistical/identifiable distinction 10
    utilitarian perspective 239
identification of ethical problems 312
    table 3
idursulfase 189
implantable cardiac defibrillator
    (ICD) 188–89
implicit bedside rationing, and law 129–31
    as amalgam of clinical and financial
        factors 129, 132–33
    and Hippocratic obligation 129
    and judicial passivity 131–34
    and merciful lies 131
implicit bias 342–47, 430
implicit prioritization 423
    risk of personal and professional
        biases 423
incentives for overtreatment 356
individual-oriented medical law 125
inefficiency, health care 211–16
    type A 213, 215, 217–18
    type B 213, 215
inequalities between socioeconomic
    groups 391
Institute of Medical Ethics 425
insurance as a shared communal
    resource 417
Intermountain Health Care 369
International Society on Priorities in
    Health Care 251
Italian health care system 88
    basic moral principles 88
    equalization fund 93
    financing health care, out of
        pocket 95–96

Italian health care system (*Cont.*)
    financing health care, public 93–95
    GPs and cost control 97–98
    inpatient care, DRGs 91
    LEA decree, establishing essential
        levels of health care 89
    mixed rationing approach 91–93
    pharmaceutical policy 95–96, 99–100
    primary care 90
    regionalization 98
    risk sharing schemes 96–97
    specialist ambulatory services 90
Italian National Health Service 88

Jehovah's Witness case 186, 198
Jevon's paradox 156
justice as fairness 253–54

Kahneman, D. 402
Kaiser Permanente 358
knowing how, and ethics 306
knowing that, and ethics 306
knowing why, and ethics 306
Kraus, Hannah case 185–87, 196

Larrey, Baron Dominique Jean 148
last chance therapies 182
legal realism 128
LeGrand, Julian 110–11, 379
Levinas, Emmanuel 258–60
    Levinasian tradition 259
Levinsky, Norman 171–72, 257, 261
likelihood of treatment denial based on
        group identity by country 33fig. 4
Lønning, Inge 76
Lønning II Commission 77–78, 80

MacIntyre, Alistair
    After Virtue 257
macro-level constraints 325
Mannion, Russell 111
marginal benefit 181–82, 214, 250, 284,
        294, 368–70, 412–13
Mayo Clinic 356, 369
McAllen, Texas 173–74
McLean, Gary, et al. 114–15
medical futility 207, 317

Medical Professionalism Charter 165
medically least well off 194–96
medically necessary care 139
Medicare 246, 356–58
Menzel, Paul 4, 207
METAP (Modular, Ethical Treatment
        decisions, Allocation of resources
        at the micro-level, Process)
        Project 301–03, 308–10, 317, 319–20
    checklist for collection of
        information 315
    and fairness-sensitive issues 302–04,
        312, 319
    and futility 318
    and geriatric care 310–13, 317–18
    and intensive care 313–19
mock priority setting forums 429, 434–35
moral competence 304–06, 309
moral virtues 304
myopia bias 63, 153, 158
Myozyme ruling 51–52
    and cost-effectiveness 52–53
    Pompe disease 51

National Council for Quality
        Improvement and Priority Setting in
        Health Care 82
National Council for Priority
        Setting 382–83
National Health Fund 94
National Health Service (NHS) 56–67,
        126, 137
    reform proposals 8
National Institute of Health and Clinical
        Excellence (NICE) 8, 62, 65–66,
        135, 137–39, 181–82, 427
    and Alzheimer's disease 64–65
    clinical guidelines, creation of 61–62
    equality schemes 219
    guidance 139–41
    health technology appraisals 61–62,
        65–66
National Service Frameworks 62
National Solidarity Fund 93
New Zealand: National Advisory
        Committee on Core Health and
        Disability Services 134

Newdick, Christopher 129
  and absolute clinical freedom 129
NHS and Community Care Act 59
NICE *see* National Institute of Health and
  Clinical Excellence
no-benefit interventions 205
non-ideal justice 176
non-justiciability VIII 132–34, 140
Norway 11, 403
Norway, Government Commission on
  Choices in Health Care 135
Norwegian Board of Health
  Supervision 273–74
Norwegian Council for Priority Setting
  and Quality in Health Care 375
Norwegian Directorate of Health 274,
  375
Norwegian health care system 71–78
  comprehensive approach to priority
    setting 81–82
  co-payment requirements 73–74
  drug expenses for patients 80
  elderly patient care 75–76, 80
  financing 71
  health care resources 72–73
  health spending 72
  organization 71–72
  primary care physicians as
    gatekeepers 73, 81–82
  psychiatric patient care 74–75, 79, 82
  rationing 79–80
Norwegian Knowledge Centre for the
  Health Services 81–82, 374 (*See also*
  NICE)
Norwegian Medical Association 80, 375
Norwegian Medicines Agency 73, 374
Norwegian primary prevention guidelines
  group 374
Norwegian rationing strategy 13
Norwegian risk algorithm
  (NORRISK) 375
Norwegian strategy and reduced health
  inequality 378–81
NovoSeven, and hemophiliacs 186
nudging 406–08

Oregon Health Services Commission 134

overdiagnosis and overtreatment 9,
  204–05, 207–08
overutilization 2

Pareto optimality
  and no correlation with fundamental
    values of medicine 162
parsimonious care 207, 441
participatory rational deliberation 152
participatory transparent process of
  determination of health treatments
  and services 141
patient advocacy
  limits of 177–79, 183–90
patient advocacy in Accountable Care
  Organizations (ACOs) (*See also* ACOs)
  and conversation with
    colleagues 366–68
  and conversation with patients
    366–69, 371
  and proportional advocacy 365–70
  and thresholds for marginally beneficial
    care 366–70
patient-centered care 208
patient-friendly decision aids 205
Patient Protection and Affordable
  Care Act 358
patient's best interest 172, 174–75, 177,
  181, 185–86, 191–92, 194, 197–98,
  231–33, 370, 413, 428, 430
  physician's first duty, not only
    duty 231–33
patient's loss-aversion 417–18
Patient's Rights Act of 1999 78, 265–66
pay for performance and GPs 7, 112–21
  and diabetes management 117–18
  and health inequalities 118, 120
  Quality and Outcomes Framework
    (QOF) 112–20
  rationing promoted by QOF 117–20
Peake case 184–87, 189, 196
Pegoraro, Renzo 4
Pegram v Herdrich 133, 139
Perceived Equity scale 32–34
  physician agreement with cost
    containment policies by
    country 37–38

Perceived Equity scale (*Cont.*)
  and physician recognition of
    discrimination 32–34
  scarce resources by country 37–38
Physician Charter on Medical
    Professionalism 388
physician compensation incentives 359
  and balancing of incentives 363
  and conflicts of interest 359–62, 364,
    366, 370
  and fairness of incentives 363–64
  and immediacy of incentives 362–63
  and intensity of incentives 359–62
  and risk adjustment
    methodology 362–63
physician education about bedside
    rationing 424–27
  and clinical guidelines 427
  medical student objectives regarding
    priority setting 425
  need for change of attitude 428
  and residency training 426–27
physician stewardship 387–89
physicians as bellwethers 387, 390
  as alternative form of advocacy 391–92
  and bedside rationing 388–89
  and constrained resources 387, 389, 391
  and controlling medical
    expenditures 387
  and need to promote efficiency and
    avoid waste 391
  and objections to cost-effectiveness
    data 389
physicians as gatekeepers and patient
    advocates 136–37
polycentricism and the law 132
population-focused public health
    policy 125
post code rationing 62–63
practice guidelines 374–76
  and absolute risk 375–76
  and age-related risk thresholds 376–77
  and cardiovascular disease
    guidelines 376–77
  defined 373–74
  and differentiated risk threshold 376–77
  and redistribution of life expectancy 377

  and risk of covert rationing 374
  as tools of rationing 374
pricelessness of human life 175, 181–82,
    194
Primary Care Trusts 235
principle of equality 267
  and Norway 267
principles of justice 10 (*See also*
    distributive justice)
prioritarian consideration to favor the
    worst off 290
prioritizing care versus rationing 238
priority setting as a clinical skill 395–96,
    423–31, 435
priority setting in Norway 265–73
  based on prognosis 277
  differences among regional health
    authorities 279–80
  and end-of-life decisions 272
  and evidence-based medicine 273–74
  guiding principles 270, 273–74
  and necessary care 266–68
  and Patients' Rights Act 266
  and practice guidelines 373–75, 380
  Priority Group 1, highest
    severity 271–73
  Priority Group 2, serious potential
    prognostic loss 271–73
  Priority Group 3, substantial reduction
    in quality of life 271–73
  and rationing 373
  and reduction in inequality of
    age-at-death 378–81
  Regulations on Priority Setting
    266–73, 275–76
  skepticism about criteria for priority
    setting 277–78
  and specialist health care
    services 266–67, 274, 276
Prisoner's Dilemma 236
procedural justice 140, 307–08
  criteria of 218
Propper, Carol 107
psychological barriers to rationing 400
  flaws in human judgment 400–01
  identified versus statistical lives 400
  inherent self-centeredness 400

long term benefit versus short term
gain 400, 402–03
political untenability 401
reluctance by physicians to discuss
cost 401–02
public antipathy to rationing 13
public deliberation 154–55
and non-ideal justice 176
and rational democratic
deliberation 175–83
and role of physicians in democratic
deliberation 180, 182–83
and shared understandings of fair
rationing 175–83
public democratic deliberative
process 8–9
publicity bias 155–56
publicity condition 176, 191, 196–98

Quality Adjusted Life Year (QALY) 187,
254–55, 294–95
incompatibility with the foundations of
a constitutional democracy 254
quality, and cost of end-of-life care 415–17
Quality and Outcomes Framework
(QOF) 106, 112–19

R v Cambridge Health Authority, ex parte B
133–34
R v Central Birmingham Health Authority,
ex parte Collier 130, 134
R v North Derbyshire Health Authority,
ex parte Fisher 139
R v North West Lancashire Health Authority,
ex parte A, D and G 138–39
R (Rogers) v Swindon Primary Care Trust 138
R v Secretary of State for Health, ex parte
Pfizer Ltd. 138–39
"R" word, the 244–45
rational democratic deliberation 175–83,
190–91
and non-ideal justice 176, 192
and role of physicians in democratic
deliberation 179–80, 182–83
and shared understandings of fair
rationing 175–83
rationing

accountability 395–404
definition of 211, 396
need for explicit discussion 395–99,
403–06, 408–11
reasonableness 395, 404, 411
transparency 395, 404, 411
as universal need 409
rationing by clinical judgment 11, 285–96
based on reciprocity as cooperative
fairness 288–89, 292–93
choosing what matters most versus
taking care away 409–410
conditions for fairness and
legitimacy 287
and consistency of application 289–91
as an explicit process 289, 291
and general considerations of
justice 288, 290–91
incremental gain and thresholds 293–94
and institutional policy 411–412
and judging expected benefit 294
and judging expected
cost-effectiveness 294–96
need for iterative re-examination 289,
292
and need for public deliberation
408–11 (*See also* rational democratic
deliberation)
and respect for individual
variation 288, 290, 294–96
risk of subjectivity and bias 177, 180,
198, 253
Rawls, John X 9–10, 14, 45; XV 2
Theory of Justice 257
realistic prioritizing 246
reciprocity XVII 288–89, 291
redistribution of life expectancy 376
reflective equilibrium 198 (*See also*
Rawls, John)
Regional Health Authorities 265, 270,
272, 274, 279–80
Reiter-Theil, Stella 5
resource allocation and bedside rationing
defined intro 3–4
and fairness and equity 5–6
and need for professional education
14–15

resource allocation and bedside
    rationing (*Cont.*)
  and the political sphere 11
  as priority setting 396, 403, 405–11
  in relation to inefficiencies in health
    care 9–10
resource allocation and the law 125–27
  ensured transparency in allocative
    decisions 138–39
  facilitative functions of law 128–29
  judicial independence 127–28
  judicial passivity 131–34
  judicial review versus contractual
    agreement 127
  precedent and the law 127–28
  publicity condition 140
risk adjustment methodology 363
risk of medicalizing the healthy elderly 380
risk thresholds 375–78
Roland, Martin 113–15
role play with simulated patients 436
Royal College of General Practitioners
    (RCGP) 426
Rule of Rescue 149–50, 157

Sarkisyan, Nataline case 186–87, 195
Schiavo case 187
Schwartz, William 225
shared decision making 208, 336–37
Slowther, Anne 5
Smith & York 113
social determinants of health 429
social diversity and multiculturalism 334
social inequities 345
social stratification 325–26, 328
socially disadvantaged populations 12,
    325–331
  and bedside rationing 327–328
  defined 326
  and empirical research 328–29
  global perspective 331–32
  and impaired communication 328
  and low income countries 342–45
  and physician bias 327–28, 345
  and practical strategies for ethical
    health resource allocation 332–42
  and stereotypes 325–26, 330, 345

solidarity 10
  with the worst off 79
status quo bias 158
Steel, N. & Willems, S. 115, 117
stereotypes and unconscious
    biases 327–28
stewardship of resources 212, 214, 216,
    232, 254, 284, 387–89
stigma and stereotyping, and
    physicians 324
stigmatized patient groups 12
stop-loss provisions 362–63
strategies to promote physician
    fairness 332–42
  addressing sources of ambiguity 336–38
  appreciating group and individual
    differences 334–36
  articulating reasoning process for
    resource allocation 336–38
  committee for equitable care 340–41
  and cultural competence training
    programs 335–36
  and exposure to
    counter-stereotypes 341–42
  feedback mechanisms and potential
    physician bias 339–41
  and prioritarian motives and
    beliefs 340, 346–47
  promoting physician awareness of
    implicit bias 333–34, 341–42,
    344–45
  reducing stressors affecting implicit
    biases 338–39
student debates on rationing/priority
    setting 435
substantial criteria of distributive
    justice 317
substantial justice 310
Sutton, Matt et al. 116
Sweden, Swedish Parliamentary Priorities
    Commission 134
Swiss Academy of Medical Sciences 43,
    48–49
  and health technology assessment 50
  Rationing Working Group 48–50
  Sustainable Medicine report 50
Swiss health care system

and Choosing Wisely 49
compulsory universal coverage 44–45
and diagnosis-related groups 50–51
and directions for reform 50–51
and free choice of providers 50
highly decentralized system 51
and limits on provider numbers 51
out of pocket payments 45, 47
priority setting 47–49
public-private financing 43–45
regressive financing 45
scope of coverage 44
and selective contracting 52
Switzerland 404

Take Home Messages (THMs) 193
congruence of social and bedside
rationing judgments 194–96
no gaming the system by
physicians 196–97
physician creation of bedside rationing
protocols 193–94
physician need to reduce excessive
care 194
public reasons must justify bedside
rationing 197–98
transparency about rationing protocols
is essential 197
Thaler, Richard and Sunstein, Cass 406
theories of distributive justice 211
(See also distributive justice)
tragedy of the commons 224, 400,
409–10
tragic choices 175
transparency 197–98, 301, 310, 375, 388,
435–36
triage,
conventional 148, 154
non-conventional 148
T-wave alternans test 188–89
two-tier health system 120

Ubel, Peter 199
UK health care system 56–57

basic principles 56, 63
best value for taxpayer money 67
Clinical Commissioning Groups 62,
64–67
financing of 56–58
GP practices as fundholders 59
long term care financing 56–58, 60–61
organizational structure 58–61
Primary Care Trusts IV 60–62
resource allocation strategies 59,
61–62
targets for health care delivery 60
UK physicians
equity concerns 61
insufficiency of resources 61
Ulysses contracts 158–164
and Odysseus 164
uncoordinated care 356

Values at the Bedside study 24–25, 29, 43,
244, 302, 388, 390
characteristics of physician responders
26 table 1
four countries studied 19
interventions reported rationed
27 fig. 2
limitations of 24–25
strategies used to limit interventions
23 fig. 3
values based commissioning 435–36
values based practice, defined 435
varied nature of costs of illness 397
and financial burden of illness 398
veil of ignorance 177 (See also
Rawls, John)
veil of risk 244–45, 247

Wennberg, John 79
Whitehall studies of British civil
servants 330
Wickline case 183–84, 186–87, 193, 203
Williams, Bernard 149

zero-benefit interventions 208

CPSIA information can be obtained
at www.ICGtesting.com
Printed in the USA
BVOW09s0727260418
513926BV00003B/7/P